A PRACTICAL ENGLISH—CHINESE LIBRARY OF TRADITIONAL CHINESE MEDICINE

PUBLISHING HOUSE OF SHANGHAI UNIVERSITY OF TRADITIONAL CHINESE MEDICINE

EDITOR—IN—CHIEF ZHANG ENQIN

PRESCRIPTIONS OF TRADITIONAL CHINESE MEDICINE

Written by Li Dunqing, Shi Lanhua, Gao Yi
Jiang Jingxian

Revised by Zou Jilong, Zhang Enqin
Zhang Jidong

Translated by Cui Jipin, Zuo Lianjun

Revised by Zhang Enqin, Li Yulin
Yu Wenping, Wen Hongrui

英汉对照
实用中医文库

主　编　张恩勤

方剂学

编著　李敦清　史兰华　高毅　姜静娴
审校　邹积隆　张恩勤　张继东
翻译　崔继聘　左连君
审校　张恩勤　李玉麟　于文平　温洪瑞

上海中医药大学出版社

THE GUIDING COMMITTEE OF THE LIBRARY

CHIEF AUTHORS OF THE LIBRARY

《英汉对照实用中医文库》编审指导委员会

《英汉对照实用中医文库》顾问、主编及副主编

THE EDITING AND TRANSLATING COMMITTEE OF THE LIBRARY

《英汉对照实用中医文库》编译委员会

Preface

The books in series, entitled ***"A Practical English-Chinese Library of Traditional Chinese Medicine"***, are edited with a view to disseminating the theory and knowledge of traditional Chinese medicine (TCM) across the world, promoting academic exchanges on medical science between China and other countries, and meeting with the ever-increasing international interest in TCM, so as to make it serve the interests of all nations and benefit entire mankind. This library is the first of its kind in China.

The library is composed of 12 books: ***Basic Theory of TCM*** (in two volumes), ***Diagnostics of TCM, The Chinese Materia Medica, Prescriptions of TCM, Clinic of TCM*** (in two volumes), ***Health Preservation and Rehabilitation, Chinese Acupuncture and Moxibustion, Chinese Massage, Chinese Medicated Diet*** and ***Chinese Qigong.*** The two other English-Chinese books —— ***Rare Chinese Materia Medica*** and ***Highly Efficacious Chinese Patent Medicines*** —— chiefly edited by me are also published simultaneously along with this library.

The authors and editors of the series strive to abide by the following principles: maintaining the systematism, integrity, practicability and adaptability in terms of TCM theory; paying full attention to the organic connection between basic theory and clinical treatment, taking in the available results of scientific researches carried out at home and abroad in the field of TCM; and being concise, precise, and easy to understand in the Chinese version, and correct and fluent in the English one. Some of the books mentioned above contain figures and coloured photos. It is our sincere hope that the books will turn out to be good teachers and reliable friends of those abroad who have begun to learn and practise TCM and Chinese, and provide help for those at home who wish to study TCM documents in English.

The component books of this library are written, translated, and edited through joint efforts of professors, associate professors, lecturers and medical research workers from Shandong TCM College and its affiliated hospital, Shandong Medical University and its affiliated hospital, Shandong University, Shandong Teachers Training University, Shandong Medical Academy, Shandong Provincial Anti-epidemic Station, China Academy of TCM, Nanjing TCM College, Shanghai TCM College, Beijing TCM College, etc.

In order to ensure that the present library is of good quality, we have sent its Chinese version for revision to Professor Zhou Fengwu, Professor Li Keshao who was once my tutor when I was a postgraduate student, Professor Xu Guoqian and Professor Zhang Zhenyu at Shandong TCM College, Professor Qiu Maoliang at Nanjing TCM College, and Professor Lu Tongjie, director of the Affiliated Hospital of Shandong TCM College; and the English version for proofreading to Professor Huang Xiaokai of Beijing Medical University, Professor Lu Chengzhi, head of the Foreign Languages Department of Shandong Medical University, Professor Huang Jiade of Shandong University, Mr. Huang Wenxing, professor of pharmacology, Mme. Zou Ling, professor of gynecology and obstetrics, both working in Shandong Medical University, and our foreign friends, Ms. Beth Hocks, Australian teacher of English, Mr. Howard G. Adams, American teacher of English, and some others working in Jinan.

I am deeply indebted to Mr. Li Dichen, Editor-in-Chief of Publishing House of Shanghai TCM College, and his colleagues, Mme. Xu Ping, director of the Editorial Department, and Mr. Yao Yong, responsible editor, for their advice about drawing up an outline for compiling the library to ensure a success of it; to Mr. Chen Keji, professor of China Academy of TCM and advisor on traditional medicine to WHO, Professor Zhang Zhiyuan and Associate Professor Shao Guanyong of Shandong TCM College, Mr. Liu Chonggang, deputy head of the Yellow River Publishing House, for their valuable, instructive suggestions; and to responsible members at various levels, such as Mr. Hu Ximing, Chairman of the World Acupuncture and Moxibustion Association, vice-minister of the Ministry of Public Health and chief of the Administrative Bureau of TCM and Pharmacy of the People's Republic of China, Mr. Zou Jilong, president of Shandong TCM College, Mr. Yan Shiyun, vice-president of Shanghai TCM College, Mr. Gao Heting, president of Beijing TCM College, Mr. Xiang Ping, vice-president of Nanjing TCM College, and Mr. Shang Zhichang, president of Henan TCM College for their warm encouragement and indispensable support as well as their personal participation in compiling and checking the books.

TCM, which dates back to ancient times, has a unique and profound theoretical system. The greater part of its terminology has particular denotations, and is matter-of-factly difficult to understand and translate. Inaccuracies in the library, therefore, are unavoidable. I hope that my friends in the TCM circle will oblige me with timely corrections.

May TCM spread all over the world and everyone under the heaven enjoy a long happy life.

May 20th, 1988 Dr. Zhang Enqin

Editor-in-Chief of ***A Practical English-Chinese Library of Traditional Chinese Medicine,*** Director of the Advanced Studies Department of Shandong TCM College

前 言

为扩大中医学在国际上的影响，促进中外医学学术交流，适应国外日趋发展的“中医热”形势，使传统的中医学走向世界，造福人类，我们编写了这套《英汉对照实用中医文库》。在国内，这尚属首部。

该文库包括《中医基础理论》(上、下册)、《中医诊断学》、《中药学》、《方剂学》、《中医临床各科》(上、下册)、《中医养生康复学》、《中国针灸》、《中国推拿》、《中国药膳》和《中国气功》，共十二个分册。与《文库》同时出版的还有其配套书——英汉对照《中国名贵药材》和《中国名优中成药》。

《英汉对照实用中医文库》的编译宗旨是：在理论上，努力保持中医学体系的系统性、完整性，突出实用性和针对性；在内容上，充分注意基础理论与临床治疗的有机联系，汲取国内外已公布的科研成果，以反映当代中医学术水平；在文字上，力求中文简明扼要，通俗易懂，译文准确流畅，并配有图表、彩照。我们竭诚希望《英汉对照实用中医文库》能成为国外读者学习中医、汉语的良师益友，同时也为国内读者学习中医专业英语提供帮助。

负责文库编写、翻译和审校的主要是山东中医学院及其附属医院、山东医科大学及其附属医院、山东大学、山东师范大学、山东省医学科学院、山东省卫生防疫站、中国中医研究院、南京中医学院，上海中医学院和北京中医学院等单位的部分教授、副教授、讲师和科研人员。

为确保文库质量，各分册中文稿还先后承蒙山东中医学院周凤梧教授、李克绍教授、徐国仟教授、张珍玉教授，南京中医学院邱茂良教授，山东中医学院附属医院院长吕同杰教授等审阅；英文稿先后承蒙北京医科大学英语教研室黄孝楷教授，山东医科大学英语教研室主任卢承志教授，山东大学外文系黄嘉德教授，山东医科大学药理教研室黄文兴教授、妇产科教研室邹玲教授以及澳大利亚籍教师 Beth Hocks 女士和美籍教师 Howard G. Adams 先生等审阅。

上海中医学院出版社总编辑李迪臣、编辑部主任徐平和责任编辑姚勇，亲自帮助我们修订编写大纲，指导编译工作；世界卫生组织传统医学顾问、中国中医研究院陈可冀教授，山东中医学院张志远教授、邵冠勇副教授，黄河出版社副社长刘崇刚，也为本文库的编译工作提出了许多宝贵的指导性意见；编译工作还得到了各级领导的支持和帮助，世界针灸学会联合会主席、中华人民共和国卫生部副部长兼国家中医药管理局局长胡熙明先生，山东中医学院院长邹积隆先生，上海中医学院副院长严世芸先生，北京中医学院院长高鹤亭先生，南京中医学院副院长项平先生和河南中医学院院长尚炽昌先生等，亲自参加编审并给予指导，在此一并表示衷心感谢！

由于中医学源远流长，其理论体系独特，不少名词术语深奥难解，译成英文，难度较大。故书中错误、欠妥之处在所难免，敬希国内外同道指正。

愿中医流传世界，求普天下人健康长寿。

主编　张恩勤

1988年5月20日

CONTENTS

目　录

Prescriptions of Traditional Chinese Medicine

方 剂 学

INTRODUCTION

The prescriptions of traditional Chinese medicine (TCM) can be defined as a preparation which, on the basis of the differentiation of syndromes and the establishment of therapeutic methods, organically combines various drugs for the prevention and treatment of diseases in accordance with a certain principle of formulating a prescription. Pharmacology of traditional Chinese medicinal formulae is a science that studies and interprets the theories of prescriptions and their administrations.

The formation and development of prescriptions have undergone a very long historical period. As far back as in the early period of slavery society, man began to use a single drug to prevent and treat diseases. In the Shang Dynasty, because of the increased variety of drugs and the enrichment of knowledge about diseases, more drugs were selected according to the different symptoms of illness to formulate compound prescriptions for clinical uses. People began to use compound drugs instead of a single one, thus greatly improving the curative effect. This is the embryonic form of prescriptions of TCM. A prescription book entitled "*The Prescriptions for Fifty-two Kinds of Disease*" was unearthed in 1979 from the No.3 Han Tomb at Ma Wang Dui, Changsha, Hunan Province. It is the earliest extant medical formulary in China.

With the development of traditional Chinese medicine, the prescription itself has also become perfected and enriched. Around the Warring States period and in the Qin and Han Dynasties, a classical writing of TCM entitled "*The Yellow Emperor's Canon of Internal Medicine*" came out. This is the earliest book dealing with the basic theories of the science

绪　言

方剂是在辨证立法基础上，按照一定的组方原则，将药物有机地组合在一起，用于防治疾病的制剂。方剂学则是研究并阐明方剂理论及其运用的科学。

方剂的形成与发展经历了一个漫长的历史过程。早在奴隶社会初期，人类就运用单味药来防治疾病。到了商代，由于药物品种的增多和对疾病认识的提高，人们便根据不同病情，选择多种药物配成复方，应用于临床。由单味药转向复味药，大大提高了疗效，这就是方剂的雏型。1979年在长沙马王堆三号汉墓中发现的《五十二病方》，是中国现存最古老的一部方书。

随着中国医学的发展，方剂本身也趋于完善和丰富。约在战国、秦汉时期，中医理论经典著作《黄帝内经》问世。该书最早论述

of TCM formulae, such as the principle of formulating a prescription, incompatibility of drugs in a prescription, some dosage forms and their usages. The book consisting of 13 prescriptions has laid a solid foundation for the formation and the development of the science of TCM formulae. Zhang Zhongjing, an outstanding physician in the Eastern Han Dynasty, after diligently seeking the ancient experience and book knowledge and extensively collecting numerous prescriptions, compiled ***"Treatise on Febrile and Miscellaneous Diseases"*** which containes 269 prescriptions. This book gives interpretions in detail to the modification of the prescriptions and their administrations. The dosage forms are also quite excellent. Therefore, the book has been honoured as the "forerunner of prescription books" by all the later physicians. In the prosperous period of the Tang Dynasty, more voluminous prescription writings came out one after another and promoted the development of science of TCM formulae, such as "*The Prescriptions Worth a Thousand Gold for Emergencies*" and "*A Supplement to the Essential Prescriptions Worth a Thousand Gold for Emergencies*", compiled by Sun Simiao, and "*The Medical Secrets of an Official*" compiled by Wang Tao consisting of more than six thousand prescriptions. The three medical formularies representing the major achievements made before the Tang Dynasty collected famous earlier prescriptions in the previous historical periods and some foreign prescriptions used in the Tang Dynasty and preserved the materials on prescriptions. In the Song Dynasty, the government once organized outstanding physicians to compile "*Peaceful Holy Benevolent Prescriptions*" (with 16834 prescriptions), "*General Collection for Holy Relief*" (with approximately 20000 prescriptions, and "*Prescription of Peaceful Benevolent Dispensary*" (with 788 prescriptions). The last one was compiled on the basis of the revision and supplement to the formularies collected by the Official Pharmaceutic Bureau. It is one of the earliest formulary in the world compiled by the National Pharmaceutic Bureau.

了方剂学的基本理论，如组方原则、配伍宜忌、某些剂型及用法等，并载方13首，为方剂学的形成与发展奠定了基础。东汉医家张仲景“勤求古训，博采众方”，著成《伤寒杂病论》，载方269首，对方剂的加减、用法等做了详细说明，剂型亦较完备，被后世医家誉为“方书之祖”。盛唐时期，大型方书相继问世，促进了方剂学的发展，如孙思邈的《备急千金要方》、《千金翼方》。王焘的《外台秘要》，载方6000余首。三书集唐以前方书之大成，汇集了历代名方及当时的一些外国医方，保存了丰富的方剂资料。至宋代，政府曾组织医家编撰了《太平圣惠方》(载方16834首)、《圣济总录》(载方约2万首)以及《太平惠民和剂局方》(载方788首)。其中《太平惠民和剂局方》是将官药局所收医方加以校订、增补而成，是世界最早的国家药局方之一。每方均详述其主治证、药物

Each prescription gives interpretations in detail to its indications, ingredients and preparation of drugs. This prescription book — a "legal" formulary of Chinese patent medicines in the Song Dynasty and also the first pharmacopeia of the Chinese patent medicines is a big step towards the standardization of prescription. "***Expoundings on the Treatise on Febrile Diseases***" compiled by Cheng Wuji, a physician in the Jin Dynasty, selected 20 prescriptions from the book "***Treatise on Febrile Diseases***" and analysed them in detail, especially clearly described the different roles of the principal, assistant, adjuvant and guiding drugs. It is the first theoretical book on the interpretations of prescriptions and contributes a great deal to the development of theoretical prescription treatises of later periods. Dr. Zhu Su of the Ming Dynasty and others collected almost all the medical formularies having been used before the fifteenth century and compiled the most voluminous medical book "***Prescriptions for Universal Relief***" with as many as 61739 prescriptions in it. In the Qing Dynasty, with the emergence and development of the schools of epidemic febrile diseases, numerous famous prescriptions for epidemic febrile diseases came into being, enriching and perfecting the contents of pharmacology of TCM formulae. In addition, in the Ming and Qing Dynasties a lot of monographs on prescriptions were published such as "***Textual Criticism on Prescriptions***" and "***Collection of Prescriptions with Notes***", thus further promoting the development of the theoretical research of the science of TCM formulae.

Since the founding of the People's Republic of China, a great number of prescription books have come out. Many ancient prescriptions, secret prescriptions, proved prescriptions have been collected, systematized, researched and widely applied to different clinical departments; their therapeutic mechanism and compatible properties have been explored by experimental researches. Meanwhile a lot of new effective prescriptions have been created and the reformation in the dosage forms of pres-

及药物的炮炙、修制法等，是宋代“法定”的中成药处方配本，使方剂向着标准化、规范化前进了一大步，为我国第一部中成药药典。金代成无己的《伤寒明理论》，选录20首《伤寒论》方进行详尽分析，于君臣佐使之义，阐发尤明，是方论之首创者，对后世方论专著的发展有一定贡献。明朝，朱橚等几乎收集了15世纪以前的所有方书，著成《普济方》，载方多达61739首，是我国现存最大的方书。至清代，随着温病学派的崛起，出现了许多治疗温热病的名方，充实和完善了方剂学的内容。此外，明清时期方论专著兴起，如《医方考》、《医方集解》等，使方剂学的理论研究得到进一步发展。

中华人民共和国建立以来，大量方书不断涌现，不仅收集、整理、研究古方、秘方和验方，将其广泛应用于临床各科，而且通过实验研究进一步探讨方剂的作用机制及配伍实质，同时创制

criptions have been carried out. As a result, a new prospect in the development of science of TCM formulae has been opened up.

To sum up, the formation and development of pharmacology of TCM formulae have undergone a very long historical process from the elementary stage to the advanced one, with forms from simple to complex and has gradually become an independent science with a relatively perfect theoretical system.

了众多有效新方，并进行了剂型改革，开创了方剂学发展的新局面。

综上所述，方剂学的形成与发展经历了一个由低级到高级、由简至繁的漫长历史过程，逐步成为一门有较完整理论体系的独立学科。

PART ONE

Outline

Chapter I

Formation of a Prescription

The formation of a prescription is neither simply to pile up drugs with similar functions and effects nor "to treat the head when the head aches and to treat the foot when the foot hurts", that is to say, only to treat the symptoms but not the syndrome (*zheng*) in TCM or the disease. It is on the basis of the differentiation of syndromes and establishment of the therapeutic methods, to pick out proper drugs and organically constitute them in the light of the principles of forming a prescription.

Section 1

The Principle of Forming a Prescription

By the principle of forming a prescription is mainly meant the compitible theory of principal, assistant, adjuvant, and guiding drugs in the prescription of TCM. To form a prescription in accordance with this theory, it is necessary to make a clear distinction between the principal drug and the secondary ones and make them supplement and restrict one an-

上篇　总　　论

第　一　章

方剂的组成

方剂的组成，既不是功效相近药物的简单堆砌，也不是"头痛医头、脚痛医脚"的对症治疗，而是在辩证立法的基础上，选出适当药物，并按照一定组成原则的有机组合。

第一节　组成原则

所谓组成原则，主要是指中医的主、辅、佐、使配伍理论。按照这一理论，既主次分明，又相辅相约，因而能发挥最佳的治

other, thereby, producing the most effective result in the treatment of diseases.

Principal drug: A principal drug is one which is aimed at producing the leading effects in treating the cause or the main symptom of a disease. It holds sway in the whole prescription.

Assistant drug: An assistant drug is firstly meant the drug which helps strengthen the effect of the principal drug and is secondly meant the drug which is aimed at producing the leading effect in the treatment of the accompanying symptoms.

Adjuvant drug: An adjuvant drug can be divided into three types, the first type assists the principal and assistant drugs to strengthen their therapeutic effects or treats less important symptoms by itself; the second reduces or clears away the toxicity of the principal and assistant drugs so as to prevent the toxic effect and side effect of the drugs from coming into existence; the third, aimed at dealing with possible vomiting in serious cases after taking decoction with too potent effect, possesses the properties opposite to those of the principal drug in compatibility, but produces supplementing effects in the treatment of diseases.

Guiding drug: A guiding drug can be subdivided into two types: one is known as the medicinal guide leading the other drugs in the prescription to the affected site; the second is known as a mediating drug coordinating the effects of various ingredients in the prescription.

As mentioned above, a principal ingredient should be used as the dominator in a prescription, with the assistant, adjuvant and guiding drugs subordinate to it and the four kinds of drugs supplementing one another and playing the curative roles together. The formation of various famous prescriptions reflects this principle. "Ephedra Decoction" by Zhang Zhongjing is a very good example. This pre-

疗效果。

主药：是针对病因或主证起主要治疗作用的药物。在全方中占主导地位。

辅药：意义有二，①辅助主药以加强其治疗作用的药物；②针对兼证起主要治疗作用的药物。

佐药：意义有三，①佐助药，配合主、辅药以加强其治疗作用，或直接治疗次要症状的药物；②佐制药，减弱或消除主、辅药毒性，以防机体产生不良反应的药物；③反佐药，是针对病重邪甚、服药后可能格拒，配伍与主药性味相反，而在治疗中又起相成作用的药物。

使药：意义有二，①引经药，即引方中诸药至病所的药物；②调和药，具有调和方中诸药作用的药物。

上述可知，一首方剂应以主药为核心，辅、佐、使药为从属，各药之间相互配合，共同发挥治疗作用。许多名方的组成即体现

scription is composed of ephedra, cinnamon twig, bitter apricot kernel and licorice and is aimed at treating exterior syndrome due to affection by exogenous wind-cold. Ephedra in the prescription, pungent in flavor and warm in nature, can produce the effects of inducing diaphoresis, expelling cold and facilitating the flow of the lung-*qi* to relieve astham. It is used as a principal drug which is aimed at dealing with the cause of a disease and the main symptoms. Another ingredient, cinnamon twig, pungent in flavor, sweet in taste and warm in nature, not only can relieve the exterior syndrome, expel cold and help ephedra to induce diaphoresis to expel the exopathogens but also can warm the channels to ensure the flow of *yang-qi* so as to reduce headache and pantalgia. It is used as an assistant drug. Bitter apricot kernel, with a bitter taste and warm nature, can produce the effects of lowering the adverse flow of the lung-*qi* and strengthen the asthma-reducing effect of ephedra as an adjuvant drug. Prepared licorice root, as a guiding drug with a sweet taste and a mild nature, can produce the effects of coordinating the other ingredients in the prescription and reducing the dry and drastic reactions of both ephedra and cinnamon twig so as to prevent impairment of the vital *qi*. When combined, the four drugs clearly show their respective effects, primary or secondary, supplementing and restricting one another, thus forming a prescription which is rigorous in its formation and, though composed of simple drugs, has great therapeutic effects. Of course, not every prescription is invariably composed of the principal, assistant, adjuvant and guiding drugs but according to the condition of the illness, it is either composed of only one principal drug, or composed of the principal drug and assistant drug or of the principal drug and adjuvant or of the principal drug and guiding drug such as Ginseng Decoction; and Decoction of Ginseng and Prepared Aconite for emergency cases,

了这一原则。如张仲景的麻黄汤，就是一个很好的例证。该方由麻黄、桂枝、杏仁、甘草四药组成，主治风寒表实证。方中麻黄辛温，能发汗散寒，宣肺平喘，是针对病因、主证而设，为主药；桂枝辛甘而温，既解表散寒，助麻黄发汗解表，又温经通阳，以缓解头身疼痛，为辅药；杏仁苦温降肺气，可加强麻黄平喘作用，为佐药；炙甘草甘温性缓，能调和诸药，又缓和麻、桂燥烈之性，以防其过汗伤正，为使药。四药配伍，主次分明，相辅相约，组方严谨，药简效宏。当然，每首方剂并非主、辅、佐、使皆备，而是根据其具体病情，或单用主药，或主辅相配，或主佐相合，或主使同用，如用于急救的独参汤，参附汤以及适应证较单

and Decoction of Platycodon Root for some simple minor indications.

The establishment of principal, assistant, adjuvant and guiding drugs in a prescription should be based on their respective importance of effect, potency and dosage in a prescription. Of course, the dosage of an ingredient in a prescription is not the only basis for the determination of the principal drug. Its habitual dosage should be taken as reference. Drugs such as metals, stones, shells of oysters and the like, usually used in large dosage are not necessarily the principal drugs while some poisonous drugs, used in small dosage may be the principal drugs rather than assistant, adjuvant or guiding drugs.

Section 2

Modification of a Precscription

The formation of a prescription is not only based on a definite principle but should also be accommodated in the light of the concrete conditions such as the state of illness, sex, age, the patient's constitution, the occurring season of a disease and the circumstances. Especially when a set prescription is used, the above-mentioned conditions should be taken into serious consideration to accommodate the formation of a prescription so as to suit the drugs to the illness and ensure their therapeutic effects. The modification of a prescription is usually seen as follows:

1. **Modification of drugs**: It refers to modifying less important ingredients in accordance with the difference of the secondary symptmos or the accompanying symptoms without any change of the main symptoms and the principal drugs to meet the need of complicated conditions of illness. In this

纯的桔梗汤等。

在分析确立某一方剂的主、辅、佐、使时，应以该药在方中所起作用的主次、药力大小、药量轻重为依据。当然，药量的轻重并不是确立主药的唯一依据，还应参照药物的习惯用量来进行具体分析。如金石介壳类一般用量均较大，并不一定是主药；而某些有毒之品，用量一般较小，但不一定是辅药、佐药、使药等。

第二节 组成变化

方剂的组成不仅要遵循一定的原则，而且应针对患者的病情、性别、年龄、体质、发病季节及环境等具体情况进行灵活变通。特别在选用成方时更应如此，使方药与病证完全吻合，以确保其疗效。方剂组成变化一般见于以下三种情况：

1．药味加减的变化 是指一首方剂在主证、主药不变的情况下，随着次要症状或兼夹症的不同，加减其次要药物，以适应

way, new drugs can be added to a prescription or the original drugs be taken away from it or new drugs be added to a prescription with some of the original drugs taken away from it at the same time. For instance, the indication of Cinnamon Twig Decoction is for the exterior deficiency syndrome due to affection of pathogenic wind-cold marked by fever, headache, perspiration, aversion to wind, white and thin fur, floating and slow pulse. If the patient also has a cough or asthma, magnolia and apricot kernel can be added to lower the adverse flow of *qi* and relieve asthma. It is named Decoction of Cinnamon Twig with Magnolia and Apricot Kernel. If the patient has the accompanying symptoms such as a fullness sensation in the chest and abrupt pulse, which show impairment of the heart-*yang*, peony with sour, cold, *yin* and soft nature should be excluded from the prescription. It is named Decoction of Cinnamon Twig minus Peony. If the patient has the symptoms of oppressed sensation in the chest and slight cold, which indicate that the *yang-qi* has been impaired seriously, peony should be excluded from the prescription and prepared aconite roots should be added so as to warm the channels to ensure the flow *yang-qi*. It is obvious that the modification of the drugs in the same prescription in accordance with the difference of the accompanying symptoms reflects the adaptability in forming a prescription.

2. **Modification of dose**: It refers to increasing or decreasing the dose of a drug in a prescription without any change in its ingredients. This method can either change the potency of the original prescription or extend the scope of the treatment, sometimes the dominant and the subordinate roles of the drugs in a prescription may be changed so as to suit them to new indications. For example, Decoction for Resuscitation and Decoction for Promoting Blood Circulation and Relieving Cold are both composed of prepared aconite roots, dried ginger, prepared licorice. Their functions are to recuperate

复杂的病情需要。此种变化既有单纯的加或减，又有加减同时进行。例如桂枝汤主治外感风寒表虚证，症见发热头痛、汗出恶风、舌苔薄白、脉浮缓等，若兼有咳喘者，可加厚朴、杏仁以降逆平喘，名桂枝加厚朴杏子汤；若伴见胸满、脉促者，此为心阳已伤，宜减去酸寒阴柔之芍药，名桂枝去芍药汤。如果在脉促胸闷的同时，又有微寒，说明伤阳已重，不但要去芍药，还要加附子以温经助阳。可见同一首方剂，由于兼症的不同，药味则随之而变，反映了组方的灵活性。

2．药量增减的变化　是指方中的药物组成不变，仅增减其药物用量而言。此种变化或改变原方药力，或扩大治疗范围，有时尚能更换方中药物的主次地位，以改变其适应证。如四逆汤与通脉四逆汤皆由附子、干姜、炙甘草三味组成，功能回阳救逆。

depleted *yang-qi* and save the patient from collapse. The difference between them is that the latter, consisting of a larger dose of aconite roots and dried ginger than the former, produces a stronger effect of recuperating depleted *yang-qi* and can treat more severe causes. For another instance, Decoction of Cinnamon with Peony is a revised prescription of the original Cinnamon Decoction plus Doubled dose of peony, and the scope of its treatment also extends in a certain degree. It is indicated for syndromes indicated for Mannamon Decoction accompanied by fullness and occasional pain in the abdomen. For instance, Minor Decoction for Purging Down Digestive *Qi* and Decoction of Three Drugs Containing Magnolia are both composed of rhubarb, immature bitter orange, and magnolia. Just because the doses of their ingredients are different and their principal drugs are different, their indications change accordingly.

3. **Modification of dosage forms:** It means that the same prescription should be used differently just because of its dosage forms. A prescription can be prepared into various dosage forms, each having its own characteristics. Doctors can select the most suitable dosage form to meet the need of the patient's illness and make it convenient for administration so as to raise the curative effect. For instance, pill or bolus and powder are of slow-acting and lasting effects; decoction is of speedy and drastic effect; injection produces effect more quickly and is convenient to use. Let us take Bolus for Regulating the Function of Middle-warmer as an example. It is used to treat insufficiency of the spleen-*yang* but if the condition of the illness is mild and chronic, bolus is preferable; if the case is serious and acute, it is better to take the decoctions instead. There is one more example. Decoction for Resuscitation is usually taken for the treatment of moderate cases of *yang* deficiency due to excess of *yin* but in the first-aid of shock due to *yang* insufficiency. Injection for Resuscitation is more effective.

不同的是后者附、姜用量加大，所以其回阳作用更强，所治之证亦较重。再如，桂枝加芍药汤，为桂枝汤原方倍芍药用量而成，其治疗范围也有所扩大，主治桂枝汤证兼腹满时痛者，又如均由大黄、枳实、厚朴组成的小承气汤与厚朴三物汤，只因用量分配不一样，主药不同，所以主治证亦随之而变。

3．剂型更换的变化　即同一首方剂，由于剂型不一样，在运用上亦有所区别。方剂的剂型品种繁多，特点各异，医者可根据患者病情需要，选择最适宜者，以方便病人，提高疗效。例如：丸、散剂作用较缓慢而持久，汤剂则较速而力峻，针剂就更速且又方便。以理中丸（汤）为例，对于脾胃虚寒证，凡病情较轻、较缓，宜用丸剂；若病情较重、较急，则应改用汤剂。再如四逆汤，如果治疗一般的阴盛阳虚证，口服汤剂即可，但若用于抢救阳虚型休克，四逆注射液则更为合适。

The above-mentioned three modifications of prescriptions can either be applied separately or be made simultaneously. Clinically it depends on the concrete condition of the patient's illness.

以上三种变化形式，既可分别运用，又可同时进行，临床上应根据具体病情灵活掌握。

Chapter II

Dosage Forms of a Prescription

The dosage forms of TCM prescriptions refer to the definite forms of drugs prepared according to their properties and the needs of treatment. Here are several commonly used forms of prepared drugs:

Section 1

Decoction

By decoction we mean the medicinal solution obtained by boiling for some time the selected drugs which have been soaked in an appropriate amount of water or yellow rice wine and then removing the dregs. It is the most commonly used form of prepared drugs with the characteristics of being easily absorbed, able to produce quick curative effects with mild poisonous or side effect. Its recipe can be modified to meet the needs of treating diseases, moderate or emergent. The decoction can be used as drugs for oral administration, enemas and external application-drugs, such as fumigant, lotion.

Section 2

Powder

It refers to a preparation of drugs ground into dry powder and well mixed. There are two types, the powder for

第 二 章

方剂的剂型

方剂在使用前，根据药性特点和治疗需要，将其加工制成一定的制剂形式，称为剂型。这里仅将常用的剂型简介如下：

第一节 汤 剂

药物配齐后，用水或黄酒浸透，然后煎煮一定时间，去滓取汁，称为汤剂。汤剂是最常用的一种剂型，其特点是吸收快，能迅速发挥疗效，毒副作用小，并可根据治疗需要灵活加减。适用于一般疾病或急性病。内服、灌肠以及外用熏洗均可。

第二节 散 剂

散剂是将药物碾碎后均匀混合而成的干燥粉末，有内服和外

oral administration and the powder for external application. The former is either a preparation of drugs ground into fine powder and small in dosage to be taken orally with water or a prescription of drugs ground into coarse granules and large in dosage, which should be first boiled in water and then filtered to remove the residue with the medicinal solution to be taken orally. The latter is a preparation of drugs ground into fine powder sprinkled or applied topically to the affected part after being mixed. Powder is easy to prepare, convenient to use, not liable to go bad and economical in useing drugs, so it is also one of the commonly used forms of prepared drugs.

Section 3

Pill and Bolus

Pill or bolus refers to round medicinal mass of various sizes prepared by grinding drugs into powder, mixing it with excipients such as honey, water, rice paste, flour paste, wine, vineger, drug juices, or bee-wax. Clinically, the following are commonly used.

Honeyed bolus or honeyed pill: It refers to pills or boluses prepared by grinding drugs into fine powder, mixing it with the excipient, refined honey, usually prepared into large round masses for oral administration, each weighing about 3 to 9 grams; it can also be prepared into small-sized round masses named honeyed pills for oral administration. Because honeyed boluses and honeyed pills contain some honey, they are soft and moist in property and moderate in action, and can produce flavoring, replenishing and restoring effects, fit for the treatment of many acute and chronic diseases. Bolus for Tonifying the Kidney-*qi* and Bezoar Bolus for Resurrection are good examples.

用两种。内服散剂之末细而量少者，可直接冲服；末粗而量多者，则须加水煮沸，然后去滓取汁服用。外用散剂是将药物研成极细粉末，撒布或调敷患处。散剂制作简单、服用方便、节省药材、不易变质，亦是常用剂型之一。

第三节　丸　剂

丸剂是根据配方要求，将药物研成粉末，以蜜、或水、或米糊、或面糊、或酒、或醋、或药汁、或蜂蜡等为赋形剂制成的圆形固体制剂。临床常用的有以下四种。

蜜丸：是指将药物研成细粉，以炼过的蜂蜜作赋形剂制成的丸剂。一般多制成大丸使用。每丸约3～9克；亦可制成小丸使用。蜜丸因含有蜂蜜，故性质柔润，作用缓和，并具矫味和补益作用，适用多种急慢性疾病。常用的有肾气丸、安宫牛黄丸等。

Water-paste pill: It refers to medicinal pills prepared manually or mechanically by grinding drugs into fine powder, mixing it with excipients such as cold boiled water, wine, vinegar, or some drug juices. Usually it is made into small-sized mass for oral administration. Water-paste pills are small in size, easy to be swallowed, decomposed and quick to be absorbed. It is also a relatively common form of prepared drugs. Commonly used Lenitive Pill and Pill of Six Ingredients with Magical Effects are examples.

Paste-pill: It refers to a medicinal mass prepared by grinding drugs into fine powder, mixing it with excipients such as rice paste and flour paste. Paste-pill is of a very strong stickiness, so after being taken, it is decomposed and absorbed more slowly than honeyed bolus, heonyed pill and water-paste pill. Some strong irritant ingredients or poisonous drugs are better prepared into paste-pill so as to be absorbed slowly in the body after being taken, thus prolonging the therapeutic effect as well. as reducing the drugs' stimulus to the gastro-intestinal tract, such as Pill of Cow-bezoare, etc.

Concentrated pill: It refers to medicinal pill prepared by decocting drugs until their decoction is condensed to extract, then mixing the extract with the powder of other drugs, drying the mixed material and grinding it into powder, mixing the powder with some excipients such as water, wine, and decoction of some durgs in the recipe. The characteristics of the concentrated pills are as follows: containing very effective components, small in size and dosage, convenient to use and fit for treating various diseases. The commonly used Concentrated Pill of Bezoar for Detoxicating is one of them.

水丸：是指将药物研成细粉，用冷开水或酒、或醋、或方中部分药物的煎汁作赋形剂，以人工或机械泛制而成的丸剂，一般多制成小丸使用。水丸具有丸粒小，易于吞服和易于崩解、吸收快的特点，亦是一种比较常用的剂型。常用的有保和丸、六神丸等。

糊丸：是指将药物研成细粉，用米糊或面糊为赋形剂制成的丸剂。糊丸粘性大，服用后崩解和吸收较蜜丸、水丸缓慢。某些毒性药或刺激性强的药物宜制成糊丸使用，使其服后在体内徐徐吸收，既可延长药效，又减少药物对胃肠道的刺激。常用的有犀黄丸等。

浓缩丸：是指将方中某些药物煎汁浓缩成膏，再与方中其他药物的细粉混合，经干燥、粉碎，以水或酒或方中部分药物的煎出液为赋形剂制成的丸剂。其优点是有效成分高、体积小、剂量小、服用方便，适用于治疗各种疾病。常用的有牛黄解毒浓缩丸等。

Section 4

Extract, Ointmen and Plaster

They are medicinal preparations made by decocting drugs in water or plant oil and then concentrating them. These preparations are divided into two kinds, extract for oral administration and ointment and adhesive plaster for external application. Extract for oral administration is subdivided into liquid extract, half-solid or dry extract and soft extract while those for external application are subdivided into two kinds, ointment and plaster.

Liquid extract: It refers to a liquid-soaking form of preparation made by using appropriate solvent to soak out the effective part of the drugs, then distilling out some solvent of the extract at low temperature, and adjusting its concentration and the alcohol content to a formulated standard. Usually a milligram effective component of liquid extract equals a gram of drugs except in specific cases. Commonly used are Licorice Liquid Extract and Motherwort Liquid Extract.

Half-solid or dry extracts: They are half-solid or solid froms of preparation made by using solvents to soak out the effective components of the drugs, then removing all the solvents by means of distillation at low temperature. In accordance with the formulated standard, one gram extract is as effective as two to five grams of drugs. Half–solid extract tends to be used to make pills or tablets, such as Hairy Holly Root Extract, while dry extract is a kind of dry fine powder which may be taken orally after being infused with boiling water or put into capsules for oral administration such as Gentian Root Extract.

Soft extract: It refers to a thick, half-solid form of preparation made by decocting the drugs in water repeatedly

第四节 膏 剂

膏剂是将药物用水或植物油煎熬浓缩而成的剂型，分内服、外用两种。内服膏剂有流浸膏、浸膏、煎膏三种；外用膏剂有软膏剂、硬膏剂两种。

流浸膏：是指用适当溶媒浸出药物中的有效成分后，将浸出液中部分溶媒用低温蒸发除去，并调整浓度及含醇量至规定的标准而成的液体浸出剂型。除特别规定者外，流浸膏1毫升的有效成分相当于1克的药物。常用的有甘草流浸膏、益母草流浸膏等。

浸膏：是指用溶媒将药物中的有效成分浸出后，低温将溶媒全部蒸发除去而成的半固体或固体浸出剂型。按规定标准，每1克浸膏相当于2～5克药物。浸膏又分为两种，其中软浸膏为半固体，多供制片或制丸使用，如毛冬青浸膏；干浸膏为干燥细粉，可直接冲服或装入胶囊使用。如龙胆草浸膏等。

煎膏（又称膏滋）：是指将药物反复煎煮至一定程度，去滓取

to a certain extent, discarding the residue, then concentrating it, adding appropriate honey, crystal sugar or granulated sugar in the decoction. Soft extract is small in size, convenient to use and contains a great deal of honey and sugar and of better nourishing effect. It is fit for the debilitiated patients who have been ill for a long time. Of the commonly are used Motherwort Extract and Loquat Extract.

Ointment: It refers to a half-solid form of preparation made by mixing appropriate matrix and drugs. The ointment is easy to apply to the skin and mucous membrane. The ground substance of the ointment is solid at normal temperature and is of a certain stickiness. After being applied to the skin and mucous membrane, it gradually becomes softer or melted, its effective components being absorbed slowly, producing moderate effect in the treatment. Ointment of Three Yellow Drugs, and Green Chiretta Ointment are good examples.

Plaster: It refers to a form of preparation made by using lead soap and others as ground substance with drugs mixed or dissolved in it, spreading it over a piece of cloth or some other material to be stuck on the skin for the treatment. One of them is named black plaster for its dull black colour. This preparation remains in a solid state at normal temperature, while at 36 to 37°C, it becomes softer and begins to work, acting on the affected local region or on the whole body. Dogskin Plaster and Plaster for Rheumatic Pain are examples of this kind.

Section 5

Dan

Dan in TCM refers to a chemical preparation made by heating the medicinal mineral containing mercury and sulphur to sublimation. Its properties are as follows: It is small

汁，再浓缩，加入适量蜂蜜、冰糖或砂糖煎熬而成的稠厚半固体浸出剂型。煎膏体积小，服用方便，并且含有大量蜂蜜或糖，滋补作用较强，适合于久病体虚者。常用的有益母草膏、枇杷膏等。

软膏(又称药膏)：是指用适当的基质与药物均匀混合制成的一种容易涂于皮肤、粘膜的半固体外用剂型。软膏的基质在常温下是固体的，具有一定的粘稠性。涂于皮肤或粘膜上以后，能渐软化或溶化，有效成分被缓慢吸收，呈现缓和的治疗作用。常用的有三黄软膏、穿心莲软膏等。

硬膏：是指以铅肥皂等为基质，混有或溶有药料，涂于布或裱背材料上，供贴敷于皮肤上使用的剂型。其中呈暗黑色者，称膏药或黑膏药，常温时呈固体状态，36～37℃时则软化释放药力，起到局部或全身治疗作用。常用的有狗皮膏、伤湿止痛膏等。

第五节 丹 剂

丹剂多系指用含有汞、硫磺等成分的矿物药进行加热升华所

in dosage but very effective as a preparation for external application, such as *Baijiang Dan* and *Hongsheng Dan*. In addition, some pills, powder and troche which contain rare drugs or produce specific effect are also known as *dan* such as Pill for Saving Children, Bolus for Activating Energy Flow in the Channels and Collaterals, Purple Snow Powder and *Yushu* Powder.

Secton 6

Medicated Wine

It refers to a transparent medicated liquid obtained by using wine as a solvent to soak out the effective components of the drugs. The medicated wine is fit for the treatment of general asthenia, rheumatic pain and traumatic injury. Commonly used are Wine of Ten Powerful Tonics and Medicated Wine for Rheumatism.

Section 7

Medicated Tea

It is a solid preparation made of coarse-powdered drugs and adhesive excipients and drunk as tea after being infused with boiling water in a vessel with a lid. So it is named Medicated Tea, such as *Wushi* Tea.

Section 8

Distilled Medicinal Water

It refers to distilled water obtained by distilling fresh drugs

得到的化合制剂，其特性是剂量小而作用大，为外用制剂，如白降丹、红升丹等。此外，对某些含有贵重药品或有特殊功效的丸、散、锭剂，习惯上也称丹，如小儿回春丹、活络丹、紫雪丹、玉枢丹等。

第六节　酒　　剂

酒剂是以酒为溶媒，浸取药物中有效成分，所得到的透明浸出液制剂，又称“药酒”。酒剂适用于体质虚弱、风湿疼痛、跌打损伤等病证。常用的十全大补酒、风湿药酒等。

第七节　茶　　剂

茶剂是以药物粗末与粘合剂混合而制成的固体制剂。使用时将其放入有盖容器内，以沸水浸泡，代茶饮之，故名茶剂，如午时茶。

第八节　药　　露

将新鲜、含有挥发成分的药物，放在水中加热蒸馏，所收集

containing components with volatility in water by heating. Distilled medicinal water is bland in flavor, delicately aromatic and colorless and convenient to take orally. Usually it is used as beverage, especially in summer, such as Distillate of Honeysuckle Flower.

Section 9

Troche and Medicated Cake

Troche and medicated cake belong to solid preparations with different shapes made of the fine powder of drugs and an appropriate excipient or only made of powder drugs without excipients. They are preparations for oral administration or external application such as *Zijin* Troche and Toad Venon Troche。

Section 10

Slender Roll of Medicated Paper

It is a form of preparation made by twisting medicated paper into a slender roll or by twisting paper into a slender roll and then medicating it, so it is called "slender roll of medicated paper", which is commonly used in surgery of TCM to help draw out pus by inserting it into the opening of a sore.

Section 11

Medicated Thread

It refers to a form of preparation for external use made by

的蒸馏液即为药露。药露气味清淡，芳洁无色，便于口服。一般用作饮料，夏季尤为常用，如金银花露。

第九节　锭剂、饼剂

锭剂、饼剂是将药物研成细粉，单独或与赋形剂混合而制成的不同形状的固体制剂。可供外用或内服，如紫金锭、蟾酥锭等。

第十节　条　剂

条剂是将桑皮纸粘药粉后捻成细条，或捻成细条后再粘药粉而成，故又称纸捻。用于插入疮口，化腐排脓，是中医外科常用的制剂。

第十一节　线　剂

线剂是将丝线或棉线浸泡于药液中，并与药液同煮，经干燥

soaking silk or cotton thread in medicated liquid and decocting it and then drying it, which is mainly used to ligate fistula or vegetation.

Section 12

Moxa-preparation

It is a form of preparation for external use made by pulverizing Chinese mugwort leaves into mugwort floss and rolling it into a certain shape. When used, the lighted end of it is kept a certain distance from the skin of a specific acupoint or the affected part to heat them for the therapeutic purpose.

Section 13

Syrup

It is a saturated solution of sugar with or without drugs. The one that doesn't contain drugs is known as simple syrup, usually used as excipient or condiment while the other that contains drugs is made by decocting the drugs to obtain the juice and then decocting the juice until it becomes concentrated, and finally adding into it some cane sugar. Syrup tastes sweet and is suitable for children.

Section 14

Infusion

It is a form of preparation prepared by making an extract of the drugs into medicated granule, mixing the granule with

而成的外用制剂。主要用于结扎瘘管或赘肉。

第十二节 灸 剂

灸剂是将艾叶碾成绒状，捻成一定的形状而制成的外用制剂。使用时将其置于体表某一俞穴或患处，点燃熏灼，以达到防治疾病的目的。

第十三节 糖 浆 剂

糖浆剂是含有药物或不含药物的蔗糖饱和水溶液。不含药物者称为单糖浆或糖浆，一般用作赋形剂或调味剂；含药物者是将药物煎煮取汁，并煎熬成浓缩液，加入适量蔗糖溶解而成。糖浆剂有甜味，尤适宜于儿童服用。

第十四节 冲 服 剂

冲服剂是将药物浓缩浸膏与适量辅料（淀粉、糊精、糖粉）混

an appropriate amount of excipient materials (starch, dextrin, powdered sugar). It is a new preparation for oral administration originating from decoction and syrup. It has the characteristics of being quick-acting, convenient to use, easy to carry about and fit for the treatment of many different diseases. Infusion for Soothing the Liver and Infusion for Reducing Fever due to the Common Cold are examples.

Section 15

Tablet

Tablet is a form of preparation made of refined drugs and some excipients by pressing. It is convenient in use, accurate in content, low in production cost, easy to store and transport. Bitter drugs and drugs with an offensive odour can be made into sugar-coated tablets. If it is aimed at acting only on the diseases of the intestinal tract or if the drugs in it is apt to lose the curative effect when affected by the gastric acid, enteric coasting can be used so as to enable it to break down in the intestine. Commonly used tablets are Mulberry Leaf and Crysanthemum Tablet for Cold and Antiinfective Tablet of Lonicera and Forsythia.

Section 16

Injection

Injection is a kind of germ-free solution obtained by refining the drugs. It is used for subcutaneous, muscular or

合制成的颗粒状剂型，它是在汤剂和糖浆剂的基础上发展起来的一种新型内服剂，具有作用迅速、服用方便、易于携带等优点，适用于多种疾病。常用的有疏肝冲剂、感冒退热冲剂等。

第十五节　片　　剂

片剂是将药物加工提炼并与辅料混合均匀后，加压制成的片状剂型，具有食用方便、含量准确、生产成本低、易于贮运等优点。味苦或有恶臭的药物，还可外加糖衣；如需要在肠道内起作用或遇胃酸有效成分易被破坏的药物，可外包肠溶衣，使之在肠道内崩解。常用的有桑菊感冒片、银翘解毒片等。

第十六节　针　　剂

针剂即注射剂，是将中药经提取、精制、配制而成的无菌溶

intravenous injections. It has the characteristics of being accurate in dosage, quick in action, convenient to use and of not being affected by food and digestive juice. Injection of Oriental Warmwood and Rhubarb as well as Composite Red Sage Injection are good examples.

液，主要供皮下、肌肉、静脉注射之用。它具有剂量准确、作用迅速、给药方便、药物不受食物或消化液的影响等优点。常用的有茵黄注射液、复方丹参注射液等。

Chapter III

Methods of Decocting and Taking Drugs

In the above-mentioned dosage forms of preparation, decoction is the most commonly used. The method of using a decoction refers to the methods of making and taking it. Whether the methods of decocting and taking drugs are right or not is directly related to the therapeutic effect. They are introduced in detail as follows:

Section 1

The Methods of Decocting Drugs

The method of decocting drugs refers to the appropriate way to make a decoction, to which the medical men through the ages have devoted their great attention and effeorts, just as Xu Lingtai, a famous physician in the Qing Dynasty, once described: "The methods of decocting medicinal herbs must be delt with seriously, which is closely related to the therapeutic effectiveness of a prescription." (See ***Treatise on Origin and Development of TCM***). The following should be taken into serious consideration:

1. Utensil for Decocting Drugs

Ceramic clay pot with lid is universally used at present to avoid the chemical reaction of the drugs with the utensil in the course of decocting the drugs, thus maintaining the original

第三章

煎服法

在上述剂型中，汤剂最为常用。汤剂的使用包括煎法和服法两个方面。煎服法正确与否，能直接影响疗效。现分述如下：

第一节 煎法

煎法即煎药方法。历代医家都对煎法十分重视，如清代名医徐灵胎说："煎药方法，最宜深讲，药之效不效，全在乎此。"（见《医学源流论》）。煎药时应注意以下几点：

1.煎药用具

目前通用有盖的陶瓷砂锅。因其化学性质比较稳定，能避免在煎煮过程中与药物发生化学反应，从而使方剂保持原有的功效。

curative potency of the drugs. Metal vessels such as tin or iron vessels are forbidden to prevent sediment, lower solubility of the drugs and the toxic or side effects caused by the chemial reaction with the drugs.

2. Water for decocting drugs

The water to be used must be pure and clean except some special need. Tap water, well water or distilled water can be used. Usually the drugs are put in the utensil and then water is added until the drugs are 30 mm underwater.

3. Fire for decocting drugs

The fire for decocting drugs is divided into two types: soft fire and strong fire. Qucik fire for decocting drugs is called" "strong fire" while slow fire is called "soft fire". Usually strong fire is used prior to slow fire. Besides, sometimes soft fire or strong fire is alone used to decoct drugs. The former is used to decoct tonic drugs while the latter to decoct the drugs for relieving exterior syndrome.

4. Methods for decocting drugs

Drug-decocting methods are divided into two types, the routine method and the special method.

1) **The Routine method:** This refers to the method of putting the drugs into a drug-decocting pot first, then adding water until the drugs are slightly submerged under the water surface and decocting them after the drugs are soaked through. When the drugs are decocted, strong fire should be first used until the water is boiling, and then soft fire is used instead to prevent the medicinal solution from overflowing or drying up quickly meanwhile it must not take the pot lid off too frequently so as to reduce the loss of the volatile components. Drugs for

忌用锡、铁等金属器皿煎煮，以免发生沉淀、溶解度降低，或与药物发生化学反应而产生毒、副作用。

2.煎药用水

除特殊规定者外，用水以水质纯净为原则，如自来水、井水或蒸馏水等均可。一般将药物放在煎药容器内，加水至漫过药物约30毫米为度。

3.煎药火候

有"文火"、"武火"之分。急火煎之为武火，慢火煎之为文火。一般是先武后文。此外，也有单纯用文火或武火煎煮者。前者如补益剂，后者如解表剂。

4.煎药方法

有一般煎药法与特殊煎药法两种。

1)一般煎药法　将药物放入煎药容器内，加冷水浸过药面，待药物充分浸透后再行煎煮。煎时先用武火，沸后改用文火，以免药汁溢出或过快熬干；不要频揭锅盖，以尽量减少挥发性成分

relieving exterior syndrome and drugs for clearing awag heat are preferably decocted on strong fire to avoid the volatilization of the effective components. It is better to decoct the tonic drugs with strong flavor on soft fire so that their effective components may be completely released. Some poisonous drugs such as prepared lateral aconite, aconite root, *langdu* root should also be decocted on soft fire for a longer period of time so as to reduce their toxicity.

2) **The special method:** This refers to the method for decocting some special drugs. All those that need decocting in a special way should be noted in a prescription.

(1) **To be decocted first:** Some drugs, strong in flavor and heavy in nature with active constituents difficult to extract, such as minerals and shells, should be smashed and decocted first for about ten minutes before adding other drugs. Some crude drugs with sand and mud, such as baked yellow earth and glutinous rice root, should be decocted first to obtain their juice, then other drugs are decocted in the juice instead of water.

(2) **To be decocted later:** Those drugs with fragrance and active constituents ready to diffuse or evaporate, such as peppermint and costus root, should be added and decocted for four or five minutes when the decoction is nearly done.

(3) **To be decocted in packet:** Some drugs such as plantain seed, red holloysite and inula flower should be wrapped in a piece of cloth before they are decocted with other drugs in case they may cause the decoction turbid and produce irritation to the throat.

(4) **To be simmered or decocted alone:** Some rare and expensive drugs should be simmered or decocted alone so as to avoid the destruction of their effective constituents from being absorbed by other drugs when decocted together. For example, ginseng should be sliced into pieces and then decocted in a separate vessel in a clay pot with lid for two or three hours,

的散失。解表药、清热药等气薄药物，宜武火急煎，以免药性挥发，药效降低；味厚滋补药，宜文火久煎，以使药力尽出。有毒的药物，如附子、乌头、狼毒等，亦宜用文火久煎，以减其毒性。

2)特殊煎法　是指对某些特殊药物所采取的煎煮方法。凡方中有需特殊煎煮的药物，应在处方时加以注明。

(1)先煎　味厚质重的药物，如介壳类、矿石类等，因其有效成分难以煎出，故应打碎先煎，煮沸10分钟左右后，再下其他药物。泥沙较多的药物，如灶心土、糯稻根等，宜先煎取汁，再以其汁代水煎煮其他药物。

(2)后下　凡气味芳香、有效成分易挥发的药物，宜在其他药物即将煎好时投入，煎煮4～5钟即可，如薄荷、木香等。

(3)包煎　某些药物，因其煎煮时易致药液混浊，或服药时对咽喉有刺激，须用纱布包好后再行煎煮，如车前子、赤石脂、旋覆花等。

(4)另炖或另煎　某些贵重药物，为避免其有效成分在同煎时被其他药物吸附，可另炖或另煎。如人参，应切成小片，放入

Some rare drugs, such as antelope's horn and rhinoceros horn with active constituents difficult to decoct out, should be planed into small thin pieces and decocted alone for two hours.

(5) **To be melted by heating:** Some gluey, viscous, easy-dissolved drugs, when decocted along with other drugs, are so easy to adhere to the pot as to be charred, or so easy to adhere to the other drugs as to inhibit the dissolution of their effective constituents or the filtration of the medicinal solution, that they should be put into the decocted solution of other drugs (after removal of the residue), dissolved by gently boiling or stirring, and then taken orally. Donkey-hide gelatin, malt sugar are typical drugs of this kind.

(6) **To be taken after being soaked in hot water or in decoction:** Some drugs contain volatile oil and their efiective constituents are easy to dissolve, so they should be soaked with boiling water or decoction in a vessel (with lid on) to collect the solution for oral administration.

(7) **To take drug following its infusion:** Powder, *dan*, small pill, natural medicinal juice and other fragrant or expensive drugs should be taken after being infused with boiling water, hot decoction or wine, such as fine amber powder, notoginseng powder, Purple Snowy Powder, Pill of Six Ingredients with Magical Effects, cow-bezore, musk, juice of lotus root.

Section 2

Methods of Taking Drugs

Methods of taking medicines include both the time and the method of taking medicines.

加盖盅内，隔水炖2～3小时。对贵重而又难于煎出气味的药物，如羚羊角、犀角等，则应刨成小薄片，另煎2小时。

（5）溶化（烊化） 胶质、粘性大且易溶的药物，同煎时易粘锅而被烧焦，或易粘附他药，以致影响有效成分的溶解或药汁的滤出，故应在煎好他药后，将其置于去滓的药汁中微煮或趁热搅拌，待溶解后服用，如阿胶、饴糖等。

（6）泡服 含有挥发油或药性易溶解的药物，可用开水或药汁趁热浸泡（须加盖），取汁服用，如藏红花、肉桂等。

（7）冲服 散剂、丹剂、小丸剂、自然药汁以及某些芳香或贵重药物，宜冲服。如琥珀末、三七末、紫雪丹、六神丸、牛黄、麝香、生藕汁等。

第二节 服 法

服法包括服药时间或服药方法。

1. Time of taking medicine

1) Usually drugs are recommended to be taken before meals while drugs irritant to the gastro-intestinal tract should be taken after meals.

2) Tonic drugs should be taken with an empty stomach.

3) Antimalarial drugs should be taken two hours before the attack of malaria.

4) Sedative drugs should be taken before going to bed.

5) The drugs for acute diseases should be taken at any time while those for chronic cases should be taken at regular time.

6) Drugs can be taken many times a day to meet the need of the condition of the illness and can also be decocted and taken as a drink in multiple doses.

2. Methods of taking medicine

A drug is usually taken one dose a day, with each dose being divided into two or three equal portions and taken twice or three times. It can also be taken at one draught in an emergency case, and meantime, if necessary, the patient should take the medicine in small portions at frequent intervals so as to maintain the effective dose in the body.

Generally speaking, decoction should be taken warm, especially the decoction for relieving exterior syndrome should be taken when it is hot, and then the patient must be kept warm to induce slight sweat. Cold-natured decoction for heat syndrome should be taken cool while hot-natured decoction for cold syndrome should be taken hot. But for the treatment of cold syndrome with pseudo-heat syndromes, the hot-natured decoction should be taken cool while for the treatment of heat syndrome with pseudo-cold syndrome, the cold-natured decoction should be taken warm so as to avoid vomiting after taking the medicines.

1.服药时间

1)一般药物，宜在饭前服。对胃肠有刺激的药物，宜在饭后服。

2)滋补药，宜空腹服。

3)治疟药，宜在寒热发作前两小时服。

4)安神药，宜在睡前服。

5)急性病服药不拘时间；慢性病宜定时服。

6)根据病情，可1天数服，也可煎汤代茶频服。

2.服药方法

服药一般是1日1剂，每剂分2～3次服。病急者，可一次顿服，同时还需根据病情需要，采用持续服药法，以使药物在体内保持有效浓度。

汤剂一般应温服，解表药尤应趁热服，且服后还须温覆取微汗。热证用寒药，宜冷服；寒证用热药，宜热服。但对真寒假热或真热假寒者，则应热药寒服，或寒药热服，以防发生格拒。服

Patients apt to vomit after taking medicine should take some ginger juice or take the medicine in small doses at short intervals. For unconscious patients or patients who have difficulty in swallowing, nasal feeding should be used. Drastic or poinsonous drugs should be taken in small dosage before its dose is increased gradually until the curative effect is achieved.

药呕吐者，宜先服少量姜汁，或采取频服少进的办法。昏迷病人、吞咽困难者，宜鼻饲给药。对峻热、有毒的药物，宜先进少量，后逐渐增加，得效即止，不可久服。

Part Two

Chapter IV

Prescriptions for Relieving Exterior Syndrome

The prescriptions for relieving exterior syndrome refer to those that are chiefly composed of traditional Chinese drugs having the therapeutic effects of inducing diaphoresis, expelling pathogenic factors from the muscles and skin as well as promoting eruption. They are preferred for the treatment of exterior syndrome.

As exterior syndrome involves the difference between wind-cold type and wind-heat type, and the human body covers the distinction between *yin* and *yang*, and between dificiency and excess, the prescriptions for relieving exterior syndrome are subdivided into the pungent and warm recipes for relieving exterior syndrome, pungent and cool recipes for relieving exterior syndrome, and tonic recipes for relieving exterior syndrome.

Section 1

Pungent and Warm Recipes for Relieving Exterior Syndrome

This group of prescriptions is chiefly made up of traditional Chinese drugs pungent in flavor and warm in property.

下篇 各 论

第四章

解表剂

凡以解表药为主组成，具有发汗、解肌、透疹等作用，用以治疗表证的方剂，称为解表剂。

由于表证有风寒、风热之不同，人体有阴阳虚实之差异，故解表剂又分为辛温解表剂、辛凉解表剂和扶正解表剂等。

第一节 辛温解表剂

辛温解表剂主要由辛温解表药组成，有发散风寒的作用，适

Possessing the function of dissipating wind-cold, they are usually indicated for the treatment of wind-cold exterior syndrome.

Ephedra Decoction

(Mahuang Tang)

SOURCE: ***Treatise on Febrile Diseases***

INGREDIENTS:

No. 1 Ephedra, *Herba Ephedrae* (with joints removed) 6g

No. 2 Cinnamon twig, *Ramulus Cinnamomi* 4g

No. 3 Bitter apricot kernel, *Semen Armeniacae Amarum* (with its skin removed) 9g

No. 4 Prepared licorice root, *Radix Glycyrrhizae Praeparata* 3g

DIRECTIONS: All the drugs should be decocted in water for roal dose. After administration, it is necessary for the intaker to stay in warm bed to induce slight perspiration.

FUNCTIONS: Inducing sweat to relieve exterior syndrome, facilitating the flow of the lung-*qi* to relieve asthma.

INDICATIONS: Exterior syndrome of excess type due to exopathic wind-cold marked by aversion to cold, fever without perspiration, headache, pantalgia, dyspnea, thin and white coating of the tongue, superficial and tight pulse.

Moreover, the recipe can be modified to deal with cold, influenza, bronchitis, bronchial asthma and others that are ascribed to exterior syndrome of excess type caused by exopathic wind-cold.

INTERPRETATION: In the recipe, Ingredient No.1, pungent and bitter in flavour and slight warm in nature, acts as a principal drug with the effect of inducing sweat to dispel exogenous evils and facilitating the flow of the lung-*qi* to relieve asthma. No.2, pungent and sweet in flavour and warm

用于风寒表证。

麻 黄 汤

【来源】 《伤寒论》

【组成】 麻黄(去节)6克，桂枝4克，杏仁(去皮尖)9克，甘草(炙)3克。

【用法】 水煎服，服后盖被取微汗。

【功用】 发汗解表，宣肺平喘。

【主治】 外感风寒表实证，表现为恶寒发热，头痛身痛，无汗而喘，苔薄白，脉浮紧等。

感冒、流行性感冒、支气管炎、支气管哮喘等表现为风寒表实证者，可以用本方加减治疗。

in nature, has the effects of warming and dredging the blood vessels and activating the heart-*yang* and serves as an assistant drug that helps strengthen the effect of the principal drug. Possessing bitter and pungent flavour and warm nature, No. 3 is used as an adjuvant drug with the effect of arresting cough and relieving asthma. No. 4 is an ingredient sweet in flavour and warm in nature and functions as a guiding drug, having the effects of reinforcing the middle-warmer, replenishing *qi*, moistening the lung to relieve cough and tempering the effect of other drugs.

Clinically and experimentally, it is ascertained that this recipe can relieve of the troubles by producing the effects of inducing sweat, removing fever, arresting cough, relieving pain and promoting diuresis.

CAUTIONS:

1. Being warm and pungent, the recipe is drastic in its effect of inducing sweat, so it should not be administered for cases that have nothing to do with exterior syndrome of excess type due to exopathic wind-cold such as spontaneous perspiration caused by exterior syndrome of deficiency type, general debility with exogenous diseases, blood deficiency after giving birth, etc.

2. As soon as sweat is induced out and the illness is cured, the administration should be withdrawn immediately. Prolongation of intake is of no benefit.

Cinnamon Twig Decoction

(Guizhi Tang)

SOURCE: ***Treatise on Febrile Diseases***

INGREDIENTS:

No. 1 Cinnamon twig, *Ramulus Cinnamomi* 9g

No. 2 Peony root, *Radix Paeoniae* 9g.

No. 3 Prepared licorice root, *Radix Glycyrrhizae Praeparata* 6g

【方解】 方中麻黄辛苦微温，能发汗解表，宣肺平喘，为主药。桂枝辛甘温，能温通心脉，振奋心阳，与麻黄合用则发汗解表作用更强，为辅药。杏仁苦辛温，能宣肺利气，止咳平喘，为佐药。炙甘草甘温，能补中益气，润肺止咳，调和诸药，为使药。

现代研究证实，本方具有发汗、解热、镇咳、平喘、镇痛、利尿等作用。

【使用注意】

1．本方辛温，为发汗峻剂，凡表虚自汗、外感风热、体虚外感、产后血虚等非风寒表实证禁用。

2．服本方后，一经汗出病愈，即应停服，不宜久用。

桂枝汤

【来源】《伤寒论》

【组成】 桂枝9克，芍药9克，甘草(炙)6克，生姜9克，大枣4枚。

No. 4 Fresh ginger, *Rhizoma Zingiberis* 9g.
No. 5 Chinese dates, *Fructus Ziziphi Jujubae* 4 pcs.

DIRECTIONS: All the above drugs are decocted together in water for oral administration. After taking the decoction, the patient is required to drink a small quantity of hot water or hot porridge and then lie in warm bed to induce slight perspiration.

FUNCTIONS: Expelling pathogenic fators from the muscles and skin and regulating *ying* and *wei* to relieve exterior syndrome.

INDICATIONS: Exterior deficiency syndrome due to pathogenic wind and cold, manifested by fever, headache, perspiration with aversion to wind, nasal catarrh, retching, thin and white coating of the tongue, and floating and moderate pulse.

Equally, the recipe can be modified to deal with the common cold, influenza and others that are attributable to exterior syndrome of deficiency type caused by pathogenic wind and cold, as well as urticaria, cutaneous pruritus, eczema, neuralgia, myalgia, etc.

INTERPRETATION: Of the ingredients in the recipe, No. 1 is a drug with pungent, sweet and warm properties and acts as a principal drug to relieve exterior syndromes by expelling pathogenic wind and cold from the muscles and skin. No.2 is a drug with sour, bitter and slight cold properties and is used as an assistant drug for replenishing *yin* to astringe *ying*. The combination of No. 1 and No.2 results in the double roles of both being diaphoretic and astringent for regulating *ying* and *wei* so as to induce sweat without impairmet of *yin* and arrest sweat without interference in dispelling exopathogens. They are opposite and complementary to each other. No. 4, possessing pungent and warm properties, can not only aid No.1 in expelling pathogenic factors from the muscles and skin but also warm the stomach and arrest vomiting. No.5, with sweet and mild properties, is used as tonics of stomach and blood

【用法】 水煎服。服后饮少量热粥或开水，覆被取微汗。

【功用】 解肌发表，调和营卫。

【主治】 外感风寒表虚证，表现为发热头痛，汗出恶风，鼻鸣干呕，舌苔薄白，脉浮缓。

感冒、流行性感冒等证属风寒表虚者，以及荨麻疹、皮肤瘙痒症、湿疹、神经痛、肌肉痛等，可用本方加减治疗。

【方解】 方中桂枝辛甘温，能解肌发表，外散风寒，为主。芍药酸苦微寒，能益阴敛营，为辅药。桂、芍相合，一散一收，调和营卫，使发汗而不伤阴，止汗而不恋邪，起“相反相成”之功用。生姜辛温，既助桂枝解肌，又能暖胃止呕。大枣甘平，能益

for supplementing *qi* and reinforcing the middle-warmer, nourishing *yin* and tonifying blood; and, used in combination with No. 4 as an adjuvant drug, it can regulate *ying* and *wei*. No. 3, a guiding drug, is used to tonify the middle-warmer and replenish *qi* and to coordinate the effect of the above drugs in the recipe.

Modern researches have proved that the recipe possesses the efficacies of inducing sweat, reducing fever, removing phlegm, relieving convulsion and pain, promoting digestion and absorption, nourishing the body and consolidating the constitution.

CAUTIONS:

1. The recipe is not advisable for the exterior syndrome of excess type due to pathogenic wind and cold.

2. Patients with exterior syndrome of wind-heat type marked by aversion to wind, perspiration as well as thrist and rapid pulse are prohibited from taking the recipe.

Notopterygium Decoction of Nine Ingredients

(Jiuwei Qianghuo Tang)

SOURCE: Prescription by Zhang Yuansu, quoted from the book ***Medical Problems***

INGREDIENTS:

No. 1 Notopterygium root, *Rhizoma seu Radix Notopterygii* 6g
No. 2 Ledebouriella root, *Radix Ledebouriellae* 6g
No. 3 Atractylodes rhizome, *Rhizoma Atractylodis* 6g
No. 4 Asarum herb, *Herba Asari* 2g
No. 5 Chuanxiong rhizome, *Rhizoma Ligustici Chuanxiong* 3g
No. 6 Dahurian angelica root, *Radix Angelicae Dahuricae* 3g
No. 7 Dried rehmannia root, *Radix Rehmanniae* 3g
No. 8 Scutellaria root, *Radix Scutellariae* 3g
No. 9 Licorice root, *Radix Glycyrrhizae* 3g

DIRECTIONS: All the above drugs are to be decocted in water for oral use.

FUNCTIONS: Relieving exterior syndrome, clearing

气补中，滋阴补血，与生姜为伍，能调和营卫，并为佐药。炙甘草益气和中，调和诸药，为使药。

现代研究证实，本方具有发汗、解热。祛痰、镇痉、镇痛、促进消化吸收、滋养强壮等作用。

【使用注意】

1．外感风寒表实证忌用。

2．虽有恶风、自汗，但兼口渴、脉数等风热表证者禁用。

九味羌活汤

【来源】《此事难知》引张元素方

【组成】羌活、防风、苍术各6克，细辛2克，川芎、白芷、生地黄、黄芩、甘草各3克。

【用法】水煎服。

【功用】解表，清里，止痛。

interior heat and alleviating pain.

INDICATIONS: Syndrome due to the attack of exogenous wind, cold and dampness on the body surface with interior heat, manifested by chill and fever, absence of perspiration, headache with stiff neck, aching pain of the extremities, bitter taste in the mouth with thirst, white and slippery coating of the tongue, floating pulse, etc.

The recipe can be modified to deal with influenza, lumbago, sciatica rheumatic arthritis that are ascribable to the attack of exogenous wind-cold-dampness on the body surface with interior heat.

INTERPRETATION: Of all the ingredients in the recipe, No. 1, possessing pungent, bitter and warm properties, acts as a principal drug for inducing diaphoresis, expelling pathogenic wind and dampness, removing stagnation of blood and *qi* and arresting pain; No.2 and No.3, with the effects of inducing sweat and dispelling dampness, act as assistant drugs to reinforce the effect of No.1 in dispelling exogenous evils; Nos. 4,5 and 6 are used together to dispel pathogenic cold and wind, promoting the flow of *qi* and blood and treating headache and pantalgia. As No.8 exerts the effect of purging heat from the *qi* system and No.7 produces the effect of purging heat from the blood system, both of them are used as adjuvant drugs not only for the treatment of interior heat but also for the control of dryness due to punget and warm properites of the drugs. No.9 is used as a mediator for tempering the effect of other drugs in the recipe, playing the role of a guiding drug.

Modern researches have confirmed that the recipe has the efficacies in inducing diaphoresis, reducing fever, tranquilizing the mind, alleviating pain, promoting diuresis, and relieving inflammation.

CAUTIONS: Patients with weakness of the vital energy and deficiency of *yin* are prohibited from taking the recipe.

【主治】 风寒湿邪在表兼有内热证，表现为恶寒发热，无汗，头痛项强，肢体痠痛，口苦而渴，苔白滑，脉浮等。

流行性感冒、腰痛、坐骨神经痛、风湿性关节炎表现为风寒湿在表兼里热者，可用本方加减治疗。

【方解】 方中羌活辛苦温，能发汗解表，祛风胜湿，通痹止痛，为主药。防风、苍术发汗祛湿，可助羌活解表，为辅药。细辛、川芎、白芷散风寒、行气血、除头身痛。黄芩泄气分之热，生地泄血分之热，既治兼证之热，又制辛温之燥，均为佐药。甘草调和诸药，为使药。

现代研究证实，本方具有发汗、解热、镇静、镇痛、利尿、消炎等作用。

【使用注意】 阴虚气弱之人禁用。

Minor Decoction of Green Dragon

(Xiao Qinglong Tang)

SOURCE: ***Treatise on Febrile Diseases***

INGREDIENTS:

No. 1 Ephedra *Herba Ephedrae* (with joins removed) 9g
No. 2 Peony root, *Radix Paeoniae* 9g
No. 3 Asarum herb, *Herba asari* 3g
No. 4 Dried ginger, *Rhizoma Zingiberis* 3g
No. 5 Prepared licorice root, *Radix Glycyrrhizae Praeparata* 6g
No. 6 Cinnamon twig, *Ramulus Cinnamomi* 6g
No. 7 Pinellia tuber, *Rhizoma Pinelliae* 9g
No. 8 Schisandra fruit, *Fructus Schisandrae* 3g

DIRECTIONS: All the above ingredients are to be decocted in water for oral administration

FUNCTIONS: Relieving superficial syndrome by means of inducing diaphoresis, removing fluid-retention, arresting cough and relieving asthma.

INDICATIONS: Exterior cold due to exopathogen, and excessive fluid in the body, marked by chill and fever, absence of perspiration, cough, asthma with watery and copious sputum, or thirst with little predilection for drinks or retching, or dysphagia, or diarrhea, or dysuria, and white and slippery coating of the tongue, and floating and tight pulse.

In addition, the recipe can be modified to deal with the above symptoms and signs as seen in the common cold, influenza, asthmatic bronchitis, bronchial asthma at its stage of attack, etc.

INTERPRETATION: In the recipe, Ingredients No.1 and No.6 act in combination as principal drugs used for inducing sweat to relieve superficial syndrome, dispelling pathogenic cold and facilitating the flow of the lung-*qi* to relieve

小青龙汤

【来源】《伤寒论》

【组成】麻黄(去节)9克，芍药9克，细辛3克，干姜3克，甘草(炙)6克，桂枝6克，半夏9克，五味子3克。

【用法】水煎服。

【功用】解表蠲饮，止咳平喘。

【主治】外感表寒，内停水饮，表现为恶寒发热，无汗，咳嗽气喘，痰多而稀，口不渴或渴不多饮，或干呕，或噎，或下利，或小便不利，苔白滑，脉浮紧等。

感冒、流感、喘息型支气管炎、支气管哮喘发作期等见本证候者可用本方加减治疗。

【方解】方中麻黄、桂枝发汗解表，散寒宣肺，为主药。干姜、细辛温肺化饮，并助麻黄、桂枝解表散寒，为辅药。芍药养

asthma. No.3 and No.4 possess the properties of warming the lung and removing fluid retention from interior and, therefore, share the role of an assistant drug for reinforcing No.1 and No.6 in dispelling pathogenic cold from exterior to relieve superficial syndrome. No.2 has the effects of nourishing *ying* and astringing *yin* and, when used in combination with No.6, can produce the effects of regulating *ying* and *wei*, and preventing No.1 and No.6 from inducing too much perspiration; No.8 has the ability to astringe the lung to relieve cough and can prevent exhausting and injuring of the lung-*qi* due to the dispersing effect and pungent warm property of the drugs. No.7 is a drug with the effect of expelling phlegm and fluid-retention and regulating the stomach to relieve vomiting and dysphagia, contributing its effort together with No.8 as an adjuvant drug. Regarded as a guiding drug, No.5 has the capacity of replenishing *qi* and regulating the middle-warmer, and coordinating the actions of various drugs in the recipe.

Modern researches have ascertained that this recipe possesses the effects of inducing sweat, reducing fever, relieving dyspnea and cough, removing phlegm, promoting diuresis, relieving allergic reaction and promoting blood circulation.

CAUTIONS: This recipe should not be administered to patients with dry cough, dry mouth and throat accompanied by thick yellow-coloured sputum.

Section 2

Pungent and Cool Recipes for Relieving Exterior Syndrome

This group of recipes is chiefly composed of drugs pungent in flavour and cool in property and possesses the thera-

营敛阴，与桂枝配伍，可调和营卫，防麻黄、桂枝发汗太过；五味子敛肺止咳，防辛温发散而耗伤肺气；半夏祛痰和胃散结，而止呕噎，共为佐药。甘草益气和中，调和诸药，为使药。

现代研究证实，本方具有发汗、解热、改善呼吸困难、镇咳、祛痰、利尿、抗过敏、促进血液循环等作用。

【使用注意】 凡干咳无痰，或痰色黄稠，咽干口燥者忌用。

第二节　辛凉解表剂

辛凉解表剂主要由辛凉解表药组成，有发散风热的作用，适

peutic effect of expelling pathogenic wind-heat. It is preferred for the treatment of exterior syndrome due to exogenous wind-heat.

Powder of Lonicera and Forsythis

(Yinqiao San)

SOURCE: ***Treatise on Differentiation and Treatment of Epidemic Febrile Diseases***

INGREDIENTS:

No. 1 Forsythia fruit, *Fructus Forsythiae* 9g
No. 2 Honeysuckle flower, *Flos Lonicerae* 9g
No. 3 Peppermint, *Herba Menthae* 6g
No. 4 Schizonepeta spike, *Spica Schizonepetae* 5g
No. 5 Prepared soybean, *Semen Sojae Praeparatum* 5g
No. 6 Arctium fruit, *Fructus Arctii* 9g
No. 7 Platycodon root, *Radix Platycodi* 6g
No. 8 Licorice root, *Radix Glycyrrhizae* 5g
No. 9 Lophatherum, *Herba Lophatheri* 4g
No.10 Reed rhizome, *Rhizoma Phragmitis* in proper dosage

DIRECTIONS: All the above drugs are to be decocted in water for oral administration.

INDICATIONS: Affection by exogenous wind-heat with superficial syndrome marked by fever with anhidrosis or with disturbed hidrosis, mild chilly sensation, headache, thirst, cough, sore throat, red tip of the tongue with thin white or yellowish coating on it, and floating and rapid pulse.

Besides, this recipe can be modified to treat such conditions as infection of upper respiratory tract, acute tonsillitis, encephalitis B, epidemic cerebrospinal meningitis, parotitis and so on that pertain to exterior syndrome caused by exogenous wind-heat.

INTERPRETATION: Of all the ingredients in the above

用于外感风热表证。

银 翘 散

【来源】《温病条辨》

【组成】 连翘9克，银花9克，薄荷6克，荆芥穗5克，淡豆豉5克，牛蒡子9克，苦桔梗6克，生甘草5克，竹叶4克，加芦根适量。

【用法】 水煎服。

【功用】 辛凉解表，清热解毒。

【主治】 外感风热表证，表现为发热无汗，或汗出不畅，微恶风寒，头痛口渴，咳嗽咽痛，舌尖红，苔薄白或薄黄，脉浮数。

上呼吸道感染、急性扁桃体炎、乙型脑炎、流行性脑脊髓膜炎、腮腺炎等表现为风热表证者，可用本方加减治疗。

【方解】 方中银花、连翘辛凉透表，清热解毒。薄荷、荆芥、

recipe, No.1 and No.2, pungent in flavor and cool in property, are used to relieve the exterior syndrome and clear away pathogenic heat and toxic material. Nos. 3, 4, and 5 are used to expel exogenous evils and induce diaphoresis for the treatment of chill, fever without sweating, and headache; Nos. 6, 7 and 8 used to relieve sore throat and cough by clearing away toxins and removing phlegm and, furthermore, the pungent and cool properties of No.6 is good for dispelling exterior heat; the last two drugs, No.9 and No.10, being sweet in flavor and cool in property with mild effect, are used to remove pathogenic heat and promote the production of body fluid and to relieve thirst and restlessness. Especially, No.9 can induce diuresis, which helps to drive pathogenic factor out of the body by passing water.

Modern researches have ascertained that this recipe possesses the efficacies of inducing diaphoresis, bringing down fever, relieving pain and cough, resisting bacteria and viruses, subduing inflammation, etc.

CAUTIONS:

1. The recipe is not advisable for cases ascribable to exterior syndrome caused by exogenous wind-cold.

2. The recipe should not be decocted long in case the effective components are destroyed.

Decoction of Mulberry Leaf and Chrysanthemum

(Sang Ju Yin)

SOURCE: ***Treatise on Differentiation and Treatment of Epidemic Febrile Diseases.***

INGREDIENTS:

No. 1 Mulberry leaf, *Folium Mori* 7.5g

No. 2 Chrysanthemum flower, *Flos Chrysanthemi* 3g

淡豆豉发散表邪，透热外出，以除寒热、头痛、无汗。牛蒡子、桔梗、甘草解毒利咽，祛痰止咳，以治咽痛、咳嗽，且牛蒡子性味辛凉，能发散表热。竹叶、芦根甘凉轻清，能清热生津，除烦止渴，其中竹叶尤可利小便，使邪从下出。

现代研究证实，本方具有发汗、解热、镇痛、祛痰、镇咳、抗菌、抗病毒、消炎等作用。

【使用注意】

1. 属风寒表证者，不宜用本方。

2. 本方不宜久煎，以防有效成分挥发。

桑 菊 饮

【来源】 《温病条辨》

【组成】 桑叶7.5克，菊花3克，杏仁6克，连翘5克，薄荷

No. 3 Bitter apricot kernel, *Semen Armeniacae Amarum* 6g
No. 4 Forsythia fruit, *Fructus Forsythiae* 5g
No. 5 Peppermint, *Herba Menthae* 2.5g
No. 6 Platycodon root, *Radix Platycodi* 6g
No. 7 Licoricc root *Radix Glycyrrhizae* 2.5g
No. 8 Reed rhizome *Rhizoma Phragmitis* 6g

DIRECTIONS: All the above ingredients are to be decocted in water for oral administration.

FUNCTIONS: Relieving the exterior syndrome with drugs pungent in flavor and cool in property, facilitating the flow of the lung-*qi* to relieve cough.

INDICATIONS: The onset of cough due to wind-heat, marked by cough, mild feverish body, slight thirst, thin and white coating of the tongue and floating pulse.

The modification of the above recipe can be adopted for the treatment of such diseases as the common cold, influenza, acute bronchitis, bronchial pneumonia and acute tonsillitis that indicate the exterior syndrome due to wind-heat.

INTERPRETATION: Among the drugs of the recipe, No.1 and No.2, sweet in flavor and cool in property with mild effect, act in combination as principal drugs for expelling pathogenic heat from the lung and *wei* system to relieve cough. No.5 with the effect of dispelling wind-heat acts as an assistant drug together with No. 3 and No.6 to promote the dispersing function of the lung to relieve cough. No.4, pungent and bitter in flavor and cold in property, possesses the effect of dispelling wind-heat from exterior and is used as an adjuvant drug with No.8 which is sweet in flavor and cold in property and has the effect of clearing away heat, and promoting the production of body fluid to quench thirst. No.7 is used as a mediator for coordinating various effects of the drugs in the recipe.

Clinically and experimentally, it is ascertained that the above recipe has the functions of relieving cough, removing phlegm, resisting bacteria, subduing inflammation as well

2.5克，桔梗6克，生甘草2.5克，苇根6克。

【用法】 水煎服。

【功用】 辛凉透表，宣肺止咳。

【主治】 风热咳嗽初起证，表现为咳嗽，身热不甚，口微渴，苔薄白，脉浮。

感冒、流行性感冒、急性支气管炎、支气管肺炎、急性扁桃体炎表现为风热表证者，可用本方加减治疗。

【方解】 方中桑叶、菊花甘凉轻清，疏散肺卫之热而止咳，并为主药。薄荷疏散风热，杏仁、桔梗宣肺止咳，均为辅药。连翘苦辛寒而质轻，清热透表；苇根甘寒，清热生津而止渴，共为佐药。甘草调和诸药，为使药。

现代研究证实，本方具有镇咳、祛痰、抗菌、消炎以及轻度

as inducing mild sweat and allaying fever.

CAUTIONS:

1. Those with cough due to exogenous wind-cold are prohibited from taking this recipe.

2. Since the drugs in the recipe are of dispelling effect, they should not be decocted for a long time.

Decoction of Ephedra, Apricot Kernel, Gypsum and Licorice

(Ma Xing Shi Gan Tang)

SOURCE: ***Treatise on Febrile Diseases***

INGREDIENTS:

No. 1 Ephedra, *Herba Ephedrae* (with joints removed) 6g

No. 2 Bitter apricot kernel, *Semen Armeniacae Amarum* (with its skin and tip removed) 9g

No. 3 Prepared licorice root, *Radix Glycyrrhizae Praeparata* 6g

No. 4 Gypsum, *Gypsum Fibrosum* 30g

DIRECTIONS: All the above drugs are to be decocted in water together and then taken orally.

FUNCTIONS: Expelling pathogenic heat with pungent and cool drugs, clearing away lung-heat to relieve asthma.

INDICATIONS: Cough and dyspnea due to wind-heat manifested by persistent feverish body with or without sweat, cough with dyspnea or even accompanied by nares flaring, thirst, thin white or thin yellow coating of the tongue, slippery and rapid pulse, etc.

The recipe can be modified for the treatment of acute bronchitis, bronchial pneumonia, bronchial asthma in the stage of attack and other diseases associated with cough and dyspnea caused by lung-heat.

发汗、解热作用。

【使用注意】

1. 风寒咳嗽禁用。

2. 本方药物系轻清之品，不宜久煎。

麻黄杏仁石膏甘草汤

【来源】《伤寒论》

【组成】 麻黄(去节)6克，杏仁(去皮尖)9克，甘草(炙)6克，石膏30克。

【用法】 水煎服。

【功用】 辛凉泄热，清肺平喘。

【主治】 风热喘咳证，表现为身热不解，有汗或无汗，咳逆气急，甚则鼻煽，口渴，舌苔薄白或薄黄，脉滑数等。

急性支气管炎、支气管肺炎、支气管哮喘发作期等表现为肺热咳嗽而喘者，可用本方加减治疗。

INTERPRETATION: In the recipe, Ingredient No. 1 acts as a principal drug, exerting the effect of facilitating the flow of the lung-*qi* to relieve asthma, and its pungent flavor is good at dispelling exogenous factors. No.4, with its dosage five times that of No.1, plays the role of an assistant drug with the effect of both clearing and purging lung-heat and restricting the warm property of No.1. No.2, a drug with a bitter taste and warm propety, is used as an adjuvant drug to reinforce No.1 and No.4 in facilitating the flow of the lung-*qi* to relieve asthma. No.3 is used as a guiding drug for replenishing *qi* and regulating the middle-warmer, and coordinating the effect of various drugs in case the cold and heavy property of No.4 impairs the stomach.

Clinically and experimentally, it is ascertained that this recipe has the efficacies of subduing inflammation, removing phlegm, relieving cough and dyspnea, and resisting viruses.

CAUTIONS: This recipe is only advisable for cases with dyspnea of excess type due to lung-heat; and it is not suitable for those associated with dyspnea of excess type due to wind-cold as well as those with dyspnea of deficient type.

Bupleurum and Pueraria Decoction for Dispelling Pathogens from Superficial Muscles

(Chai Ge Jieji Tang)

SOURCE: *Six Books on Febrile Diseases*

INGREDIENTS:

No. 1 Bupleurum root, *Radix Bupleuri* 9g

No. 2 Pueraria root, *Radix Puerariae* 9g

No. 3 Scutellaria root, *Radix Scutellariae* 9g

No. 4 Licorice root, *Radix Glycyrrhizae* 3g

【方解】 方中麻黄能宣肺平喘，辛散表邪，为主药。石膏辛甘大寒，其用量五倍于麻黄，既可清泄肺热，又可制约麻黄的温性，为辅药。杏仁苦温，泄肺降逆，助麻黄、石膏清肺平喘，为佐药。炙甘草益气和中，调和诸药，以防石膏寒凉沉重而伤胃，为使药。

现代研究证实，本方具有消炎、镇咳、祛痰、缓解呼吸困难、抗病毒等作用。

【使用注意】 本方只适用于肺热实喘，若属风寒实喘以及虚证之喘者，皆不宜使用。

柴葛解肌汤

【来源】 《伤寒六书》

【组成】 柴胡、葛根、黄芩各9克，甘草、芍药、羌活、白

No. 5 Peony root, *Radix Paeoniae* 3g

No. 6 Notopterygium root, *Rhizoma seu Radix Notopterygii* 3g

No. 7 Dahurian angelica root, *Radix Angelicae Dahuricae* 3g

No. 8 Platycodon root, *Radix Platycodi* 3g

No. 9 Gypsum, *Gypsum Fibrosum* 9g

No.10 Fresh ginger, *Rhizoma Zingiberis* 3 slices

No.11 Chinese dates, *Fructus Ziziphi Jujubae* 2 pcs.

DIRECTIONS: All the above drugs are to be decocted in water for oral administration.

FUNCTIONS: Expelling pathogenic factors from the muscles and skin and reducing fever.

INDICATIONS: Affection due to exogenous pathogenic wind-cold with heat in the interior resulting from stagnated pathogens, manifested as slight aversion to cold, high fever, headache, soreness and pain in the extremities, eye pain, dry nose, orbit pain, restlessness, insomnia, thin and yellowish coating of the tongue, and superficial and slightly full pulse.

Besides, other cases ascribed to the above syndrome such as the common cold, influenza, bronchitis and toothache can be dealt with with the modified recipe.

INTERPRETATION: In the recipe, No. 1 and No.2 both possess the effect of expelling pathogenic factors from the muscles and skin and reducing fever and therefore share the role of the principal drug. No.6 and No. 7, both acting as assistant drugs, are able to reinforce the action of the principal drugs in expelling pathogenic factors from the muscles and skin and able to relieve pain. No. 3 and No.9 with the effect of clearing away stagnated heat exerts the role of an adjuvant drug along with No.8 used for relieving disturbances of the lung-*qi* to benefit in scattering and purging exopathogens and No.5 used for regulating *ying* and purging heat. No.10 and No. 11 are capable of regulating *ying* and *wei* as well as regulating the stomach; No. 4 is capable of coordinating the actions of various drugs in the recipe, acting as a guiding drug.

芷、桔梗各3克，石膏9克，生姜三片，大枣二枚。

【用法】 水煎服。

【功用】 解肌，清热。

【主治】 外感风寒，郁而化热，表现为恶寒渐轻，身热增盛，头痛肢楚，目痛鼻干，眼眶痛，心烦不眠，舌苔薄黄，脉浮微洪等。

感冒、流行性感冒、支气管炎、牙痛等证属外感风寒、郁而化热者，可用本方加减治疗。

【方解】 方中葛根、柴胡解肌清热共为主药。羌活、白芷能助柴、葛解肌并除诸痛，为辅药。黄芩、石膏清郁热，桔梗宣肺气以助疏泄外邪，芍药和营泄热，为佐药。生姜、大枣调和营卫，并能和中；甘草兼能调和诸药，而为使药。

Modern researches have proved that this recipe possesses the efficacies in inducing sweat, allaying fever, resisting bacteria and viruses, subduing inflammation, alleviating pain, tranquilizing the mind and so on.

CAUTIONS:

1. The recipe is contraindicated in patients with symptoms of exterior wind-cold but without interior heat.

2. The recipe should not be administered for cases associated with *yangming fu*-organ disease marked by abdominal pain and constipation.

Section 3

Recipes for Strengthening the Body Resistance and Relieving Exterior Syndrome

This group of recipes is mainly composed of diaphoretics and tonifying drugs possessing the effect of strengthening the body resistance and relieving exterior syndrome, and indicated in the treatment of exterior syndrome due to general debility and attack of exopathogens.

Antiphlogistic Powder

(Baidu San)

SOURCE: *Key to Therapeutics of Children's Diseases*

INGREDIENTS:

No, 1 Bupleurum root, Radix Bupleuri 30g

No. 2 Root of purple-flowered peucedanum, *Radix Peucedani*
Peucedanum root 30g

现代研究证实，本方具有发汗、解热、抗菌、抗病毒、消炎、镇痛、镇静等作用。

【使用注意】

1．风寒在表，尚未化热者忌用。

2．若病入阳明之府，症见便秘、腹痛者忌用。

第三节　扶正解表剂

扶正解表剂主要由补益药与解表药组合而成，具有扶正、解除表证的作用，适用于体质素虚又感受外邪所致的表证。

败毒散

【来源】《小儿药证直诀》

【组成】柴胡、前胡、川芎、枳壳、羌活、独活、茯苓、桔

No. 3 Chuanxiong rhizome, *Rhizoma Ligustici Chuangxiong* 30g
No. 4 Fruit of citron or trifoliate orange, *Fructus Aurantii* 30g
No. 5 Notopterygium root, *Rhizoma seu Radix Notopterygii* 30g
No. 6 Pubescent angelica root, *Radix Angelicae Pubescentis* 30g
No. 7 Poria, *Poria* 30g
No. 8 Platycodon root, *Radix Platycodi* (parched) 30g
No. 9 Ginseng, *Radix ginseng* 30g
No.10 Licorice root, *Radix Glycyrrhizae* 15g

DIRECTIONS: All the above drugs are to be ground into powder and administered 6g each time for one dosage, to be decocted in water with a small amount of fresh ginger and peppermint for oral dose.

FUNCTIONS: Relieving the exterior syndrome by replenishing *qi* and dispelling pathogenic wind and dampness.

INDICATIONS: Exopathic diseases caused by weakened body resistance and pathogenic wind-cold-dampness, manifested as loathing of cold with high fever, headache and stiffness of the neck, soreness of the extremities, absence of perspiration, stuffy nose with low speaking voice, fullness and stuffiness in the chest, white and greasy coating of the tongue, floating and soft pulse which turns faint on hard pressure, etc.

The modified recipe can be adapted for the treatment of the common cold, influenza, epidemic parotitis, bronchitis, chronic rheumatic arthritis, urticaria, eczema and pyesis in its primary stage and other diseases that belong to the type of deficiency of genuine energy and attack of exogenous wind-cold-dampness on the body surface.

INTERPRETATION: Administered as principal drugs, both No. 5 and No. 6 have the function of dispersing the pathogenic wind-cold-dampness all over the body with their pungent flavour and warm property. No.3 is capable of promot ing the flow of blood and expelling pathogenic wind, and No.1, having a pungent flavor, is able to dispel pathogenic factors from the muscle and skin; Both are used as assistant drugs

梗(炒)、人参各30克，甘草15克。

【用法】 上药为末，每次6克，入生姜、薄荷少许，水煎服。

【功用】 益气解表，散风祛湿。

【主治】 正气不足，外感风寒湿邪，症见憎寒壮热，头痛项强，肢体痠痛，无汗，鼻塞声重，咳嗽有痰，胸膈痞满，舌苔白腻，脉浮濡而重取无力等。

感冒、流行性感冒、流行性腮腺炎、支气管炎、慢性风湿性关节炎、荨麻疹、湿疹、化脓症初期等证属正气偏虚、风寒湿邪在表者，可用本方加减治疗。

【方解】 方中羌活、独活辛温发散，通治一身上下之风寒湿邪，为主药。川芎行血祛风，柴胡辛散解肌，二药并助羌、独活

for their efficacy in reinforcing the action of the principal drugs in expelling exogenous factors and relieving pain. The following ingredients are all referred to as adjuvant drugs according to their functions: No.4 has the effect of sending down abnormally ascending *qi*; No.8 has the effect of promoting the functional activity of the lung; No. 2 has the effect of removing phlegm; No.7 has the effect of excreting dampness and No.9 has the effect of strengthening genuine energy so as to force pathogenic factors out through perspiration. In addition to being a mediator of various drugs, No, 10 is contributive to replenishing *qi* and regulating the middle-warmer, and is used as adjuvant and guiding drugs along with fresh ginger and peppermint which are able to disperse wind-cold.

Clinically and experimentally, it has been confirmed that the recipe is effective for inducing sweat, allaying fever, alleviating pain, reducing sputum, relieving cough, promoting urination and blood circulation, subduing inflammation, resisting bacteria and viruses and so on.

CAUTIONS: On account of its being warm and dry in property, the recipe is indicated for cases affected by exogenous wind-cold-dampness complicated with general deficiency, but it is not fit for those whose pathogens are dampness-heat.

Modified Decoction of Fragrant Solomonseal Rhizome

(Jiajian Weirui Tang)

SOURCE: *Revised Popular Treatise on Febrile Diseases*

INGREDIENTS:

No. 1 Fragrant solomonseal rhizome, *Rhizoma Polygonati Odorati* 9g

祛外邪、止疼痛，均为辅药。枳壳降气，桔梗开肺，前胡祛痰，茯苓渗湿，人参扶正气，以鼓邪从汗而解，均为佐药。甘草调和诸药，兼以益气和中；生姜、薄荷发散风寒，皆为佐使之药。

现代研究证实，本方具有发汗、解热、镇痛、祛痰、镇咳、利尿、促进血液循环、消炎、抗菌、抗病毒等作用。

【使用注意】 本方性偏于温燥，适用于外感风寒挟湿并兼体虚者，若湿而兼热者，则不宜用。

加减葳蕤汤

【来源】《重订通俗伤寒论》

【组成】 生葳蕤9克，生葱白6克，桔梗5克，白薇3克，

No. 2 Chinese green onion, *Bulbus Allii Fistulosi* 6g
No. 3 Platycodon root, *Radix Platycodi* 5g
No. 4 Swallowwort root, *Radix Cynanchi Atrati* 3g
No. 5 Prepared soybean, *Semen Sojae Praeparatum* 9g
No. 6 Peppermint, *Herba Menthae* 5g
No. 7 Prepared licorice root, *Radix Glycyrrhizae Praeparata* 2g
No. 8 Chinese dates, *Fructus Ziziphi Jujubae* 2 pcs.

DIERCTIONS: All the above drugs are to be decocted in water and the decoction is to be taken warm and in separate portions.

FUNCTIONS: Nourishing *yin* and clearing away heat, induing sweat to relieve exterior syndrome.

INDICATIONS: Original *yin*-deficiency with re-affaction due to exopathogen, manifested by headache, fever, light aversion to wind-cold, dry throat with cough, sputum too viscous to be coughed out, absence of sweat or little sweat, thirst and restlessness, reddened tongue and rapid pulse.

Moreover, the recipe can be modified to deal with the common cold, influenza, bronchitis and others that indicate exopathic diseaseas due to *yin* deficiency with re-affection by exopathogens after giving birth or bleeding.

INTERPRETATION: Acting as a principal drug in the recipe, Ingredient No. 1 sweet in flavor and mildly moist in property, provides the effect of nourishing *yin*, promoting the production of body fluid in order to enrich the source of perspiration, moistening the lung to relieve cough, and eliminating pathogenic heat from the throat so as to allay pain. No. 2, No.3, No.5 and No.6 togehter play the role of assistant drugs for relieving the exterior syndrome and facilitating the flow of lung -*qi* to relieve cough and sore throat. Ingredients No. 4 and No.8 are used in combination as adjuvant drugs; the former, having a bitter and salty taste and cold property, is used to quench thirst and get rid of irritability by cooling the blood and removing heat, and the latter, with a sweet flavour, exterts

淡豆豉9克，薄荷5克，甘草(炙)2克，红枣2枚。

【用法】 水煎，分温再服。

【功用】 滋阴清热，发汗解表。

【主治】 素体阴虚，复感外邪，表现为头痛身热，微恶风寒，咳嗽咽干，痰稠难出，无汗或汗出不多，口渴心烦，舌赤脉数等。

感冒、流行性感冒、支气管炎等表现为阴虚外感证者，以及产后、出血后又患外感者，可用本方加减治疗。

【方解】 方中葳蕤甘平柔润，滋阴益液以资汗源，润肺止咳，清利咽喉，为主药。葱白、淡豆豉、薄荷、桔梗解表宣肺，止咳利咽，均为辅药。白薇苦咸寒，凉血清热而除烦止渴；红枣甘润

the effect of moistening and nourishing the spleen. No.7 is administered as a guiding drug for coordinating the effect of various drugs in the recipe.

Modern studies have confirmed that this recipe is qualified as tonics for consolidating the constitution and a curative one for inducing sweat, bringing down fever, subduing inflammation, relieving cough, expelling phlegm, etc.

CAUTIONS: This recipe is only advisable for exogenous diseases with *yin* deficiency; it is contraindicated in cases without *yin* deficiency.

滋脾，共为佐药。炙甘草调和诸药，为使药。

现代研究证实，本方具有滋养强壮以及轻微发汗、解热、消炎、镇咳、祛痰等作用。

【使用注意】 本方只用于阴虚外感证，若无阴虚证候者禁用。

Chapter V

Heat-clearing Prescriptions

Heat-clearing prescriptions refer to those that are chiefly composed of heat-clearing drugs for the treatment of interior heat syndrome, having the functions in heat-clearing, fire-purging, blood-cooling and toxin-removing.

In view of the difference in interior heat syndromes among *qi* system, blood system and the viscera, the heat-clearing prescriptions are further classified as the prescriptions for clearing away heat from *qi* system, the prescriptions for removing heat from the *ying* and blood systems, the prescriptions for clearing away heat from both *qi* and *ying* systems, the prescriptions for cleaning away heat and toxic material, the prescriptions for removing heat from the viscera and bowels, the prescriptions for allaying fever of deficiency type and the prescriptions for clearing away summer-heat and replenishing *qi*.

Section 1

Recipes for Clearing Away Heat from the *Qi* System

This kind of prescriptions is chiefly made up of drugs possessing the effects of removing heat and purging away pathogenic fire, and has the actions of clearing away heat from

第五章

清热剂

凡主要由清热药物组成，具有清热、泻火、凉血、解毒作用，治疗里热证的方剂，称为清热剂。

里热证有热在气分、血分、脏腑的不同，因此清热剂又分为清气分热、清营凉血、气血两清、清热解毒、清脏腑热、清虚热、清暑益气等七类。

第一节 清气分热剂

清气分热剂主要由清热泻火药组成，有清气分热、除烦止渴

the *qi* system and relieving thirst and restlessness. It can be applied to the syndrome of excessive heat in the *qi* system.

White Tiger Decoction

(Baihu Tang)

SOURCE: ***Treatise on Febrile Diseases***

INGREDIENTS:

No. 1 Gypsum, *Gypsum Fibrosum* (ground) 30g
No. 2 Wind-weed rhizome, *Rhizoma Anemarrhenae* 9g
No. 3 Prepared Licorice root, *Radix Glycyrrhizae Praeparata* 3g
No. 4 Polished round-grained nonglutinous rice, *Semen Oryzae Nonglutionosae* 9g

DIRECTIONS: Decoct all drugs in water until the rice is well-done. Take the decoction warm orally after removal of the residue.

FUNCTIONS: Clearing away heat and promoting the production of body fluid.

INDICATIONS: *Yangming* channel diseases (excessive heat syndrome in *yangming* channels and *qi* system) marked by high fever, flushed face, polydipsia, profuse perspiration, aversion to heat and full forceful pulse.

The recipe can be modified to deal with influenza, epidemic encephalitis B, epidemic cerebrospinal meningitis, pneumonia and septicemia indicating excessive heat syndrome in the *qi* system, and also with the treatment of stomatitis, periodontitis, gastritis, diabetes and others which pertain to stomach heat syndrome.

INTERPRETATION: In the recipe, Ingredient No.1, pungent and sweet in flavour and extremely cold in nature, acts as a principal drug effective against excessive heat in *yangming* channel. No. 2, which is bitter in taste and cold

的作用，适用于气分热盛之证。

白 虎 汤

【来源】《伤寒论》

【组成】石膏(碎)30克，知母9克，甘草(炙)3克，粳米9克。

【用法】水煎至米熟，去滓温服。

【功用】清热生津。

【主治】阳明经证(阳明气分实热证)，表现为壮热面赤，烦渴引饮，大汗出，恶热，脉洪大有力等。

流行性感冒、流行性乙型脑炎、流行性脑膜炎、肺炎、败血症等表现为气分热盛者，口腔炎、牙周炎、胃炎、糖尿病等证属胃热者，均可用本方加减治疗。

【方解】方中石膏，辛甘大寒，清阳明内盛之热，为主药。

moist in nature, serves as an assistant drug for strengthening the action of the principal drug. Ingredients No.3 and No.4 function as adjuvant and guiding drugs that can not only reinforce the function of the stomach and protect the body fluid, but also prevent the middle-warmer from being injured by bitter and cold drugs.

Modern researches have proved that the recipe has the efficacies of allaying fever, tranquilizing the mind, subduing inflammation, inhibiting hidropoiesis, quenching thirst, lowering blood sugar level.

CAUTIONS: It is not advisable for those whose exterior syndrome is not relieved, nor for those who have fever due to blood-deficiency or cold syndrome with pseudo-heat symptoms.

Lophatherum and Gypsum Decoction

(Zhuye Shigao Tang)

SOURCE: ***Treatise on Febrile Diseases***

INGREDIENTS:

No. 1 Lophatherum, *Herba Lophatheri* 15g

No. 2 Gypsum, *Cypsum Fibrosum* 30g

No. 3 Prepared pinellia tuber, *Rhizoma Pinelliae Praeparata* 9g

No. 4 Ophiopogon root, *Radix Ophiopogonis* 15g

No. 5 Ginseng, *Radix Ginseng* 5g

No. 6 Prepared licorice root, *Radix Glycyrrhizae Praeparata* 3g

No. 7 Polished round-grained nonglutinous rice, *Semen Oryzae Nonglutinosae* 15g

DIRECTIONS: All the ingredients should be decocted in water for oral dose.

FUNCTIONS: Clearing away heat and promoting the production of body fluid, replenishing *qi* and regulating the stomach.

知母，苦寒质润，助石膏清肺胃之热，为辅药。甘草、粳米既能益胃护津，又可防苦寒伤中之弊，为佐使药。

现代研究证实，本方具有解热、镇静、消炎、止汗、止渴、降血糖等作用。

【使用注意】 凡表证未解、血虚发热、真寒假热者，均不可用本方。

竹叶石膏汤

【来源】 《伤寒论》

【组成】 竹叶15克，石膏30克，制半夏9克，麦冬15克，人参5克，甘草(炙)3克，粳米15克。

【用法】 水煎服。

【功用】 清热生津，益气和胃。

INDICATIONS: Lingering heat with impairment of both the *qi* and body fluid in the later stage of exogenous febrile disease, epidemic febrile disease and summer-heat disease, marked by feverish body, hyperhidrosis, general debility and short breath, irritability, inclination to vomit, dry mouth and fondness of drink, or insomnia due to restlessness, reddened tongue with little coating, and rapid pulse.

The recipe can also be modified to deal with cases with deficiency of both *qi* and *yin* occuring in the later stage of influenza, epidemic encephalitis B, epidemic cerebrospinal meningitis, pneumonia and septicemia.

INTERPRETATION: In the recipe, Ingredients No. 1 and No.2, with the effects of clearing away heat and relieving restlessness, are used as principal drugs. No. 4 and No. 5, being effective for nourishing *yin* and promoting the production of body fluid, serve as assistant drugs. No.3 is an adjuvant drug for lowering the adverse flow of *qi* to relieve vomiting. No.6 and No.7 are guiding drugs with the functions nourishing the stomach and regulating the middle-warmer.

Clinically and experimentally, it is ascertained that the recipe is contributive not only to nourishing and strengthening the constitution to promote digestion and absorption, but also to subduing inflammation, tranquilizing the mind, bringing down fever, arresting cough, dispelling phlegm and preventing vomiting.

CAUTIONS: It is not advisable for cases with febrile disease when the vital energy is dominating with pathogens prevailing, or excessive heat existing in the body, or neither *qi* nor *yin* being impaired.

【主治】 伤寒、温病、暑病之后，余热未清，气津两伤，症见身热多汗，虚羸少气，烦闷欲呕，口干喜饮，或虚烦不寐，舌红少苔，脉数等。

流行性感冒、流行性乙型脑炎、流行性脑脊髓膜炎、肺炎、败血症等后期出现气阴两虚者，可用本方加减治疗。

【方解】 方中竹叶、石膏清热除烦，为主药。人参益气，麦冬养阴生津，共为辅药。半夏降逆止呕为佐药。甘草、粳米养胃和中为使药。

现代研究证实，本方既具有滋补强壮、促进消化吸收的作用，又有消炎、镇静、解热、镇咳、祛痰、止呕之功。

【使用注意】 热病正盛邪实、大热未衰、气阴未伤者忌用。

Section 2

Recipes for Removing Heat from the *Ying* and Blood Systems

This group of prescriptions refers to those that chiefly consist of traditional Chinese drugs with effects of clearing away heat and cooling the blood, arresting bleeding and removing blood stasis, and clearing up heat and toxic materals of any pathogenic organism. These are used to treat syndromes of invasion of both *ying* and blood systems by heat.

Decoction for Clearing Heat in the *Ying* System

(Qingying Tang)

SOURCE: ***Treatise on Differentiation and Treatment of Epidemic Febrile Diseases.***

INGREDIENTS:

No. 1 Rhinoceros horn, *Cornu Rhinocerotis* 2g
No. 2 Rehmannia root, *Radix Rehmanniae* 15g
No. 3 Scrophularia root, *Radix Scrophulariae* 9g
No. 4 Lophatherum, *Herba Lophatheri* 3g
No. 5 Ophiopogon root, *Radix Ophiopogonis* 9g
No. 6 Red sage root, *Radix Salviae Miltiorrhizae* 6g
No. 7 Coptis root, *Rhizoma Coptidis* 5g
No. 8 Honeysuckle flower, *Flos Lonicerae* 9g
No. 9 Forsythia fruit, *Fructus Forsythiae* 6g

DIRECTIONS: All the ingredients should be decocted in water for oral dose.

第二节　清营凉血剂

清营凉血剂主要由清热凉血药组成，有清营凉血、止血散瘀、清热解毒的作用，适用于热入营血之证。

清　营　汤

【来源】《温病条辨》

【组成】犀角2克，生地黄15克，玄参9克，竹叶心3克，麦冬9克，丹参6克，黄连5克，银花9克，连翘6克。

【用法】水煎服。

FUNCTIONS: Clearing and dispelling pathogenic heat from the *ying* system, nourishing *yin* and promoting blood circulation.

INDICATIONS: Invasion of the *ying* system by pathogenic heat manifested by feverish body which is aggravated in the night, delirium occuring now and then, insomnia due to vexation, or by faint skin rashes, deep-red and dry tongue and rapid pulse.

The recipe can also be modified to deal with *ying*-syndrome occuring in epidemic encephalitis B, epidemic cerebrospinal meningitis, septicemia and other infectious diseases.

INTERPRETATION: In the recipe, Ingredient No.1, being salty in flavour and cold in property, and No.2, being sweet in taste and cold in nature, both exert a role of a principal drug, having the effect of removing heat from the *ying* and blood systems. No.3 and No.5 together act as assistant drugs having the effect of nourishing *yin* and clearing heat. The rest share the role of adjuvant and guiding drugs. Ingredients Nos. 4,5,8 and 9 are used to clear and dispel pathogenic heat from the *yin* system through *qi* system, and No. 6 is used to promote blood circulation to remove blood stasis.

Clinically and experimentally, it is ascertained that the recipe possesses the efficacies of relieving inflammation, bringing down fever, tranquilizing the mind, resisting bacteria and viruses, tonifying the heart, arresting bleeding, improving immunologic function, promoting blood circulation and so on.

CAUTIONS: Cases with white and slippery coating of the tongue which suggests invasion by pathogenic dampness should not use the recipe in case it encourages pathogenic dampness.

Decoction of Rhinoceros Horn and Rehmannia

(Xijiao Dihuang Tang)

SOURCE: ***Prescriptions Worth a Thousand Gold for Emer-***

【功用】 清营透热，养阴活血。

【主治】 热入营分，表现为身热夜甚，时有谵语，心烦不眠，或斑疹隐隐，舌绛而干，脉数等。

乙型脑炎、流行性脑膜炎、败血症及其他感染性疾病出现营分证者，可用本方加减治疗。

【方解】 方中犀角咸寒，生地甘寒清营凉血，为主药。玄参、麦冬养阴清热，共为辅药。银花、连翘、黄连、竹叶清热解毒以透邪热，使入营之邪透出气分而解；丹参活血消瘀，皆为佐使药。

现代研究证实，本方具有消炎、解热、镇静、抗菌、抗病毒、强心、止血、增强免疫功能、促进血液循环等作用。

【使用注意】 舌苔白滑者，是挟有湿邪之证，不可使用本方，以防助湿留邪。

犀角地黄汤

【来源】 《千金要方》

gencies

INGREDIENTS:

No. 1 Rhinoceros horn, *Cornu Rhinocerotis* 1.5—3g

No. 2 Dried rehmannia root, *Radix Rehmanniae* 30g

No. 3 Peony root, *Radix Paeoniae* 12g

No. 4 Moutan bark, *Cortex Moutan Radicis* 9g

DIRECTIONS: All the ingredients should be decocted in water for oral dose with the exception of Ingredient No.1 which should be ground into powder first and then taken orally along with the decoction.

FUNCTIONS: Clearing away heat and toxic material and cooling blood and removing blood stasis.

INDICATIONS: Syndromes of invasion of the blood system by pathogenic heat which results in bleeding, manifested by hematemesis, epistaxis, hematuria, hemafecia, dark purple colour of rashes, deep-red tongue with prickle-like fur; or syndrome of blood retention marked by madness, a parched throat with a thirst for water, with water in the mouth but no desire to swallow it, distension in the lower abdomen, dark smooth stools.

The recipe can be modified to deal with cases whose blood system is affected by pathogenic heat, as seen in epidemic encephalitis B, epidemic cerebrospinal meningitis, typhus, epidemic hemorrhagic fever, acute yellow atrophy of liver, hepatic coma, septicemia, thrombocytopenic purpura and hemophilia.

INTERPRETATION: Of the ingredients in the recipe, No.1 acts as a principal drug having the functions of clearing away heart-fire, removing pathogenic heat from the blood and toxic material from the body; No.2 serves as an assistant drug possessing the effect of removing heat from the blood and arresting bleeding, nourishing *yin* and clearing away heat; No.3 and No.4 both sharing the part of adjuvant and guiding drugs, are provided with the effect of removing heat from

【组成】 犀角1.5～3克，生地黄30克，芍药12克，牡丹皮9克。

【用法】 水煎，犀角磨汁和服。

【功用】 清热解毒，凉血散瘀。

【主治】 热入血分证。热甚动血出现吐衄、尿血、便血、斑色紫黑、舌绛起刺等；或蓄血发狂，但欲漱水不欲咽，少腹胀满，大便黑而易解者。

流行性乙型脑炎、流行性脑膜炎、斑疹伤寒、流行性出血热、急性黄色肝萎缩、肝昏迷、败血症、血小板减少性紫斑、血友病等证属热入血分者，可用本方加减治疗。

【方解】 方中犀角清心凉血解毒，为主药。生地凉血止血，养阴清热为辅药。芍药、丹皮清热凉血，活血散瘀，使止血而无

the blood, promoting blood circulation to remove blood stasis, arresting bleeding with no formation of stasis.

Clinically and experimentally, it is ascertained that this recipe possesses the efficacies of allaying a fever, tranquilizing the mind, relieving inflammation, resisting bacteria, arresting bleeding, promoting blood circulation, strengthening the heart function, etc.

CAUTIONS: It is contraindicated in cases with bleedings caused by deficiency of *qi* or with weakness of the spleen and stomach.

Section 3

Recipes for Clearing Away Heat from Both *Qi* and Blood Systems

This type of prescriptions, which is chiefly composed of drugs with the effects of clearing *qi* and cooling blood, has the function of clearing away heat from both *qi* and blood systems and applies to the syndrome of intense heat in both *qi* and blood systems with epidemic or heat pathogens flooding both interiorly and exteriorly.

Antipyretic and Antitoxic Decoction

(Qingwen Baidu Yin)

SOURCE: *A View of Epidemic Febrile Diseases with Rashes*

INGREDIENTS:

No. 1 Gypsum, *Gypsum Fibrosum* 30g

No. 2 Dried rehmannia root, *Radix Rehmanniae* 15g

留瘀之弊，为佐使药。

现代研究证实，本方具有解热、镇静、消炎、抗菌、止血、促进血液循环、强心等作用。

【使用注意】 凡气虚失血或脾胃虚弱者忌用。

第三节 气血两清剂

气血两清剂主要由清气药和凉血药组成，有气血两清的作用，适用于疫毒或热毒充斥内外的气血两燔证。

清瘟败毒饮

【来源】 《疫疹一得》

【组成】 生石膏30克，生地黄15克，犀角3克，黄连3克，

No. 3 Rhinoceros horn, *Cornu Rhinocerotis* 3g
No. 4 Coptis root, *Rhizoma Coptidis* 3g
No. 5 Capejasmine fruit, *Fructus Gardeniae* 6g
No. 6 Scutellaria root, *Radix Scutellariae* 6g
No. 7 Platycodon root, *Radix Platycodi* 3g
No. 8 Wind-weed rhizome, *Rhizoma Anemarrhenae* 6g
No. 9 Red peony root, *Radix Paeoniae Rubra* 6g
No.10 Scrophularia root, *Radix Scrophulariae* 6g
No.11 Forsythia fruit, *Fructus Forsythiae* 6g
No.12 Licorice root, *Radix Glycyrrhizae* 3g
No.13 Moutan bark, *Cortex Moutan Radicis* 6g
No.14 Lophatherum *Herba Lophatheri* 3g

DIRECTIONS: Decoct gypsum in water to the boiling point for some dozens of times before it is mixed and decocted with other drugs. Without being decocted, rhinoceros horn is to be ground into powder and taken orally along with the decoction.

FUNCTIONS: Clearing away heat and toxic materials, removing heat from the blood and purging pathogenic fire from the body, nourishing *yin* and arresting bleeding.

INDICATIONS: Intense heat and virulent pathogen in both *qi* and blood systems occurring in the course of epidemic infectious diseases manifested by high fever, thirst, severe headache, retching, restlessness, delirium, coma, skin eruption or hematemesis, epistaxis, convulsion or coldness of the extremities, sunken and rapid pulse or sunken fine and rapid pulse, or superficial and rapid pulse, and deep redness of the tongue with cracked lips.

In addition, the recipe can be modified to deal with septicemia, encephalitis B, epidemic cerebrospinal meningitis or other febrile diseases with the above syndrome.

INTERPRETATION: In the recipe, Ingredient No.1 is dosed the most and, coordinated with No.8 and No.12, ex-

栀子6克，黄芩6克，桔梗3克，知母6克，赤芍6克，玄参6克，连翘6克，生甘草3克，丹皮6克，鲜竹叶3克。

【用法】 先煎石膏数十沸，后下诸药。犀角磨汁和服。

【功用】 清热解毒，凉血泻火，滋阴止血。

【主治】 瘟疫热毒，充斥内外之气血两燔证，表现为大热口渴，剧烈头痛，干呕狂燥，谵语神昏，或发斑疹，或吐血、衄血，四肢抽搐，或厥逆，脉沉数，或沉细而数，或浮大而数，舌绛唇焦等。

败血症、乙型脑炎、流行性脑脊髓膜炎或其他热病表现为热毒炽盛者，可用本方加减治疗。

【方解】 方中重用石膏并配知母、甘草取法白虎汤，以清热

erts the role of clearing away heat and promoting the production of body fluid, having an effect similar to White Tiger Decoction. As an adoption of Antidotal Decoction of Coptis, No.4, No.5, and No.6, are used in combination to purge the pathogenic fire and heat in the tri-warmer. The combination of No. 2, No. 3, No. 9 and No. 13, the right formula for Decoction of Rhinoceros Horn and Rehmannia, yields the effect of clearing away heat and toxic materials, and cooling blood and removing blood stasis. No. 10 and No.11 are boosters for dispelling wandering fire. No. 7 and No. 14 are used for their function of guiding drugs. The combination of three recipes dominates the effect of clearing thoroughly the heat in the *yangming* channesl, and in coorperation with drugs of purging fire and cooling blood, it may achieve desirable antipyretic and antitoxic effect.

Modern researches have ascertained that the recipe is strong in its effect for relieving inflammation, allaying fever, tranquilizing the mind and resisting pathogens. Meanwhile, it can play a part in preventing bleeding and strengthening the function of the heart.

CAUTIONS: Being extremely cold in nature, the recipe must not be prescribed for those without exuberant and noxious heat.

Section 4

Recipes for Clearing Away Heat and Toxins

This type of prescriptions is chiefly composed of traditional Chinese drugs having the effect of removing pathogenic fire, heat and toxic materials and is indicated for the treatment of domination of toxic heat in the interior and the attack of epidemic pathogens on the head or face.

保津。黄连、黄芩、栀子共用，仿黄连解毒汤之义，以通泻三焦火热。犀角、生地、赤药、丹皮相配，即犀角地黄汤原方，以清热解毒，凉血散瘀。再配连翘、玄参解散浮游之火，桔梗、竹叶取其载药上行之功。三方合用，以大清阳明经热为主，配以泻火凉血药相辅而成，共奏清瘟败毒之效。

现代研究证实，本方具有很强的消炎、解热、镇静、抗菌作用，同时还有止血，强心等功效。

【使用注意】 本方药性大寒，非属热极毒盛者，不可以妄用。

第四节 清热解毒剂

清热解毒剂主要由泻火、清热、解毒药组成，具有清热、泻火、解毒的作用。适用于热毒内盛以及疫毒发于头面等证。

Antidotal Decoction of Coptis

(Huanglian Jiedu Tang)

SOURCE: ***The Medical Secrets of an Official*** (but the prescription was made by Dr. Cui)

INGREDIENTS:

No. 1 Coptis root, *Rhizoma Coptidis* 9g
No. 2 Skutellaria root, *Radix Scutellariae* 6g
No. 3 Phellodendron bark, *Cortex Phellodendri* 6g
No. 4 Capejasmine fruit, *Fructus Gardeniae* 9g

DIRECTIONS: All the ingredients should be decocted in water for oral administration.

FUNCTIONS: Purging pathogenic fire and lessening virulence of any pathogenic organism.

INDICATIONS: All the syndromes of fire-toxin by excessive heat or intense heat in the tri-warmer manifested by high fever, fidgetiness, dry mouth and lips, delirium, insomnia, hematemesis or epistaxis in the course of febrile diseases or skin eruptions due to intense heat, dysentery with fever, jaundice due to damp-heat, sore and carbuncle, deep-coloured urine, reddened tongue with yellow coating, and rapid and forceful pulse.

The recipe can also be modified to treat many other disorders. For example, influenza, encephalitis B, epidemic cerebrospinal meningitis, septicemia, pyogenic infection of skin, acute infectious hepatitis, acute gastroenteritis, bacillary dysentery, infection in the urinary tract, acute cholecystitis and others that belong to syndromes of fire-toxin and excessive heat, disorder of vegetative nervous function, menopausal syndrome, neurosis, insomnia, hypertension, stomatitis, toothache, and nervous gastritis which indicate the syndrome

黄连解毒汤

【来源】《外台秘要》引崔氏方

【组成】黄连9克，黄芩6克，黄柏6克，栀子9克。

【用法】水煎服。

【功用】泻火解毒。

【主治】一切实热火毒、三焦热盛之证，表现为大热烦躁，口燥唇干，谵语不眠，或热病吐衄，或热甚发斑，身热下痢，湿热黄疸，疮痈疔毒，小便黄赤，舌红苔黄，脉数有力等。

流行性感冒、乙型脑炎、流行性脑脊髓膜炎、败血症、皮肤化脓性感染、急性传染性肝炎、急性胃肠炎、细菌性痢疾、泌尿道感染、急性胆囊炎等证属实热火毒者；植物神经失调、更年期综合征、神经官能症、失眠、高血压、口腔炎、牙痛、神经性胃

of intense heat in the heart and stomach or excessive fire in the liver and gallbladder; as well as various inflammatory bleedings or rashes.

INTERPRETATION: In the recipe, Ingredient No. 1 is used as a principal drug which plays a significant role in purging pathogenic fire in the heart and stomach. No. 2 acts as an assistant drug with the effect of clearing away heat in the lung and purging fire in the upper-warmer. No. 3 and No. 4 are used in combination as both adjuvant and guiding drugs, the former providing the effect of purging pathogenic fire in the lower-warmer and the latter having the effect of removing pathogenic fire in the tri-warmer by inducing diuresis. The combination of the four ingredients results in the disappearance of both fire-pathogen and heat-toxin. The health condition thus becomes normal.

Modern researches have confirmed that the recipe can exert the function of relieving inflammation, allaying fever, resisting bacteria and viruses, and tranquilizing the mind. In addition, it has the virtue to normalize the function of the gallbladder, arrest bleeding, promote diuresis, and reduce blood pressure.

CAUTIONS: The recipe is fit for cases with overabundance of heat-toxin in the tri-warmer but no impairment of the body fluid. So it is not advisable for those with injury of the body fluid by heat manifested as deep-red and uncoated tongue.

Universal Relief Decoction for Disinfection

(Puji Xiaodu Yin)

SOURCE: *Dongyuan's Effective Prescriptions*

INGREDIENTS:

No. 1 Scutellaria root, *Radix Scutellariae* (parched with wine) 15g

炎等呈现心胃火盛、肝胆火旺者；各种炎症性出血或发疹者，均可用本方加减治疗。

【方解】 方中黄连泻心胃之火，为主药。黄芩清肺热，泻上焦之火，为辅药。黄柏泻下焦之火，栀子通泻三焦之火，导热下行，共为佐使之药。四药合用，能使火邪去而热毒解，故诸症可愈。

现代研究证实，本方除有消炎、解热、抗菌、抗病毒、镇静作用外，尚有利胆、止血、利尿、降压等作用。

【使用注意】 本方适用于三焦热毒炽盛而阴液未伤者，凡热伤阴液，舌质光绛者，不宜使用。

普济消毒饮

【来源】 《东垣试效方》

【组成】 黄芩(酒炒)、黄连(酒炒)各15克，陈皮(去白)、生

No. 2 Coptis root, *Rhizoma Coptidis* (parched with wine) 15g
No. 3 Tangerine peel, *Pericarpium Citri Reticulatae* (white part removed) 6g
No. 4 Licorice root, *Radix Glycyrrhizae* 6g
No. 5 Scrophularia root, *Radix Scrophulariae* 6g
No. 6 Bupleurum root, *Radix Bupleuri* 6g
No. 7 Platycodon root, *Radix Platycodi* 6g
No. 8 Forsythia fruit, *Fructus Forsythiae* 3g
No. 9 Isatis root, *Radix Isatidis* 3g
No. 10 Puff-ball, *Lasiosphaera Seu Calvatia* 3g
No. 11 Arctium fruit, *Fructus Arctii* 3g
No. 12 Peppermint, *Herba Menthae* 3g
No. 13 Batryticated silkworm, *Bombyx Batryticatus* 2g
No. 14 Cimicifuga rhizome, *Rhizoma Cimicifugae* 2g

DIRECTIONS: All the above ingredients should be decocted in water for oral use.

FUNCTIONS: Clearing away heat and toxic material, and dispelling wind and other exopathogens.

INDICATIONS: Infection with swollen head marked by chill and fever, flushed swollen face, heavy eyes, sore throat, dryness of the tongue, thirst, reddened tongue with yellow coating and rapid forceful pulse.

The modified recipe can be used for treatment of diseases with the above symptoms as seen in facial erysipelas, acute parotitis and tonsillitis, carbuncle and other infectious swelling in the face.

INTERPRETATION: In the recipe, Ingredients No. 1 and 2 play the role of principal drugs having the effect of dispelling heat-toxin originally affecting the face and head. Being pungent in flavour and cool in nature, No. 11, No. 8, No. 12 and No. 13 as assistant drugs in combination, have the effect of dispelling pathogenic wind-heat in the face and head. Nos. 4 5,7,9 and 10, used in combination as adjuvant drugs, have the

甘草、玄参、柴胡、桔梗各6克，连翘、板蓝根、马勃、牛蒡子、薄荷各3克，僵蚕、升麻各2克。

【用法】水煎服。

【功用】清热解毒，疏风散邪。

【主治】大头瘟，症见恶寒发热，头面红肿焮痛，目不能开，咽喉不利，舌燥口渴，舌红苔黄，脉数有力等。

颜面丹毒、急性腮腺炎、急性扁桃体炎以及头面痈疮肿毒等出现上述症候者，可用本方加减治疗。

【方解】方中黄芩、黄连能清降发于头面之热毒，为主药。牛蒡子、连翘、薄荷、僵蚕辛凉，能疏散头面风热，共为辅药。

function of removing heat-toxin from the throat, face and head. The rest play the part of guiding drugs in combination. No. 3 is used to promote the circulation of *qi* and digestion, Nos. 14 and 6 to dispel pathogenic wind-heat and to assist the other drugs in reaching the face and head to remove heat pathogens from them.

Modern researches have ascertained that the recipe has the function of relieving inflammation, resisting bacteria and viruses, allaying fever, tranquilizing the mind and alleviating pain.

CAUTIONS: As the majority of the drugs are bitter and pungent in flavour and cold in nature, patients with *yin*-deficiency should be cautious when taking this recipe.

Section 5

Recipes for Removing Heat from the Viscera

This sort of prescriptions is chiefly made up of drugs effective for removing pathogenic heat and fire and is indicated for the treatment of fire-heat syndrome caused by overabundance of pathogenic heat in the viscera or bowels.

Powder for Treating Dark Urine

(Daochi San)

SOURCE: ***Key to Therapeutics of Children's Diseases***

INGREDIENTS:

No. 1 Dried rehmannia root, *Radix Rehmanniae* 18g

No. 2 Fiveleaf akebia stem, *Caulis Akebiae* 12g

玄参、马勃、板蓝根、桔梗、甘草能清解咽喉、头面热毒，皆为佐药。陈皮理气而疏通壅滞，升麻、柴胡疏散风热，并协诸药上达头面，以清头面热毒，共为使药。

现代研究证实，本方具有抗菌、消炎、抗病毒、解热、镇痛、镇静、止痛等作用。

【使用注意】 本方药物多苦寒辛散，阴虚者慎用。

第五节　清脏腑热剂

清脏腑热剂主要由清热泻火药组成，适用于热邪偏盛于某一脏腑所产生的火热证。

导　赤　散

【来源】《小儿药证直诀》

【组成】 生地黄 18 克，木通 12 克，生甘草 6 克，淡竹叶12

No. 3 Licorice root, *Radix Glycyrrhizae* 6g

No. 4 Lophatherum, *Herba Lophatheri* 12g

DIRECTIONS: All the ingredients should be decocted in water for oral administration.

FUNCTIONS: Removing pathogenic heat from the heart and nourishing *yin*, inducing diuresis for treating stranguria.

INDICATIONS: Domination of heat in the heart channel manifested as irritable feverish sensation in the chest, thirst, flushed face, predilection for cold drinks, oral ulceration; or transfer of heart-heat to the small intestine from the heart channel, marked by scanty and dark urine and difficulty and pain in micturition.

Besides, the recipe can be modified to deal with stomatitis, vegetative nerve functional disturbance, cystitis, pyelitis and insomnia which pertain to the domination of heat in the heart channel.

INTERPRETATION: In the recipe, Ingredient No. 1 is indicated for removing pathogenic heat, cooling blood and nourishing *yin*; No.2 is for purging pathogenic fire from the heart and promoting urination; No. 4 is for reducing pathogenic heat from the heart, relieving restlessness, inducing heat downward and out through urination; No. 3 for clearing heat and toxic materials and relieving painful urination as well as for coordinating the actions of various ingredients in the recipe.

Modern researches have ascertained that the prescription possesses the functions of relieving inflammation, allaying fever, inducing diuresis and tranquilizing the mind.

CAUTIONS: Being bitter in flavour and cold in nature, Ingredient No. 2 should be carefully administered in patients with weakness of the spleen and stomach.

克。

【用法】 水煎服。

【功用】 清心养阴，利水通淋。

【主治】 心经热盛证，表现为心胸烦热，口渴面赤，意欲冷饮，口舌生疮，或心热移于小肠，小溲赤涩刺痛等。

口腔炎、植物神经失调、膀胱炎、肾盂炎、失眠等证属心经热盛者，可用本方加减治疗。

【方解】 方中生地清热、凉血、养阴。木通降心火、利小便。竹叶清心除烦，引热下行，从小便而出。生甘草清热解毒而止淋痛，并调和诸药。

现代研究证实，本方具有消炎、解热、利尿、镇静等作用。

【使用注意】 方中木通性味苦寒，脾胃虚弱者当慎用。

Decoction of Gentian for Purging Liver-fire

(Longdan Xiegan Tang)

SOURCE: ***Collection of Prescriptions with Notes***

INGREDIENTS:

No. 1 Gentian root, *Radix Gentianae* (parched with wine) 6g

No. 2 Scutellaria root, *Radix Scutellariae* (parched with wine) 9g

No. 3 Capejasmine fruit, *Fructus Gardeniae* (parched with wine) 9g

No. 4 Oriental water plantain, *Rhizoma Alismatis* 12g

No. 5 Fiveleaf akebia stem, *Caulis Akebiae* 9g

No. 6 Plantain seed, *Semen Plantaginis* 9g

No. 7 Chinese angelica root, *Radix Angelicae Sinensis* (washed with wine) 3g

No. 8 Dried rehmannia root, *Radix Rehmanniae* (parched with wine) 9g

No. 9 Bupleurum root, *Radix Bupleuri* 6g

No.10 Licorice root, *Radix Glycyrrhizae* 6g

DIRECTIONS: All the above drugs should be decocted in water for oral administration.

FUNCTIONS: Purging excessive fire from the liver and gallbladder and removing damp-heat from the lower-warmer.

INDICATIONS: Upward attack of excessive fire in the liver and gallbladder or downward flow of damp-heat from the liver channel manifested as headache, conjunctival congestion, hypochondriac pain, bitter taste, deafness, pain and bulge of ear; or marked by pruritus and swelling of vulva, impotence, polyhidrosis around the external genitals, stranguria with turbid urine, and damp-heat leukorrhagia.

Equally, the recipe can be modified to cure diseases

龙胆泻肝汤

【来源】《医方集解》

【组成】 龙胆草(酒炒)6克，黄芩(酒炒)9克，栀子(酒炒)9克，泽泻12克，木通9克，车前子9克，当归(酒洗)3克，生地黄(酒炒)9克，柴胡6克，生甘草6克。

【用法】 水煎服。

【功用】 泻肝胆实火，清下焦湿热。

【主治】 肝胆实火上扰或肝经湿热下注，表现为头痛目赤，胁痛口苦，耳聋耳肿；或阴肿阴痒，阴痿阴汗，小便淋浊，妇女湿热带下等。

高血压病、植物神经失调、急性结膜炎、急性中耳炎、鼻前

marked by extreme fire in the liver and gallbladder, such as hypertension, vegetative nerve functional disturbance, acute conjunctivitis, acute otitis media, furuncle of nasal vestibule or furuncle of external auditory canal, acute cholecystitis and acute hepatitis; and to deal with cases with downward flow of damp-heat as seen in acute infection in the urinary system, acute orchitis, epididymitis, acute eczema, acute pelvic inflammation, acute prostatitis, vaginitis and herpes zoster.

INTERPRETATION: In the recipe, Ingredient No. 1 extremely bitter in flavour and cold in nature, is used to purge excessive fire in the liver and gallbladder and clear damp-heat in the lower-warmer, providing the principal curative efficacy. No. 2 and No. 3, being bitter in flavour and cold in nature, are used in combination to reinforce the effect of the Ingredient No. 1, playing the role of an assistant drug. Functioning together as adjuvant and guiding drugs, No. 4, No. 5 and No. 6 have the effect of removing heat and inducing diuresis to dispel damp-heat while No. 7 and No. 8 possess the effect of nourishing *yin* and blood so as to soothe the liver. No. 9 and No. 10 work in combination as guiding drugs, with the former having the effect of soothing the liver and regulating the circulation of *qi* in the liver and gallbladder and inducing the efficacy of all the medicines into the liver and gallbladder, and the latter having the effect of coordinating the effect of various ingredients in the recipe so as to prevent the stomach from being hurt by the bitter and cold property of the drugs.

Clinically and experimentally, it is ascertained that the recipe has the effect of bringing down the fever, tranquilizing the mind, relieving inflammation, inducing diuresis, resisting bacteria, promoting the function of gallbladder, protecting the liver, arresting bleeding and decreasing blood pressure.

CAUTIONS: Since most of the drugs in the recipe are bitter in flavour and cold in property, constant and long-term administration of it is not advisable. Great care should be

庭或外耳道疖肿、急性胆囊炎、急性肝炎等证属肝胆火旺者；急性泌尿系感染、急性睾丸炎、附睾炎、急性湿疹、急性盆腔炎、急性前列腺炎、阴道炎、带状疱疹等证属湿热下注者，可用本方加减治疗。

【方解】 方中龙胆草大苦大寒，泻肝胆实火，清下焦湿热，为主药。黄芩、栀子苦寒泻火，助龙胆草泻肝胆实火，为辅药。泽泻、木通、车前子清热利湿，使湿热从小便排除，生地、当归滋阴养血以柔肝，为佐使药。柴胡疏畅肝胆之气，并引诸药入肝胆，甘草调和诸药，以免苦寒伤胃之弊，共为使药。

现代研究证实，本方具有解热、镇静、消炎、利尿、抗菌、利胆、保肝、止血、降血压等作用。

【使用注意】 本方多苦寒药，易伤胃气，不宜多服久服，脾

taken when exhibiting the drugs for those whose spleen-stomach functions are weak, otherwise the stomach-*qi* might be easily hurt.

Lung-heat Expelling Powder

(Xiebai San)

SOURCE: *Key to Therapeutics of Children's Diseases*

INGREDIENTS:

No. 1 Wolfberry bark, *Cortex Lycii Radicis* 30g

No. 2 Mulberry bark, *Cortex Mori Radicis* 30g

No. 3 Prepared licorice root, *Radix Glycyrrhizae Praeparata* 3g

DIRECTIONS: All the above ingredients should be ground into powder first and then mixed with a little polished round-grained nonglutinous rice and two small cups of water, decocted until one third of the water is evaporated. Its decoction should be taken before meals.

FUNCTIONS: Purging pathogenic heat accumulated in the lung to relieve cough and asthma.

INDICATIONS: Cough and asthma due to lung-heat, manifested by feverish skin which is aggraviated in the afternoon, reddened tongue with yellow coating and fine rapid pulse.

The recipe can be modified to deal with bronchitis, measles pneumonia, pulmonary tuberculosis and others which pertain to the syndrome of cough and asthma due to lung-heat.

INTERPRETATION: In the recipe, Ingredient No. 2, sweet in taste and cold in property, acts on the lung and has the effect of dispelling lung-heat, functioning as a principal drug. No. 1 serves as an assistant drug which is effective for purging latent fire in the lung and simultaneously reducing fever of deficiency type. No. 4 and polished round-grained

胃虚弱者尤当慎用。

泻白散

【来源】 《小儿药证直诀》

【组成】 地骨皮、桑白皮各30克，炙甘草 3 克。

【用法】 上药挫散，入粳米一撮，水二小盏，煎七分，食前服。

【功用】 泻肺清热，止咳平喘。

【主治】 肺热咳喘，皮肤蒸热，日哺尤甚，舌红苔黄，脉细数等。

支气管炎、麻疹肺炎、肺结核等表现为肺热咳喘者，可用本方加减治疗。

【方解】 方中桑白皮甘寒入肺，清泻肺热，为主药。地骨皮泻肺中伏火兼退虚热，为辅药。炙甘草、粳米养胃和中，补土生

nonglutinous rice in combination are used as adjuvant and guiding drugs, giving the effects of nourishing and regulating the stomach and promoting the function of the spleen and lung in order to strengthen the lung-*qi*.

As it is ascertained clinically and experimentally, the recipe has the effects of reducing fever, relieving inflammation, preventing cough and removing sputum.

CAUTIONS: The recipe is not advisable for those suffering from cough with dyspnea caused by exopathic wind-cold nor for those with cough of deficiency-cold type.

Spleen-heat Expelling Powder

(Xiehuang San)

SOURCE: ***Key to Therapeutics of Children's Diseases***

INGREDIENTS:

No. 1 Agastache, *Herba Agastachis* 21g,
No. 2 Capejasmine fruit, *Fructus Gardeniae* 6g
No. 3 Gypsum, *Gypsum Fibrosum* 15g
No. 4 Licorice root, *Radix Glycyrrhizae* 90g
No. 5 Ledebouriella root, *Radix Ledebouriellae* 120g

DIRECTIONS: All the ingredients should be broken into pieces first, then stir-baked with honeyed wine until they become powder and sweet-smelling. Administer 3-6g of the powder for each dosage. If the ingredients are to be decocted in water, the dosage of each can be modified with reference to the proportion of original prescription.

FUNCTIONS: Purging latent fire in the spleen and stomach.

INDICATIONS: Latent fire syndrome in the spleen and stomach characterized by oral ulceration, foul breath, excessive thirst, inclination to hunger, dryness of the mouth and lips,

金以扶肺气，为佐使药。

现代研究证实，本方具有解热、消炎、镇咳、祛痰等作用。

【使用注意】 外感风寒引起的喘咳，或虚寒性咳嗽，均不可使用本方。

泻 黄 散

【来源】《小儿药证直诀》

【组成】 藿香叶21克，山栀仁6克，石膏15克，甘草90克，防风120克。

【用法】 原方锉，同蜜酒微炒香，为细末，每次服3～6克。如水煎服，其用量可参照原方比例酌情增减。

【功用】 泻脾胃伏火。

【主治】 脾胃伏火证，表现为口疮口臭，烦渴易饥，口燥唇

reddened tongue and rapid pulse, as well as unusual movement of the tongue seen in children which is indicative of excessive heat in the spleen.

Equally, the recipe can be modified to deal with recurrent aphthae, aphthae in children and other diseases indicating latent heat in the spleen and stomach.

INTERPRETATION: In the recipe, No. 3 and No.2 are used in combination as principal drugs, the former having the effect of clearing pathogenic heat of the stomach and *yang-ming* channel and the latter possessing the function of purging pathogenic fire in the tri-warmer to get heat out of the body along with urination. No.5, having the advantage of dispelling latent fire in the spleen channel and being able to exert adroitly guiding function according to circumstances, is often used in combination with No. 2 as assistant drugs to dispel spleen-fire by both upward and downward ways. No. 1, fragrant in odour, is used as an adjuvant drug for its effect of enlivening the spleen, regulating the flow of *qi* and promoting the function of the middle-warmer, strengthening functional activities of *qi* of the spleen and stomach as well as reinforcing the effect of No.5 for dispelling the latent fire. No. 4, acting as a guiding drug, is used for regulating the function of the middle-warmer to purge pathogenic fire, coordinating the effect of various drugs in the recipe so that spleen-fire could be purged without hurting the spleen itself.

It is proved clinically and experimentally that the recipe possesses the efficacies of allaying fever, relieving inflammation, tranquilizing the mind, promoting diuresis, promoting the secretion of gastric juice and digestion.

干，舌红脉数，以及小儿脾热弄舌等。

复发性口疮、口疳等表现为脾胃伏火证者，可用本方加减治疗。

【方解】 方中石膏清阳明胃火，山栀子泻三焦之火，使热从小便排出，共为主药。防风疏散脾经伏火，因势利导，与山栀子合用以上下分消，为辅药。藿香芳香醒脾，理气和中，振复脾胃气机，并助防风升散脾胃伏火，为佐药。甘草为使药，能和中泻火，调合诸药，使脾火泻而无伤脾之虑。

现代研究证实，本方具有解热、消炎、镇静、利尿、促进胃液分泌和助消化的作用。

Powder for Clearing Stomach-heat

(Qingwei San)

SOURCE: ***Secret Record of the Chamber of Orchids***

INGREDIEDTS:

No. 1 Dried rehmannia root, *Radix Rehmanniae* 12g
No. 2 Chinese angelica, *Radix Angelicae Sinensis* 6g
No. 3 Moutan bark, *Cortex Moutan Radicis* 9g
No. 4 Coptis root, *Rhizoma Coptidis* 3g
No. 5 Cimicifuga rhizome, *Rhizoma Cimicifugae* 6g

DIRECTIONS: All the drugs should be decocted in water for oral administration.

FUNCTIONS: Clearing stomach-heat and removing heat from the blood.

INDICATIONS: Stagnation of heat in the stomach marked by headache radiated by toothache, feverish cheeks, aversion to heat with predilection for cold, ulceration in the gum, or gingival atrophy with oozing of bloody fluid and pus, or swelling and soreness of the tongue, lips and cheeks, or hot and foul breath, dryness of mouth and tongue, reddened tongue with yellow coating, and slippery strong and rapid pulse.

The recipe can be modified to deal with periodontitis, stomatitis, gingival pustular swelling, glossitis and gastritis indicative of stomach-heat.

INTERPRETATION: In the recipe, Ingredient No. 4, being bitter in taste and cold in nature, is used as a principal drug, providing the effect of clearnig the fire in heart and stomach. No.1 and No.3 are used in combination as assistant drugs; the former possessing the effect of removing heat from the blood and nourishing *yin* and the latter having the function of removing heat from the blood, reducing pathogenic heat,

清 胃 散

【来源】《兰室秘藏》

【组成】生地黄12克，当归身6克，牡丹皮9克，黄连3克，升麻6克。

【用法】水煎服。

【功用】清胃凉血。

【主治】胃中积热证，表现为牙痛牵引头痛，面颊发热，恶热喜冷，或齿龈溃烂，或牙宣出血，或唇舌颊腮肿痛，或口气热臭，口舌干燥，舌红苔黄，脉滑大而数等。

牙周炎、口腔炎、齿龈脓肿，舌炎、胃炎等表现为胃热者，可用本方加减治疗。

【方解】方中黄连苦寒清心胃之火，为主药。生地凉血滋阴，

and expelling latent fire from the blood. No. 2, as an adjuvant drug, has the effects of nourishing the blood, promoting blood circulation and subduing swelling and alleviating pain. No.5 can dispel pathogenic fire and remove toxic substances and functions as a medicinal guide of *yangming* channel by guiding various drugs directly to the affected regions. The coordination of various drugs results in clearing stomach-heat and removing pathogenic heat from the blood.

Modern researches have proved that the recipe possesses the efficacies of resisting bacteria, subduing inflammation, arresting bleeding, bringing down fever, tranquilizing the mind, relieving pain and promoting blood circulation.

CAUTIONS: It is not fit for patients with toothache of wind-cold type and toothache caused by hyperactivity of fire due to *yin* deficiency.

Gypsum Decoction

(Yunu Jian)

SOURCE: ***Complete Works of Zhang Jingyue***

INGREDIEDTS:

No. 1 Gypsum, *Gypsum Fibrosum* 30g

No. 2 Prepared rehmannia root, *Radix Rehmanniae Praeparata* 30g

No. 3 Ophiopogon root, *Radix Ophiopogonis* 6g

No. 4 Wind-weed rhizome, *Rhizoma Anemarrhenae* 4.5g

No. 5 Achyranthes root, *Radix Achyranthis Bidentatae* 4.5g

DIRECTIONS: All the ingredients should be decocted in water for oral administration, either warm or cold.

FUNCTIONS: Clearing stomach-heat and nourishing *yin*.

INDICATIONS: Syndromes of stomach-heat and *yin*

丹皮凉血清热，除血中伏火，共为辅药。当归养血活血，消肿止痛，为佐药。升麻散火解毒，为阳明引经药，可引诸药直达病所。诸药配合，共奏清胃凉血之效。

现代研究证实，本方具有抗菌、消炎、止血、解热、镇痛、镇静、促进血液循环等作用。

【使用注意】 风寒牙痛及阴虚火旺牙痛均不宜用。

玉 女 煎

【来源】《景岳全书》

【组成】 石膏30克，熟地30克，麦冬6克，知母、牛膝各4.5克。

【用法】 水煎，温服或冷服。

【功用】 清胃滋阴。

【主治】 胃热阴虚证，症见头痛牙痛，牙齿松动，烦热口渴，

deficiency characterized by headache, toothache, odontoseisis, dysphoria with thirst, dry and reddened tongue with dry yellow coating.

The recipe can be modified for treating periodontitis, purulent swelling of gums, acute stomatitis, glossitis, chronic gastritis, indicating syndromes of stomach-heat and *yin* deficiency.

INTERPRETATION: In the recipe, Ingredient No. 1, pungent and sweet in taste and extreme cold in nature, is used as a principal drug provinding the effect of clearing stagnation of heat in the *yangming* channel. No. 2, which is sweet and warm, acts as an assistant drug, giving the effect of invigorating *yin* of *shaoyin*. When No. 1 and No. 2 are exhibited in combination, the effect of clearing pathogenic fire and nourishing the body fluid can be yielded. No.4, bitter in taste and cold and moist in property, is used to reinforce the effect of No.1 in purging pathogenic fire and heat from the stomach, and No. 3 has the effect of nourishing the stomach-*yin* and can aid No.2 in nourishing the kidney-*yin*. No.5 functions in guiding pathogenic heat downwards to reduce excessive fire and conducting the blood downwards to prevent it from running upwards.

Modern studies have revealed that this recipe possesses the efficacies of relieving inflammation, allaying fever, tranquilizing the mind, nourishing the body and consolidating the constitution.

CAUTIONS: It is not advisable for patients with loose stool.

Peony Decoction

(Shaoyao Tang)

SOURCE: *Six Medical Books* by Liu Hejian.

舌干红，苔黄而干等。

牙周炎、齿龈脓肿、急性口腔炎、舌炎、慢性胃炎等属胃热肾阴虚者，可用本方加减治疗。

【方解】 方中石膏辛甘大寒，以清阳明有余之热，为主药。熟地甘温，补少阴不足之阴，为辅药。二药相配，清火滋水并用。知母苦寒质润，助石膏泻火清胃；麦冬养胃阴，协助熟地滋肾阴；牛膝导热下行，降上炎之火，引血下行，以止上溢之血。

现代研究证实，本方具有消炎、解热、镇静、滋养强壮等作用。

【使用注意】 大便溏泄者，不宜用本方。

芍 药 汤

【来源】 刘河间《医学六书》

INGREDIENTS:

No. 1 Peony root, *Radix Paeoniae* 15g
No. 2 Chinese angelica root, *Radix Angelicae Sinensis* 9g
No. 3 Coptis root, *Rhizoma Coptidis* 9g
No. 4 Areca seed, *Semen Arecae* 5g
No. 5 Aucklandia root, *Radix Aucklandiae* 5g
No. 6 Licorice root, *Radix Glycyrrhizae* 5g
No. 7 Rhubarb root, *Radix et Rhizoma Rhei* 9g
No. 8 Scutellaria root, *Radix Scutellariae* 9g
No. 9 Cinnamon bark, *Cortex Cinnamomi* 5g

DIRECTIONS: All the ingredients should be decocted in water for oral administration.

FUNCTIONS: Clearing away damp-heat and toxic material and regulating *qi* and blood.

INDICATIONS: Diarrhea or dysentery due to damp-heat pathogen marked by abdominal pain, pus and blood in the stool, tenesmus, burning sensation in the anus, scanty deep-coloured urine, yellow greasy coating of the tongue, etc.

The recipe can be modified to treat acute enteritis, bacillary dysentery and other conditions indicative of damp-heat in the large intestine.

INTERPRETATION: Ingredient No. 1, as a principal drug, is administered in larger dosage to regulate *qi* and blood for the treatment of abdominal pain and tenesmus caused by dysentery. No.3, No.7 and No.8 share the effects of clearing away heat and removing toxic materials. No. 2 and No.9 give the effects of regulating the *ying* and promoting circulation of blood. No. 4 and No. 5 are indicated for promoting the flow of *qi* and removing stagnancy. No.6 coordinates various effects of all the drugs in the recipe.

Modern researches have confirmed the effects of this recipe in resisting bacteria, subduing inflammation, and relieving spasm and pain.

【组成】 芍药15克，当归、黄连各9克，槟榔、木香、甘草各5克，大黄、黄芩各9克，官桂5克。

【用法】 水煎服。

【功用】 清热利湿，调气和血。

【主治】 湿热泻痢证，表现为腹痛便脓血，赤白相兼，里急后重，肛门灼热，小便短赤，苔腻微黄等。

急性肠炎、细菌性痢疾等属大肠湿热者，可用本方加减治疗。

【方解】 方中重用芍药，能调和气血，以治痢疾腹痛、里急后重，为主药。黄连、黄芩、大黄清热解毒。当归、肉桂和营行血。木香、槟榔行气导滞。甘草调和诸药。

现代研究证明，本方具有抗菌、消炎、解痉、镇痛等作用。

CAUTIONS: It is not advisable for cases with external syndromes at the onset of dysentery nor for those suffering from chronic dysentery or deficiency-cold dysentery.

Pulsatilla Decoction

(Baitouweng Tang)

SOURCE: ***Treatise on Febrile Diseases***

INGREDIENTS:

No. 1 Pulsatilla root, *Radix Pulsatillae* 15g
No. 2 Phellodendron bark, *Cortex Phellodendri* 12g
No. 3 Coptis root, *Rhizoma Coptidis* 6g
No. 4 Ash bark, *Cortex Fraxini* 12g.

DIRECTIONS: All the drugs should be decocted in water for oral administration.

FUNCTIONS: Removing noxious heat and cooling the blood to treat dysentery.

INDICATIONS: Dysentery or diarrhea due to noxious heat marked by more blood and less mucus in stools, abdominal pain, tenesmus, burning sensation in the anus, feverish body, restlessness, thirst with inclination to drink, reddened tongue with yellow coating, and taut and rapid pulse.

The recipe can be modified to treat acute enteritis, bacillary dysentery, amebic dysentery and others which pertain to dysentery or diarrhea due to noxious-heat.

INTERPRETATION: In the recipe, Ingredient No. 1 plays the role of the principal drug, having the effect of removing noxious-heat from the blood system. No. 2 and No. 3, both bitter in taste and cold in property, can remove noxious-heat and consolidate *yin* to treat dysentery or diarrhea. No. 4, with its nature cold and taste bitter and puckery, is used as an astringent to clear away heat and dry dampness, to treat dysentery

【使用注意】 痢疾初起有表证者，或久痢、虚寒痢者，均不宜用本方。

白头翁汤

【来源】《伤寒论》

【组成】 白头翁 15 克，黄柏 12 克，黄连 6 克，秦皮12克。

【用法】 水煎服。

【功用】 清热解毒，凉血止痢。

【主治】 热毒血痢证，表现为下痢脓血，赤多白少，腹痛，里急后重，肛门灼热，身热心烦，渴欲饮水，舌红苔黄，脉弦数等。

急性肠炎、细菌性痢疾、阿米巴痢疾等属热痢者，可用本方加减治疗。

【方解】 方中白头翁清血分热毒，为主药。黄连、黄柏苦寒清热解毒，坚阴止痢。秦皮性寒味苦而涩，清热燥湿，收涩止痢。

diarrhea.

Modern researches have confirmed that the recipe has the effects of relieving inflammation, resisting bacteria and ameba, allaying fever, relieving spasm and arresting diarrhea and blood.

CAUTIONS: It is not advisable for cases with dysentery of deficiency type or chronic dysentery.

Section 6

Recipes for Allaying Fever of Deficiency Type

This group of prescriptions is made up of traditional Chinese drugs effective for nourishing *yin* and expelling interior and hectic heat. They are indicated for the treatment of hectic fever due to *yin*-deficiency, or persistant fever due to heat of insufficiency type.

Sweet Wormwood and Turtle Shell Decoction

(Qinghao Biejia Tang)

SOURCE: ***Treatise on Differentiation and Treatment of Epidemic Febrile Diseases.***

INGREDIENTS:

No. 1 Sweet wormwood, *Herba Artemisiae* 6g
No. 2 Fresh-water turtle shell, *Carapax Trionycis* 15g
No. 3 Dried rehmannia root, *Radix Rehmanniae* 12g
No. 4 Wind-weed rhizome, *Rhizoma Anemarrhenae* 6g
No. 5 Moutan bark, *Coretex Moutan Radicis* 9g

DIRECTIONS: All the drugs should be decocted in water for oral administration.

现代研究证实，本方具有消炎、抗菌、抗阿米巴、解热、解痉、止泻、止血等作用。

【使用注意】 虚痢、久痢均不宜用本方。

第六节 清虚热剂

清虚热剂主要由养阴清热药组成，具有滋阴透热、清热除蒸的作用。适用于骨蒸潮热，或久热不退的虚热证。

青蒿鳖甲汤

【来源】 《温病条辨》

【组成】 青蒿6克，鳖甲15克，细生地12克，知母6克，丹皮9克。

【用法】 水煎服。

FUNCTIONS: Nourishing *yin* and expelling pathogenic heat from the interior.

INDICATIONS: Latent heat in the interior of the body, manifested by fever at night and normal in the morning, absence of perspiration after fever subsides, polyphagia with emaciation, reddened tongue with little coating and rapid pulse.

The recipe is modified to deal with such diseases as pulmonary tubercolosis and other chronic consumptive diseases related to hyperactivity of fire due to *yin* deficiency.

INTERPRETATION: In the recipe, Ingredient No. 2 directly enters the *yin* system and, being salty in taste and cold in nature, has the effect of nourishing *yin* so as to reduce fever of deficiency type; No. 1 is used as an aromatic with the function of clearing heat from the channels and making it off from the body. Both the above ingredients are principal drugs and the combined application of the two yields the effect of expelling heat without injuring *yin* while replenishing *yin* with no influence on the expulsion of pathogens. No. 3, an ingredient with a sweet taste and cool nature, and No.4 which is bitter, cold and moist, both strengthen the efficacy of No. 2 in reducing fever of deficiency type. No. 5 has the effect of cooling the blood and removing heat from the body and is used to assist No. 1 in removing latent heat in the *yin* system.

Modern researches have confiremed that the recipe possesses the efficacy in tranquilizing the mind, relieving inflammation, resisting bacteria, inhibiting hyperfunction of catabolism, nourishing the body and consolidating the constitution.

CAUTIONS:

1. As Ingredient No. 1 in the above recipe is not resistant to high temperature, it should not be decocted for too long. It may be infused in boiling water for oral administration.

2. It is not advisable for cases with tendency to convulsion

【功用】 养阴透热。

【主治】 邪热内伏证，表现为夜热早凉，热退无汗，能食形瘦，舌红少苔，脉数。

肺结核、贫血、其他慢性消耗性疾病等证属阴虚火旺者，可用本方加减治疗。

【方解】 方中鳖甲直入阴分，咸寒滋阴，以退虚热；青蒿芳香清热透络，引邪外出。二药合用，透热而不伤阴，养阴而不恋邪，共为主药。生地甘凉滋阴，知母苦寒滋润，助鳖甲以退虚热。丹皮凉血透热，助青蒿以透泄阴分之伏热。

现代研究证实，本方具有解热、镇静、消炎、抗菌、抑制异化作用、滋养强壮作用。

【使用注意】

1．方中青蒿不耐高温，煎煮时间不宜太长，或用沸水泡服。

2．阴虚欲抽搐者，不宜用本方。

due to *yin*-deficiency.

Powder for Clearing Bone-heat

(Qinggu San)

SOURCE: ***Standards of Diagnosis and Treatment***

INGREDIENTS:

No. 1 Stellaria root, *Radix Stellariae* 5g

No. 2 Picrorhiza rhizome, *Rhizoma Picrorhizae* 3g

No. 3 Large-leaf gentian root, *Radix Gentianae Macrophyllae*, 3g

No. 4 Fresh-water turtle shell, *Carapax Trionycis* 3g

No. 5 Wolfberry bark, *Cortex Lycii Radicis* 3g

No. 6 Sweet wormwood, *Herba Artemisiae* 3g

No. 7 Wind-weed rhizome, *Rhizoma Anemarrhenae* 3g

No. 8 Licorice root, *Radix Glycyrrhizae* 2g

DIRECTIONS: All the drugs should be either decocted in water for oral administration or ground into powder to be taken after being infused in boiling water, 9 grams each time, three times a day.

FUNCTIONS: Clearing away fever of deficiency type and removing hectic fever due to *yin*-deficiency.

INDICATIONS: Steaming sensation in the bones and hectic fever due to *yin*-deficiency manifested by tidal fever in the afternoon or during the night, steaming sensation in the extremities, restlessness, emaciation, night sweat, flushing of cheeks, hot sensation in the palms and soles, reddened tongue with little or no coating, and thready and rapid pulse.

The recipe can be modified for the treatment of pulmonary tuberculosis as well as other chronic consumptive diseases related to the above syndrome.

INTERPRETATION: In the recipe, Ingredient No. 1,

清　骨　散

【来源】《证治准绳》

【组成】 银柴胡 5 克，胡黄连、秦艽、鳖甲、地骨皮、青蒿、知母各 3 克，甘草 2 克。

【用法】 水煎服；或研末，每日三次，每次 9 克，冲服。

【功用】 清虚热，退骨蒸。

【主治】 骨蒸潮热证，表现为午后或夜间潮热，骨蒸心烦，形瘦盗汗，两颊潮红，手足心热，舌红少苔，脉细数。

肺结核、其他慢性消耗性疾病等证属阴虚内热、虚劳骨蒸者，可用本方加减治疗。

【方解】 方中银柴胡善清虚劳骨蒸之热，而无苦泄之弊，为

as a principal drug, can quickly clear away hectic fever and steaming sensation in the bones due to consumption without giving rise to diarrhea. No. 2, No. 3, No. 7 ,No. 5 and No. 6 are used in combination to play the part of assistant drugs. Nos. 2,5 and 7 have the effect of treating hectic fever due to consumption by entering the *yin* system to reduce fever of deficiency type. No. 3 and No. 6 have the effect of removing latent heat. No. 4, salty in taste and cold in nature, acts as an adjuvant drug providing the effect of replenishing *yin*, checking exuberance of *yang* and guiding the other drugs to the *yin* system for removal of heat. No. 8 is dosed a bit as a guiding drug for the coordination of various effect of the drugs in the recipe.

Modern researches have confirmed that the recipe has the efficacies of allaying fever, tranquilizing the mind, relieving inflammation, nourishing the body and consolidating constitution, and inhibiting excitability of the vegetative nerve.

CAUTIONS: The recipe has greater effect in reducing fever but weaker effect in nourishing *yin*, therefore, it is not advisable for cases with severe *yin*-deficiency and milder hectic fever.

Section 7

Recipes for Clearing Away Summer-heat and Replenishing *Qi*

This type of prescriptions is chiefly composed of the summer-heat-clearing drugs and the *qi* and *yin*-nourishing drugs. With its virtue of clearing away summar-heat and replenishing *qi*, it is indicated for syndromes related to impairment of *qi* and *yin* caused by summer-heat.

主药。胡黄连、知母、地骨皮入阴，退虚热以治骨蒸劳热。青蒿、秦艽清伏热，共为辅药。鳖甲咸寒，滋阴潜阳，并引药入阴以清热，为佐药。少用甘草为使药，调和诸药。

现代研究证实，本方具有解热、镇静、消炎、滋养强壮、降低植物神经系统兴奋性等作用。

【使用注意】 本方退热作用较强，而滋阴作用较弱。若阴虚较甚、潮热较轻者，不宜使用。

第七节 清暑益气剂

清暑益气剂主要由清暑药和益气养阴药组成，有清暑益气之功，适用于暑伤气阴之证。

Decoction for Clearing Away Summer-heat and Replenishing Qi

(Qingshu Yiqi Tang)

SOURCE: ***Compendium on Epidemic Febrile Diseases***

INGREDIENTS:

No. 1 Root of American ginseng, *Radix Panacis Guinquefolli* 5g

No. 2 Stem of noble dendrobium, *Herba Dendrobii* 15g

No. 3 Ophiopogon root, *Radix Ophiopogonis* 9g

No. 4 Coptis root, *Rhizoma Coptidis* 3g

No. 5 Lophatherum, *Herba Lophatheri* 6g

No. 6 Lotus petiole, *Petiolus Nelumbinis* 15g

No. 7 Wind-weed rhizome, *Rhizoma Anemarrhenae* 6g

No. 8 Licorice root, *Radix Glycyrrhizae* 3g

No. 9 Polished round-grained nonglutinous rice, *Semen Oryzae Nonglutinosae* 15g

No.10 Watermelon peel, *Exocarpium Citrulli* 30g

DIRECTIONS: All the drugs should be decocted in water for oral administration.

FUNCTIONS: Clearing away summer-heat and replenishing *qi*, nourishing *yin* and promoting the production of body fluid.

INDICATIONS: Consumption of *qi* and fluid by summer-heat manifested by feverish body, profuse perspiration, restlessness, thirst, scanty and dark urine, general debility, short breath, lassitude, and feeble and rapid pulse.

The recipe can be modified for the treatment of sunstroke, heat stroke, infantile summer fever as well as other infectious diseases occurring in the summer which are related to the

清暑益气汤

【来源】《温热经纬》

【组成】西洋参5克，石斛15克，麦冬9克，黄连3克，竹叶6克，荷梗15克，知母6克，甘草3克，粳米15克，西瓜翠衣30克。

【用法】水煎服。

【功用】清暑益气，养阴生津。

【主治】暑伤气津证，表现为身热多汗，心烦口渴，小便短赤，体倦少气，精神不振，脉虚数等。

日射病、热射病、中暑、小儿夏季热及其他夏季感染性疾病

injury of *qi* and body fluid by summer-heat.

INTERPRETATION: In the recipe, No. 1 and No. 10 are used in combination as principal drugs with the former having the effects of supplementing *qi* and promoting the production of body fluid, and nourishing *yin* and removing heat, and the latter possessing the effect of clearing away summer-heat. No.6 can strengthen the effect of expelling summer-heat while No.2 and No.3 can strengthen the effects of nourishing *yin* and clearing away heat. Working together, they are referred to as assistant drugs. The rest play the role of adjuvant and guiding drugs. Among them, No.5 and No.7 are used to remove heat and restlessness; No. 8 and No. 9 are used to supplement *qi* and promote the function of the stomach.

Modern researches have confirmed that the prescription has the efficacies of relieving inflammation, allaying fever, tranquilizing the mind, resisting bacteria, nourishing the body and consolidating the constitution and protecting the body fluid.

CAUTIONS: It is not advisable for cases having summer-heat with pathogenic dampness.

证属暑热伤及气津者，可用本方加减治疗。

【方解】 方中西洋参益气生津，养阴清热，合西瓜翠衣清热解暑，共为主药。荷梗加强清热解暑作用；石斛、麦冬加强养阴清热作用，共为辅药。知母、竹叶清热除烦；甘草、粳米益气养胃，共为佐使药。

现代研究证实，本方具有消炎、解热、镇静、抗菌、滋养强壮、保护体液等作用。

【使用注意】 暑病挟湿者，不宜使用。

Chapter VI

Purgative Prescriptions

Purgative prescriptions are mainly composed of purgative drugs with the therapeutic effects of relieving constipation, evacuating gastrointestinal retention, clearing away heat of excess type, purging away excessive fluid and accumulation of cold type. They are indicated for the treatment of interior syndrome of excess type.

Interior syndrome of excess varies with the accumulation of heat, cold, dryness and fluid; the constitution of the human body differs with the strong and the weak, the old and the young, the excessive and the deficient. Purgative prescriptions, therefore, can be further divided into five types: purgative recipes of cold nature, purgative recipes of warm nature, emollient recipes for causing laxation, recipes for eliminating retained fluid and recipes for both reinforcement and elimination.

Section 1

Purgative Recipes of Cold Nature

This group of recipes chiefly consists of cold-natured cathartics with the effects of purging away heat and relieving constipation. It is associated with the treatment of excess syndrome of internal heat.

第六章

泻下剂

泻下剂主要由泻下药组成，具有通导大便、排除胃肠积滞、荡涤实热、攻逐水饮、寒积的作用。适用于里实证。

里实证有热结、寒结、燥结、水结之区别；人体素质又有强弱、老幼、虚实之差异。因此，泻下剂可分为寒下剂、温下剂、润下剂、逐水剂、攻补兼施剂等五类。

第一节 寒下剂

寒下剂主要由寒下药组成，具有泻热通便之功用，适用于里热积滞实证。

Major Decoction for Purging Down Digestive *Qi*

(Da Chengqi Tang)

SOURCE: ***Treatise on Febrile Diseases***

INGREDIENTS:

No. 1 Rhubarb, *Radix et Rhizoma Rhei* 12g
No. 2 Magnolia bark, *Cortex Magnoliae Officinalis* 15g
No. 3 Immature bitter orange, *Fructus Aurantii Immaturus* 12g
No. 4 Mirabilite, *Natrii Sulphas* 9g

DIRECTIONS: The above drugs should be decocted in water for oral administration. No.2 and No.3 are to be decocted prior to No.1. The decoction is to be taken after No.4 is infused in it.

FUNCTIONS: Expelling pathogenic heat and loosening the bowels, promoting the circulation of *qi* to purge accumulation in the bowels.

INDICATIONS:

1. Excessive-heat syndrome of *yangming-fu* organ, manifested as constipation, frequent wind through the anus, feeling of fullness in the abdomen, abdominal pain with tenderness and guarding, tidal fever, delirium, polyhidrosis of hands and feet, prickled tongue with yellow dry fur or dry black tongue coating with fissures, deep and forceful pulse.

2. Syndrome of fecal impaction due to heat with watery discharge, manifested as watery discharge of terribly foul odor accompanied by abdominal distension and pain with tenderness and guarding, dry mouth and tongue, smooth and forceful pulse.

3. Cold limbs due to excess of heat, convulsion, mania

大承气汤

【来源】《伤寒论》

【组成】大黄 12 克，厚朴 15 克，枳实12克，芒硝 9 克。

【用法】水煎服。先煎枳实、厚朴，后纳大黄，芒硝冲服。

【功用】泻热通便，行气荡积。

【主治】

1．阳明腑实证，表现为大便不通，矢气频作，脘腹痞满，腹痛拒按，按之硬，潮热谵语，手足汗出，舌苔黄燥起刺或焦黑燥裂，脉沉实等。

2．热结旁流证，表现为下利清水，臭秽异常，伴腹部胀满，疼痛拒按，按之有硬块，口舌干燥，脉滑实等。

3．热厥、痉病、发狂等，属于里热实证者。

and other symptoms belonging to excess syndrome of interior heat.

Equally, this recipe can be modified to deal with infectious or non-infectious febrile diseases in their climax marked by accumulation of heat type, and in the treatment of paralytic, simple and obliterative intestinal obstructions.

INTERPRETATION: Of the four ingredients in the recipe, No.1, bitter in flavour and cold in property, acts as a principal drug to treat the main symptom by removing and purging pathogenic heat and fire, cleaning accumulation of food and stool in the gastrointestinal tract and relieving constipation. Being salty in flavour and cold in nature, No. 4 possesses the effect of moistening the dryness, softening hard mass and purging heat, and is used in combination with No.1 as an assistant drug to reinforce its effect of drastic purgation. Both No.2 and No. 3 share the efforts to assist the above two drugs in purging away the accumulation of food and stool to accelerate the relief of pathogenic heat accumulated in the stomach and large intestine by promoting circulation of *qi* and relieving distension and fullness. So they play the role of guiding drugs.

Modern researches have ascertained that this recipe has the functions of relieving inflammation, resisting bacteria, promoting blood circulation of intestines, stimulating intestinal peristalsis, purging stool, tranquilizing the mind, bringing down fever, etc.

CAUTIONS:

1. Being a drastic recipe, it must be administered with great care to those of general asthenia, or to those whose external syndrome has not yet been relieved or to those with absence of dry stool in gastrointestinal tract.

2. The drastic effect of this recipe is harmful to the stomach-*qi*. So, immediate withdrawal is indicated once the effect attained. Over-administration is prohibited.

传染性或非传染性发热性疾病的极期表现热结者，以及麻痹性、单纯性、闭塞性肠梗阻等，可用本方加减治疗。

【方解】 方中大黄苦寒清热泻火，荡涤热结，泻下通便以治疗主证，为主药。芒硝咸寒，润燥软坚泻热，与大黄相须为用，峻下热结之力增强，为辅药。厚朴、枳实行气散结，消痞除满，并助大黄、芒硝推荡积滞，以加速热结的排泄，为使药。

现代研究证实，本方具有消炎、抗菌、改善肠循环、促进肠蠕动、泻下、镇静、解热等作用。

【使用注意】

1．本方为泻下峻剂，若体质虚弱，或表证未解，或肠胃无燥结者，慎用。

2．本方药力峻猛，易伤胃气，应中病即止，不可过服。

3. Never is it administered for pregnant women.

SUPPLEMENTARY RECIPES

1. **Minor Decoction for Purging Down Digestive *Qi*** (*Xiao Chengqi Tang*)

SOURCE: ***Treatise on Febrile Diseases***

INGREDIENTS:

No. 1 Rhubarb, *Radix et Rhizoma Rhei* 12g

No. 2 Magnolia bark, *Cortex Magnoliae Officinalis* 6g

No. 3 Immature bitter orange, *Fructus Aurantii Immaturus* 9g

DIRECTIONS: All the drugs except No.1 which is to be added later should be decocted in water for oral administration.

FUNCTIONS: Relieving heat accumulation by mild effect.

INDICATIONS: Mild cases of excess syndrome of *yang-ming-fu* organ, manifested as delirium, tidal fever, constipation, distension and fullness in the chest and abdomen, yellow shriveled tongue coating, smooth and swift pulse as well as the onset of dysentery with distending abdominal pain or epigastric fullness, tenesmus and so on.

2. **Purgative Decoction for Coordinating the Function of Stomach** (*Tiaowei Chengqi Tang*)

SOURCE: ***Treatise on Febrile Diseases***

INGREDIENTS:

No. 1 Rhubarb, *Radix et Rhizoma Rhei* 12g

No. 2 Liquorice, *Radix Glycyrrhizae* 6g

No. 3 Mirabilite, *Natrii Sulphas* 12g

DIRECTIONS: The above drugs are decocted in water with the exception of No.3 which is infused in the decoction just before the oral dose.

FUNCTIONS: Purging pathogenic heat accumulated in the gastrointestinal tract by laxative action.

INDICATIONS: *Yangming* disease marked by gastrointestinal dryness and heat, manifested by obstruction of de-

3．孕妇禁用。

【附方】

1．小承气汤(《伤寒论》)

【组成】 大黄12克，厚朴6克，枳实9克。

【用法】 水煎服，大黄后下。

【功用】 轻下热结。

【主治】 阳明腑实轻证，表现为谵语，潮热，大便秘结，胸腹痞满，舌苔老黄，脉滑而疾，或痢疾初起，腹中胀痛，或脘腹胀满，里急后重等。

2．调胃承气汤(《伤寒论》)

【组成】 大黄12克，甘草6克，芒硝12克。

【用法】 水煎服，芒硝冲服。

【功用】 缓下热结。

【主治】 阳明病胃肠燥热，表现为大便不通，口渴心烦，蒸

fecation, thirst and vexation, fever like steaming, abdominal distension and fullness, delirium, yellow tongue coating, slippery and rapid pulse as well as eruption, hematemesis, epistaxis, painful swelling of mouth, teeth and throat caused by domination of heat in the intestine and stomach. It can also be indicated for the cases with mild abdominal fullness.

Major Decoction for Removing Phlegm-heat from Chest

(Daxianxiong Tang)

SOURCE: ***Treatise on Febrile Diseases***

No. 1 Rhubarb, *Radix et Rhizoma Rhei* 10g
No. 2 Mirabilite, *Natrii Sulphas* 10g
No. 3 Kansui root, *Radix Euphorbiae Kansui* 1g

DIRECTIONS: No. 1 is decocted in water priorly, and No. 2 is dissolved posteriorly. The decoction is to be taken after No.3 is ground into fine powder and is infused in boiling water or in the decoction.

FUNCTIONS: Purging heat and removing water retention by hydragogue.

INDICATIONS: Syndrome due to accumulation of pathogenic heat with stagnancy of fluid or phlegm in the chest, manifested as fullness, pain and tenderness of the area from the epigastrium to the lower abdomen where the patient may feel too painful to be touched, constipation, mild tidal fever as well as restlessness and shortness of breath, thirst and dryness of the tongue, sunken, tense and forceful pulse.

Equally, this recipe can be modified to deal with inflammatory hydrothorax and ascites, acute edematous pancreatitis or severe cases of intestinal obstruction and others

蒸发热，或腹中胀满，或谵语，舌苔黄 脉滑数；以及肠胃热盛而致发斑吐衄、口齿咽喉肿痛等；腹满痞塞较轻者用之。

大陷胸汤

【来源】《伤寒论》

【组成】大黄 10 克，芒硝 10 克，甘遂 1 克。

【用法】水煎大黄，溶芒硝，冲甘遂末服。

【功用】泻热逐水。

【主治】结胸证，表现为从心下至少腹硬满而痛不可近，大便秘结，日晡小有潮热，或短气躁烦，舌上燥而渴，脉沉紧，按之有力。

炎症性胸水、腹水、急性水肿性胰腺炎、或危重肠梗阻等证

which pertain to the accumulation of pathogenic heat with stagnancy of fluid or phlegm in the chest.

INTERPRETATION: Being bitter in flavour and cold in property, Ingredient No.3 possesses the effects of eliminating retained fluid by hydragogue, expelling pathogenic heat and dispersing accumulation of the pathogens while No.1, bitter in flavor and cold in property, has the function of cleaning up pathogenic heat. Working in combination, the above two drugs exert the role of principal drugs indicated for purging the pathogens consisting of excessive fluid and pathogenic heat. No.2 has salty flavour and cold property and is used as an assistant drug to soften and resolve the hard mass as well as expel pathogenic heat. The three ingredients, few in variety and large in dosage, are highly drastic and specific in action, acting together as a drastic recipe for cleaning up pathogenic heat, expelling retained fluid and dispersing the accumulation of pathogens.

Clinically and experimentally, it is ascertained that this recipe has the efficacies of purgation, diuresis, antiinflammation and antisepsis.

CAUTIONS:

1. The administration should be withdrawn immediately after thorough purgation is achieved; The secondary administration is necessary for those without thorough purgation. Since the recipe is indicated for the treatment of acute diseases, the prescribed dosage should be strictly observed to avoid impairment of the vital *qi*, but the pathogens should be purged promptly so as to prevent the persistence in the body.

2. The administration is prohibited for those with weak constitution or those who have just recovered from the illness and can not bear the drastic effect of the recipe.

属结胸证者，可用本方加减治疗。

【方解】 方中甘遂苦寒逐水饮，泄热散结；大黄苦寒荡涤邪热，二药伍用，共泻水热互结之邪，均为主药。芒硝咸寒，软坚散结泻热，为辅药。三药味少量大，力专效宏，为泻热逐水散结之峻剂。

现代研究证实，本方具有泻下、利尿、消炎、抗菌等作用。

【使用注意】

1. 服用本方后“得快利”则止后服，未“得快利”可继续服药。所治证急，既要防止利下过度伤正气，又要掌握及时攻下以防留邪。

2. 若素体虚弱，或病后不任攻伐者禁用本方。

Section 2

Purgative Recipes of Warm Nature

This kind of prescriptions, composed of purgatives together with drugs of warm nature, has the effects of warming and relaxing the bowels and expelling the accumulation of cold nature. It is preferred for the treatment of syndrome of interior excess due to the accumulation of pathogenic cold.

Decoction of Rhubarb and Aconite

(Daihuang Fuzi Tang)

SOURCE: *Synopsis of Prescriptions of the Golden Chamber*

INGREDIENTS:

No. 1 Rhubarb, *Radix et Rhizoma Rhei* 9g

No. 2 Prepared aconite root, *Radix Aconiti Praeparata* 9g

No. 3 Asarum herb, *Herba Asari* 3g

DIRECTIONS: All the above drugs are to be decocted in water for oral administration.

FUNCTIONS: Warming *yang* and dispelling pathogenic cold, relieving constipation and promoting the circulation of *qi*.

INDICATIONS: Syndrome of interior excess due to the accumulation of pathogenic cold, manifested as abdominal pain, constipation, hypochondriac pain, fever, cold limbs, white and greasy coating on the tongue, taut and tense pulse.

Besides, this recipe can be modified to deal with such cases

第二节 温 下 剂

温下剂常用泻下药配温里药组成，有温散寒结、下其里实的作用。适用于因寒成结之里实证。

大黄附子汤

【来源】《金匮要略》

【组成】大黄9克，附子(炮)9克，细辛3克。

【用法】水煎服。

【功用】温阳散寒，泻结行滞。

【主治】寒结里实证，表现为腹痛便秘，胁下偏痛，发热，手足厥逆，舌苔白腻，脉弦紧。

急、慢性便秘兼寒积者，急性阑尾炎、肠梗阻属虚寒型者，

as acute or chronic constipation accompanied with accumulation of pathogenic cold, acute appendicitis, intestinal obstruction ascribable to insufficient-cold type.

INTERPRETATION: Of the three ingredients in the recipe, the first two are both referred to as principal drugs, the first of which, acrid in flavour and extremely hot in nature, has the functions of warming and recuperating the kidney-*yang* in order to remove constipation due to excessive cold as well as to relieve pain, while the second is used to remove pathogenic accumulation by purging the bowels. No.3 of acrid flavour and warm property is used as an assistant drug for expelling pathogenic cold from the channels and assisting in the functions of warming the kidney-*yang* and relieving pain. The cooperation of three drugs results in a warm nature with well preserved effects of removing retention and expelling accumulation of pathogen. So it is considered the very recipe for purging cold accumulation with drugs of warm nature.

Modern researches have proved that this recipe possesses the efficacies of promoting metabolism and blood circulation as well as cardiac stimulant, analgesia and purgation.

CAUTIONS:

1. Generally, the dosage of rhubarb should not exceed that of prepared aconite root.

2. If the administration of this recipe results in the relief of constipation, the patient can be pronounced to be out of danger; but if the patient does not respond well to the recipe marked by constipation, vomiting, cold limbs and thready pulse, it indicates that the patient is still in danger.

可用本方加减治疗。

【方解】 方中附子味辛、大热，温肾壮阳，大补真火，以破阴解凝，并有镇痛作用；大黄荡涤泻下而除积滞，均为主药。细辛辛温，温经散寒，助附子温阳、镇痛，为辅药。三药配伍，寒性减而荡积破结作用尤存，故为温下寒结之方。

现代研究证实，本方具有加强代谢、促进循环、强心、镇痛、泻下等作用。

【使用注意】

1. 大黄用量一般不超过附子。

2. 服用本方后大便通利，病可转危为安；若药后仍然大便不通，反增呕吐、肢冷、脉细者，是为危候。

Decoction for Warming Spleen

(Wenpi Tang)

SOURCE: ***Thousand Gold Remedies for Emergencies***

INGREDIENTS:

No. 1 Rhubarb, *Radix et Rhizoma Rhei* 12g

No. 2 Prepared aconite root, *Radix Aconiti Praeparata* 9g

No. 3 Dried ginger, *Rhizoma Zingiberis* 6g

No. 4 Ginseng, *Radix Ginseng* 9g

No. 5 Liquorice, *Radix Glycyrrhizae* 3g

DIRECTIONS: All drugs are to be decocted in water with No.1 decocted later so as to preserve its available composition. The decoction is for oral administration.

FUNCTIONS: Warming and invigorating the spleen-*yang* and eliminating cold accumulation.

INDICATIONS: Constipation caused by accumulation of cold due to hypofunction of the spleen, marked by peri-umbilical cold-pain which will be alleviated with a warm hand on the region; also may be used to treat protracted diarrhea accompanied by abdominal pain, epigastric fullness, cold extremities, white tongue fur, deep and taut pulse.

Equally, the recipe can also be modified to treat the following cases; constipation due to insufficiency of *yang* as seen in chronic gastritis, enteritis and other chronic illnesses; or chronic diarrhea due to insufficiency of *yang* as seen in the cases of chronic dysentery, chronic ulcerative colitis, intestinal tuberculosis, etc.

INTERPRETATION: Very acrid in flavour, extremely hot in nature and not stagnant, No.2 dominates the function of scattering accumulation of cold by warming and strengthen-

温脾汤

【来源】《备急千金要方》

【组成】 大黄12克，附子9克，干姜6克，人参9克，甘草3克。

【用法】 水煎服，大黄后下。

【功用】 温补脾阳，攻下冷积。

【主治】 脾虚寒结或下利证，表现为大便秘结，脐腹冷痛，喜得温按，或久利不止，腹痛，心下痞，手足不温，苔白，脉沉弦等。

慢性胃炎、慢性肠炎及其他慢性疾患出现阳虚便秘者；或者慢性痢疾、结肠炎溃疡、肠结核等慢性腹泻表现为阳虚者，均可用本方加减治疗。

【方解】 方中附子大辛大热，走而不守，温壮脾阳以散寒凝；

ing the spleen-*yang*; No.1 exerts the function of expelling retention of wastes in order to purge the cold accumulation. Both No.1 and No.2 act in combination as principal drugs. No.3, also acrid and hot, plays the subordinate role in warming the middle-warmer and dispelling cold. No.4 and No.5 reinforce the middle-warmer and replenish *qi*. Furthermore, No.4 is capable of strengthening the *yang*-warming function of No.2 and No.3; while No.5 is good at coordinating the nature of the above drugs. In the whole recipe tonification promotes purgation while purgation is involved in tonification.

Modern researches have verified that this is a popular recipe for anti-inflammation, antisepsis, promoting circulation, increasing physiologic function, stimulating peristalsis, exciting nervous center, promoting digestion and absorption, stimulating heart functions, etc.

CAUTIONS: Prepared aconite root should be decocted for 30 to 60 minutes in water prior to other ingredients so as to lessen its toxicity, while rhubarb should be added into the decoction posterior to all other ingredients lest its purgative action should be reduced.

Section 3

Emollient Recipes for Causing Laxation

The recipes of this kind are chiefly made up of emollient cathartics and have the function of causing laxation. They are indicated in constipation due to intestinal dryness resulting from insufficiency of body fluid.

大黄荡涤泻下而除积滞，攻逐冷积，共为主药。干姜辛热，助附子以温中散寒。人参、甘草补中益气，其中人参亦可加强干姜、附子的温阳作用；甘草又可调和药性。全方乃以补促泻，寓泻于补之剂。

现代研究证实，本方具有抗菌、消炎、改善循环、提高机能、促进蠕动、兴奋中枢、促进消化吸收、强心等作用。

【使用注意】 附子应先煎30～60分钟，以减弱其毒性。大黄后下，以防其泻下作用减弱。

第三节　润　下　剂

润下剂主要由润下药组成，具有润肠通便作用。适用于津枯肠燥便秘证。

Hemp Seed Pill

(Maziren Wan)

SOURCE: ***Treatise on Febrile Diseases***

INGREDIENTS:

No. 1 Hemp seed, *Fructus Cannabis* 500g

No. 2 White peony root, *Radix Paeoniae Alba* 250g

No. 3 Fruit of immature citron, *Fructus Aurantii Immaturus* 250g

No. 4 Rhubarb, *Radix et Rhizoma Rhei* 500g

No. 5 Magnolia bark, *Cortex Magnoliae Officinalis* 250g

No. 6 Bitter apricot kernel, *Semen Armeniacae Amarum* 250g

DIRECTIONS: The above drugs are ground into fine powder and then boluses are made out of powdered medicines mixed with honey, just the same size as a parasol seed. Nine grams is taken each time orally with warm boiled water, one or two times a day. This recipe may be decocted for internal administration, but the dosage must be reduced in proportion to that of the original recipe.

FUNCTIONS: Moistening the intestines to relieve constipation.

INDICATIONS: Syndrome of constipation due to intestinal dryness, manifested as frequency of urination, dry stool, or constipation due to dehydration after febrile diseases, and habitual constipation.

This recipe can equally be adapted for the treatment of constipation caused by intestinal dryness due to over-sweating in the febrile diseases, habitual constipation marked by rabbit-stool-like feces.

INTERPRETATION: This recipe, in fact, is the modified copy of Minor Decoction for Purging Down Digestive *Qi*, with its dosage reduced and with the addition of hemp

麻子仁丸

【来源】《伤寒论》

【组成】麻子仁500克，芍药250克，枳实250克，大黄500克，厚朴250克，杏仁250克。

【用法】上药共为细末，炼蜜为丸，如梧桐子大，每次服9克，每日1～2次，温开水送服。亦可按原方用量比例减量改汤剂煎服。

【功用】润肠通便。

【主治】肠燥便秘证，表现为大便硬，小便数，或热病后津液不足之便秘，习惯性便秘等。

热病汗过多之肠燥便秘，习惯性便秘等出现兔粪状大便者，可用本方加减治疗。

【方解】本方即小承气汤减量，加火麻仁、杏仁、白芍药、

seed, bitter apricot kernel, white peony root and honey. In the recipe, Ingredient No.1, great in dosage, sweet in flavour, mild in nature and abundant in lipid, functions as the principal drug acting on the channels of the large intestine, spleen and stomach to moisten the large intestine for treatment of constipation. The acrid and mild natured Ingredient No.6, as an assistant drug, acts on the lung channel and the large intestine channel and has the function of sending down *qi* and relaxing the bowels with its lubricant nature. All the ingredients in the Minor Decoction for Purging Down Digestive *Qi* have the effect of purging the retention of gastrointestinal dryness and heat, and thus being referred to as adjuvant drugs. The guiding drug is honey with the effect of moistening dryness and relaxing the bowels. The various ingredients of the prescription act in coorperation to moisten the intestine and loose the bowels, and pertain to the recipe of mild laxation by moistening.

Modern researches have confirmed that this recipe has the functions of moistening the intestine and softening stool.

CAUTIONS:

1. The recipe should be administered with great care for the aged and the weak or those with constipation caused by exhaustion of body fluid and blood dryness without pathogenic heat.

2. It is not advisable for the pregnant women.

Section 4

Recipes for Eliminating Retained Fluid

This group of recipes consists of drastic purgatives and functions in eliminating excessive retained fluid. It is used in the treatment of hydrothorax, ascites and edema of excess type.

蜂蜜组成。方中麻子仁量大，甘平多脂油润，入脾、胃、大肠经，润肠通便，为主药。杏仁辛性平，入肺、大肠经，能降气润肠，为辅药。小承气汤泻肠胃之燥热积滞，为佐药。蜜蜂润燥滑肠，为使药。诸药配伍，意在润肠通便，属缓下滋润之剂。

现代研究证实，本方主要具有润肠软便的作用。

【使用注意】

1．年老、体虚或津枯血燥而内无邪热的便秘证，应慎用。

2．孕妇慎用。

第四节　逐　水　剂

逐水剂主要由峻泻逐水药组成，具有攻逐水饮的作用。适用于水饮停聚于胸腹及水肿之实证。

Ten Chinese-dates Decoction

(Shizao Tang)

SOURCE: ***Treatise on Febrile Diseases***

INGREDIENTS:

No. 1 Parched genkwa, *Flos Genkwa*

No. 2 Kansui root, *Radix Euphorbiae Kansui*

No. 3 Knoxia root, *Radix Knoxiae*

All the above drugs should be equal in dosage.

DIRECTIONS: The above drugs, mixed and ground into fine powder or then put into capsules, are taken 0.5-1g each time, once a day, with the decoction of 10 Chinese-dates. When the patient has drastic watery diarrhea, it is recommended that a diet of porridge be taken to benefit recovery.

FUNCTIONS: Drastically expelling the excessive fluid.

INDICATIONS: Pleural effusion and edema, manifested by pain in the chest and hypochondrium when coughing or spitting, hardness and stuffiness in the epigastrium, retching, shortness of breath, headache with halo, difficult respiration due to pain in the thorax and back, slippery coating on the tongue, sunken and taut pulse; or edema which is more serious in the lower part of the body, abdominal fullness, dyspnea, difficulty in urination and defecation.

Moreover, the modified recipe is also used to treat hydrothorax, ascites and edema caused by exudative pleurisy, hepatic cirrhosis, acute pancreatitis, chronic nephritis and nephrotic syndrome, etc.; or simple intestinal obstruction, acute gastric dilatation and others that are ascribed to strong body resistance with exuberance of pathogenic factors.

INTERPRETATION: Collectively, all the three ingre-

十 枣 汤

【来源】《伤寒论》

【组成】 芫花(熬)、甘遂、大戟各等分。

【用法】 上三药各等分为末，或装入胶囊，每服0.5～1克，以大枣十枚煎汤送服，每日一次。得快利后糜粥自养。

【功用】 峻逐水饮。

【主治】 悬饮及水肿证，表现为咳唾胸胁引痛，心下痞硬，干呕短气，头痛目眩，胸背掣痛不得息，舌苔滑，脉沉弦，或一身俱肿，以下半身尤重，腹胀喘满，二便不利等。

渗出性胸膜炎、肝硬化、急性胰腺炎、慢性肾炎、肾病综合征等有胸水、腹水、水肿者，或单纯性肠梗阻、急性胃扩张等属正盛邪实者，可用本方加减治疗。

【方解】 方中芫花、甘遂、大戟均有显著的通便利尿作用，

dients possess the remarkable therapeutic effects of freeing the movement of the bowels and inducing diuresis. Separately, No.1 is preferred for the treatment of recurrent fluid retention and accumulation of phlegm and heat in the upper-warmer; No.2 for draining retention in the channel system; No.3 for the purgation of accumulation of pathogenic water in the gastro-intestinal tract and viscera. The three ingredients, acting in combination as principal drugs, can forcefully enhance the effect of eliminating edema and accumulated fluid. However their poisonous and drastic nature is liable to hurt the vital *qi*. For this reason, Chinese-dates are added because their functions of replenishing *qi* and invigorating the spleen can make the drastic purgation of excessive fluid effective without affecting the vital *qi*, thus reducing the toxic effect of the three ingredients.

Modern researches have confirmed that this recipe can produce drastic effect of purgation and obvious effect of diuresis by stimulating the intestinal mucosa to produce inflammatory congestion and violent peristalsis.

CAUTIONS:

1. This recipe is advisable only to those who have excessive fluid and are in stout constitution. When the rapid purgation occurs, the administration must be withdrawn. If the purgation is not thorough, which suggests incomplete removal of fluid retention, the administration may be continued depending on the health condition.

2. If the purgation is required for patients with excessiveness of pathogen and general debility, there are several methods available in accordance with the patient's conditions, such as the method of administering medicines to drive out the pathogenic factors first and then give tonics for recuperation, the method of administering tonics first to improve the patient's general condition and then give drastic drugs to drive out pathogens, and the method of administering medicines

其中芫花善理上焦胸胁伏饮痰癖，甘遂善行经隧脉络之水湿，大戟泻脏腑肠胃之水邪，三药合用共为主药，其逐水饮、消肿满之功明显增强。但三药性烈而有毒，易伤正气，故配大枣益气健脾以制水，又缓和三药毒性，使峻下水饮而不伤正气。

现代研究证实，本方药物通过对肠粘膜的强烈刺激，引起炎症性充血和剧烈蠕动而产生很强的泻下作用，同时有明显的利尿作用。

【使用注意】

1. 病水饮而体壮者方可使用，以得快利为度。若服后虽泻而不爽，水饮未尽去者，次日可视体质情况再服。

2. 若患者邪实体虚，但又非攻不可者，可据病情采用先攻

to drive out invading pathogens and give tonics to reinforce the body resistance at the same time. When the patient's general condition takes a favourable turn, the treatment should be aimed at warming and replenishing the kidney-*qi* and recuperating the spleen and stomach.

3. It is never administered for pregnant women and the patients with weak health condition without excessiveness of pathogens.

Section 5

Recipes for Both Reinforcement and Elimination

This kind of recipes is chiefly made up of purgatives and tonifying drugs and possesses double properties of reinforcement and elimination. They are usually indicated for the treatment of syndrome of interior excess due to accumulation of pathogens with interior deficiency of the vital *qi*.

Decoction of Yellow Dragon with Supplements

(Xinjia Huanglong Tang)

SOURCE: ***Treatise on Differentiation and Treatment of Epidemic Febrile Diseases***

INGREDIENTS:

No. 1 Slim dried rehmannia root, *Radix Rehmanniae* 15g

No. 2 Liquorice, *Radix Glycyrrhizae* 6g

No. 3 Ginseng, *Radix Ginseng* 4.5g

No. 4 Rhubarb, *Radix et Rhizoma Rhei* 9g

后补、先补后攻或攻补兼施之法。病情好转，即当温补真元，调养脾胃。

3．体虚无实及孕妇禁用。

第五节　攻补兼施剂

攻补兼施剂主要由泻下药与补益药组成，具有泻下与补益双重作用。适用于里实积结而正气内虚之证。

新加黄龙汤

【来源】《温病条辨》

【组成】细生地15克，生甘草6克，人参4.5克，生大黄9

No. 5 Mirabilite, *Natrii Sulphas* 9g
No. 6 Scrophularia root, *Radix Scrophulariae* 15g
No. 7 Ophiopogon root, *Radix Ophiopogonis* 15g
No. 8 Chinese angelica root, *Radix Angelicae Sinensis* 4.5g
No. 9 Sea cucumber 2 pieces
No.10 Ginger juice 6 spoonfuls

DIRECTIONS: The above drugs should be decocted in water for oral administration.

FUNCTIONS: Nourishing *yin*, replenishing the vital *qi* and purging the accumulation of pathogenic heat.

INDICATIONS: Syndrome of the accumulation of heat accompanied by weakened body resistance with such symptoms as constipation, abdominal fullness and distension, mental fatigue, shortness of breath, dryness of the mouth and throat, parched or chapped lips with fissures on the tongue, dry scorched yellow or black tongue fur.

Equally, this recipe can be modified to treat paralytic, simple and obliterative intestinal obstruction, habitual constipation, epidemic or non-epidemic febrile diseases in their climax marked by interior excess and accumulation of heat, and effective for those with deficiency of the vital *qi* and massive loss of *yin* and blood.

INTERPRETATION: In the recipe, No.4 and No.5 purge the bowels to remove heat, soften hardness and moisten dryness. No.1, No.6, No.7 and No. 9 nourish *yin* to increase the body fluid. No.2, No.3 and No.8 not only replenish the vital *qi* but also tonify *yin* and blood so as to bring the effects of the drugs into full play. As a result, the bowels are purged and pathogenic heat is expelled. Ginger juice can be used to nourish the stomach and spleen to send down the stomach-*qi* and prevent retch and vomiting.

Modern researches have confirmed that this recipe has the efficacies of relieving inflammation, resisting bacteria, improving intestinal blood circulation and intestinal peristalsis, in-

克，芒硝9克，玄参15克，麦冬15克，当归4.5克，海参2条，姜汁6匙。

【用法】 水煎服。

【功用】 滋阴益气，泻下热结。

【主治】 热结正虚证，表现为大便秘结，腹中胀满而硬，神疲少气，口干咽燥，唇裂舌焦，苔焦黄或焦黑燥裂。

麻痹性、单纯性、闭塞性肠梗阻，习惯性便秘，传染性或非传染性发热疾病的极期，表现为热结里实、正气不足而阴血大亏者，可用本方加减治疗。

【方解】 方中大黄、芒硝泻热通便，软坚润燥。玄参、生地、麦冬、海参滋阴增液。人参、甘草、当归补气益血，既扶正气，又补阴血，使药力得以发挥，而大便可通，邪热可退。姜汁可健脾胃，降胃气，并防止格拒呕逆。

现代研究证实，本方具有消炎、抗菌、改善肠循环、促进蠕

creasing the activity of gastrointestinal tract, loosing the bowels, tranquilizing the mind and bringing down fever.

CAUTIONS: Ginseng should be decocted alone, and then poured into the decoction of other ingredients before intake.

动、增强机能、泻下、镇静、解热等作用。

【使用注意】 人参另煎，兑入他药中同服。

Chapter VII

Prescriptions for Warming the Interior

The prescriptions for warming the interior refer to those that mainly consist of drugs in warm nature with the effect of warming the interior, restoring *yang*, dispelling cold and promoting blood circulation for the treatment of syndrome of interior cold.

Mostly, the syndrome of interior cold results from *yang*-deficient constitution, or cold originating from interior or from impairment of *yang* due to erroneous treatment; or from exopathic cold directly attacking the viscera, channels and collaterals. Since the syndrome of interior cold differs in degrees of severity and varies in distribution of impaired regions, the prescriptions for warming the interior is accordingly subdivided into three kinds, namely, the recipes for warming the middle-warmer to dispel cold, the recipes for recuperating depleted *yang* to rescue the patient from collapse and the recipes for warming the channels to dispel cold.

Section 1

Recipes for Warming the Middle-warmer to Dispel Cold

This group of recipes is composed of interior-warming drugs in compatibility with the drugs for strengthening the

第七章

温里剂

凡以温热药为主组成，具有温里阳、散寒通脉作用，用以治疗里寒证的方剂，称为温里剂。

里寒证多由素体阳虚，寒自内生；或因误治伤阳；或外寒直中脏腑、经络所致。但是，里寒证有轻重之别，所伤部位各异。因此，温里剂又分为温中祛寒剂、回阳救逆剂、温经散寒剂三类。

第一节 温中祛寒剂

温中祛寒剂常由温里药与健脾补气药配伍而成，具有温中祛

spleen and replenishing *qi*, having the functions of warming the middle warmer to dispel cold. The recipes are indicated in the treatment of cold syndromes due to hypofunction of the spleen and stomach.

Bolus for Regulating the Function of Middle-warmer

(Lizhong Wan)

SOURCE: ***Treatise on Febrile Diseases***

INGREDIENTS:

No. 1 Ginseng, *Radix Ginseng* 90g

No. 2 Dried ginger, *Rhizoma Zingiberis* 90g

No. 3 Bighead atractylodes rhizome, *Rhizoma Atractylodis Macrocephalae* 90g

No. 4 Prepared licorice root, *Radix Glycyrrhizae Praeparata* 90g

DIRECTIONS: Grind the above drugs into fine powder, mix it with honey and make them into boluses, take the boluses orally with warm boiled water, 9g each time, two or three times a day; or decoct the drugs for oral dose with the orignal dosage of the ingredients taken proportionally.

FUNCTIONS: Warming the middle-warmer to dispel cold and replenishing *qi* to invigorate the spleen.

INDICATIONS: Hypofunction of the spleen and stomach marked by abdominal pain with predilection for warmth and for pressure by hand, watery diarrhea, fullness of the abdomen, anorexia, vomiting, pale tongue with white coating, deep and thready pulse; or manifested by bleeding due to *yang*-deficiency; or chronic infantile convulsion; or predilection for spitting saliva after recovery from illness; or by obstruction of *qi* in the chest due to *yang*-deficiency of the middle-warmer.

寒作用。适用于中焦脾胃虚寒证。

理 中 丸

【来源】《伤寒论》

【组成】 人参、干姜、白术、甘草(炙)各90克。

【用法】 上药研末，和蜜为丸，1日2～3次，每次9克，开水送下。或按原方比例酌定用量水煎服。

【功用】 温中祛寒，益气健脾。

【主治】 脾胃虚证，表现为腹痛喜温喜按，泻利清稀，腹满食少，呕吐，舌淡苔白，脉沉细；或阳虚失血；或小儿慢惊风；或病后喜唾涎沫；或中焦阳虚所致胸痹等。

The recipe can be modified to treat cold syndromes due to hypofunction of the spleen and stomach as seen in cases of chronic gastritis, gastroduodenal ulcer, chronic colitis, indigestion, gastric dilatation, gastropotosia, or cold syndromes of excess type in the spleen and stomach as seen in cases of acute gastritis and enteritis.

INTERPRETATION: Of the ingredients in the recipe, No.2, with its pungent hot property attributing to the channels of the spleen and stomach, acts as a principal drug and is to restore the *yang* of the spleen and stomach by means of warming the middle-warmer to dispel cold, to arrest vomiting by way of regulating the stomach to send down reversed flow of *qi*. No.1, slightly bitter in flavor and slightly warm in nature, is administered as an assistant drug for tonifying *qi*, strengthening the spleen and stomach. No.3, with its sweet and bitter flavour and warm nature attributing to the channel of spleen, serves as an adjuvant drug for strengthening the spleen and eliminating dampness. No.4, sweet and mild in property, attributing to the channel of spleen, replenishes the spleen-*qi* and regulates the middle-warmer, and tempers the effect of other drugs in the recipe, playing the part of a guiding drug.

Modern researches have ascertained that this recipe has the efficacies in adjusting the functions of the stomach and intestine, promoting blood circulation, strengthening metabolism, relieving spasm, alleviating pain, arresting vomiting and diarrhea, inducing diuresis, etc.

CAUTIONS: Since the recipe tends to be warm and dry in property, it is not advisable for cases with fever due to exopathogens, or with internal heat due to *yin* deficiency.

慢性胃炎、胃及十二指肠溃疡、慢性结肠炎、消化不良、胃扩张、胃下垂等证属脾胃虚寒者，或急性胃炎、急性肠炎属脾胃虚寒者，可用本方加减治疗。

【方解】 方中干姜辛热入脾胃，温中祛寒，以恢复脾胃之阳，和胃降逆以止呕，为主药。人参甘微苦微温，补气健脾益胃，为辅药。白术甘苦温入脾，健脾燥湿，为佐药。炙甘草甘平入脾胃，益脾气和中，调和诸药，为使药。

现代研究证实，本方具有调整胃肠机能、促进循环、增强代谢、解痉、镇痛、制吐、止泻、利尿等作用。

【使用注意】 本方药性偏于温燥，故凡外感发热或阴虚内热者忌用。

Minor Decoction for Strengthening the Middle-warmer

(Xiao Jianzhong Tang)

SOURCE: ***Treatise on Febrile Diseases***

INGREDIENTS:

No. 1 Peony root, *Radix Paeoniae* 18g
No. 2 Cinnamon twig, *Ramulus Cinnamomi* 9g
No. 3 Licorice root, *Radix Glycyrrhizae* 6g
No. 4 Fresh ginger, *Rhizoma Zingiberis Recens* 10g
No. 5 Chinese-dates, *Fructus Ziziphi Jujubae* 4 pcs.
No. 6 Malt extract, *Saccharum Granorum* 30g

DIRECTIONS: The decoction is prepared by decocting all the drugs but the last one, filtering out the residue, and adding No. 6 into the already-decocted solution. It should be taken warm.

FUNCTIONS: Warming the middle-warmer, tonifying deficiency and relieving spasm and pain.

INDICATIONS: Abdominal pain due to cold of deficiency type, marked by abdominal pain which can be relieved by warming and pressing; or consumptive diseases manifested by palpitation, restlessness, pale complexion, whitish coating of the tongue, thready, taut and weak pulse; or fever due to *yang*-deficiency.

To treat gastroduodenal ulcer, administration of the above recipe by adding 30g of dahurian angelica root and increaseing of the dosage of No. 3 to 15g, created by Dr. Zhang Enqin, can yield remarkble result.

INTERPRETATION: The last ingredient in the recipe, which is dominant in dosage, is referred to as a principal drug because its sweet taste and warm nature facilitates its effect

小建中汤

【来源】《伤寒论》

【组成】芍药18克，桂枝9克，甘草6克，生姜10克，大枣4枚，饴糖30克。

【用法】水煎取汁，兑入饴糖，温服。

【功用】温中补虚，缓急止痛。

【主治】虚寒腹痛证，表现为腹中时痛，喜温喜按，按之则痛减，或虚劳心中悸动，虚烦不宁，面色无华，苔白，脉细弦弱，或阳虚发热等。

张恩勤以本方加白芷30克，甘草增至15克，治疗胃及十二指肠溃疡著效。

【方解】方中饴糖甘温入脾，益脾气而养脾阴，既能温中补

on the spleen, and it is able to replenish the spleen-*qi* and nourish the spleen-*yin*, having the functions not only in warming the middle-warmer and restoring *qi* but also in regulating the internal organs and relieving spasm. Both No. 1 and No.2 play the part of an assistant drug: the former, sour in flavour and slightly cold in nature, has the function of replenishing *yin* -blood to relieve spasm and pain, and the latter, pungent in flavour and warm in nature, is effective for supporting *yang–qi*. The combined administration of the above two drugs—one warm in nature and beneficial to *yang* and the other cold and beneficial to *yin*—helps to regulate *ying* and *wei*, *yin* and *yang*. The rest are used together as adjuvant and guiding drugs. No.4 is used to replenish *wei-yang*. No. 5 is used to tonify *ying-yin* and strengthen the spleen and stomach, and No.3 to regulate the middle-warmer and replenish *qi*. Upon analysis, the recipe is the modification of Cinnamon Twig Decoction with the dosage of peony root doubled and with the addition of malt extract. In other words, this recipe for warming the middle-warmer, tonifying *qi* and relieving spasm and pain originates from a recipe for expelling pathogenic factors from muscles and skin and regulating *ying*.

Studies in recent years have confirmed that this recipe possesses the efficacies in relieving spasm, alleviating pain, promoting blood circulation, strengthening digestion and absorption, promoting the healing of ulcers, nourishing the body, consolidating the constitution, etc.

CAUTIONS:

1. Contraindicated in cases with hyperactivity of pathogenic fire due to *yin*-deficiency.

2. Not administered to those suffering from vomiting since the sweet flavor of the drugs may induce vomiting.

3. Contraindicated in patients who vomit ascaris, because ascaris tends to reverse upwards when meeting the sweet flavor of food or drugs.

虚，又能和里缓急，药量独重，为主药。芍药与桂枝为辅药，芍药酸微寒，益阴血而缓急止痛，桂枝辛温以助阳气，二药合用，一温一寒，一助阳，一助阴，起调营卫、和阴阳作用。生姜益卫阳，大枣补营阴、益脾胃，甘草调中益气，共为佐使药。从全方用药分析，该方是桂枝汤倍芍药加饴糖而成，由原方解肌和营之剂，而变为温中补虚、缓急止痛之方。

现代研究证实，本方具有解痉、镇痛、促进血液循环、加强消化吸收、促进溃疡愈合、滋养强壮等作用。

【使用注意】

1. 阴虚火旺者忌用。

2. 呕吐者不可用，因甜能助呕。

3. 吐蛔者不可用，因蛔得甘味则逆上。

4. Contraindicated in patients with fullness in the stomach, for the sweet flavor makes the above symptoms worse by replenishing *qi*.

Decoction of Evodia Fruit
(*Wuzhuyu Tang*)

SOURCE: ***Treatise on Febrile Diseases***

INGREDIENTS:

No. 1 Evodia fruit, *Fructus Evodiae* 3g
No. 2 Ginseng, *Radix Ginseng* 6g
No. 3 Chinese-dates, *Fructus Ziziphi Jujubae* 4 pcs.
No. 4 Fresh ginger, *Rhizoma Zingiberis Recens* 18g

DIRECTIONS: All the above drugs are to be decocted in water for oral administration.

FUNCTIONS: Warming the middle-warmer and restoring *qi*, sending down the ascending reverse flow of *qi* to arrest vomiting.

INDICATIONS:

1. Cold syndrome due to *yang* insufficiency of the liver and stomach manifested by the tendency to vomiting after meals, fullness and stuffiness in the chest; or by epigastralgia and gastric discomfort with acid regurgitation.

2. Headache due to *jueyin* channel syndrome characterized by retching, salivation, and pain and cold feeling in the vertex.

3. Vomiting and diarrhea due to *shaoyin* syndrome marked by symptoms such as cold extremities, dysphoria, etc.

The modified recipe can be applied to the treatment of such diseases as chronic gastritis, acute gastritis, gastroduodenal ulcer, hepatitis, vomiting of pregnancy, migraine, Menierei's disease and others that pertain to cold syndrome due to *yang* insufficiency of the liver and stomach and with turbid

4．中满者不可用，因甘能补气填实故也。

吴茱萸汤

【来源】《伤寒论》

【组成】吴茱萸3克，人参6克，大枣4枚，生姜18克。

【用法】水煎服。

【功用】温中补虚，降逆止呕。

【主治】

1．肝胃虚寒证，表现为食谷欲呕，胸膈满闷，或胃脘作痛，吞酸嘈杂等。

2．厥阴头痛证，表现为干呕，吐涎沫，巅顶痛而冷。

3．少阴吐利证，表现为手足逆冷，烦躁欲死等证。

慢性胃炎、急性胃炎、胃及十二指肠溃疡、肝炎、妊娠呕吐、偏头痛、美尼尔氏综合征等证属肝胃虚寒、浊阴上逆者可用本方

yin reversing upwards.

INTERPRETATION: In the recipe, Ingredient No. 1, possessing pungent flavor and hot nature, attributes to the channels of the spleen, liver and kidney. As a principal drug, it is effective for the treatment of diseases in the three channels. It also has the functions of warming the stomach, sending down the reversed ascending *qi* to prevent vomiting, dispersing the depressed liver-energy to alleviate pain and warming the kidney to arrest diarrhea. No. 2 is used as tonic for tonifying primordial *qi* and replenishing *yin*, and is considered as an assistant drug. No. 4, with its pungent and warm property and its effect on the stomach, is administered as an adjuvant drug to lower the adverse flow of *qi* and reinforce the efficacy of the principal drug in arresting vomiting and scattering cold. No.3, as a guiding drug, has sweet flavor and slow effect and functions in the regulation of the middle-warmer. It not only relieves the dryness caused by the pungent and warm evodia fruit and fresh ginger, but also aids ginseng in restoring *qi* and strengthening the body's resistance.

Modern studies have showed that this recipe produces the effect of promoting blood circulation in the digestive tract, lowering tension of the smooth muscle, decreasing peristalsis, relieving spasm, preventing vomiting, alleviating pain, facilitating digestion, strengthening the functions of the whole body and so on.

CAUTIONS:

1. The recipe should never be administered to patients with stomachache or vomiting of bitter fluid due to stagnated heat, as well as acid regurgitation that is ascribed to heat syndrome.

2. For the treatment of severe vomiting, the decoction should be taken cold so as to prevent vomiting of the drug.

3. In a few patients, vomiting of the drug may become worse but it will subside by itself in half an hour. The patients should be advised to take a little rest after taking the

加减治疗。

【方解】 方中吴茱萸味辛性热，入肝、脾、肾三经，可温胃、降逆、止呕，疏肝止痛，温肾止泻，一药三经同治，为主药。人参大补元气，兼能益阴，为辅药。生姜辛散温胃，降逆止呕，加强主药降逆止呕散寒之作用，为方中佐药。大枣为使药，甘缓和中，既缓吴茱萸、生姜辛温燥性，又助人参补虚扶正。

现代研究证实，本方具有促进消化道血液循环、降低平滑肌张力、减慢蠕动、解痉、制吐、镇痛、助消化、提高全身机能等作用。

【使用注意】

1．郁热所致胃痛、吐苦水及吞酸属热者，禁用本方。

2．呕吐严重者，应采用热药冷服法，以免格拒不纳。

3．少数患者服药后反有呕吐加剧现象，一般半小时左右可

drug to alleviate the reaction.

Section 2

Recipes for Recuperating Depleted *Yang* to Rescue the Patient from Collapse

This kind of recipe is chiefly composed of the drugs of heat nature with the functions of warming the kidney and recuperating depleted *yang* to rescue the patient from collapse. It is usually indicated for the treatment of general cold syndrome due to *yang*-deficiency of the kidney or both the heart and kidney.

Decoction for Resuscitation

(Sini Tang)

SOURCE: ***Treatise on Febrile Diseases***

INGREDIENTS:

No. 1 Prepared aconite root, *Radix Aconiti Praeparata* 9g

No. 2 Dried ginger, *Rhizoma Zingiberis* 9g

No. 3 Prepared licorice root, *Radix Glycyrrhizae Praeparata* 12g

DIRECTIONS: Ingredient No. 1 is to be decocted one hour prior to the other two. The decoction should be taken warm.

FUNCTIONS: Warming the spleen and kidney, recuperating depleted *yang* to rescue the patient from collapse.

INDICATIONS: Syndrome of cold limbs due to insufficiency of *yang* marked by cold limbs, intolerance to cold, li-

自行缓解，应嘱其服药后稍事休息，以减轻服药反应。

第二节　回阳救逆剂

回阳救逆剂主要由温热药组成，具有温肾、回阳、救逆作用。适用于肾阳虚或心肾阳虚所致的全身阴寒证。

四逆汤

【来源】《伤寒论》

【组成】附子9克，干姜9克，甘草(炙)12克。

【用法】先煎附子1小时，再加余药同煎，取汁温服。

【功用】温暖脾肾，回阳救逆。

【主治】阳虚寒厥证，表现为四肢厥逆，恶寒蜷卧，下利清

enteric diarrhea, cold-pain of the abdomen, mental fatigue and sleepiness, tastelessness with no desire for drink, pale complexion, profuse sweat, deep slow and thready pulse.

In addition to the above symptoms, syndromes such as domination of cold due to *yang* deficiency as seen in cases of distinct declination of bodily strength caused by chronic disorders or hypopituitarism, hypothyroidism, hypoadrenocorticism, *yang* depletion as seen in shock due to heart failure, cardiac infarction and other diseases can respond well in treatment to the modified recipe mentioned above.

INTERPRETATION: Ingredient No. 1 in the recipe, pungent and hot in the extreme, acts on the channels of the heart, kidney and spleen, helping to warm the *yang–qi* and recuperate the depleted *yang* to rescue the patient from collapse, and therefore, it is prefered as a principal drug. No.2, an assistant drug in the recipe, functions in warming *yang* of the middle-warmer and eliminating interior cold, so it is administered to treat vomiting and diarrhea due to cold of the insufficiency type and meanwhile, it enhances the function of the principal drug in strengthening the kidney-*yang*. For this reason, there goes the saying "Without dried ginger, the hot property of prepared aconite roots can not be brought into play". The combination of No. 1 and No. 2 can develop drastic flavor to strengthen forcefully the effect of warming *yang*. The last one with the effects of strengthening the spleen and replenishing *qi*, as adjuvant and guiding drugs is used in assisting No. 1 to recuperate depleted *yang* and promote blood circulation, and in assisting No.2 in warming and restoring *yang* of the middle-warmer to reduce toxin of No. 1 and relieving the extremely pungent property of the first two drugs so as to make it possible to warm *yang* and remove *yin* cold without injuring *yin*.

Recent studies have confirmed that this recipe has the efficacies in exciting central nervous system, promoting me-

谷，腹中冷痛，神疲欲寐，口淡不渴，面色苍白，大汗淋漓，脉沉迟微细等。

慢性疾患体力明显衰退，或垂体、甲状腺、肾上腺皮质机能低下等证属阳虚寒盛者；心力衰竭、心肌梗塞和其他原因引起的休克证属亡阳者，可用本方加减治疗。

【方解】 方中附子大辛大热，入心、肾、脾诸经，温化阳气回阳救逆，为主药。干姜为辅药，温中焦之阳而除里寒，以治虚寒吐利，并能助附子壮肾阳，故有"附子无姜不热"之说。二药伍用，一走一守，气味雄厚，使温阳之力明显增强。炙甘草健脾益气，助附子回阳通脉，助干姜温复中阳，解附子毒性，缓姜、附辛烈之性，使温阳破阴而无劫阴之弊，为佐使药。

现代研究证实，本方具有兴奋中枢神经系统、促进代谢、改

tabolism, improving functions, preventing shock and so on.

CAUTIONS:

1. Since it is indicated for the treatment of cold limbs due to *yang* insufficiency, the recipe should never be administered for syndromes attributable to cold limbs caused by excess of heat.

2. Patients with flushed face and restlessness ascribed to cold syndrome with pseudo-heat symptoms, should take the decoction cool to prevent rejection of the drug.

3. Prolonged decocting aconite root is abvisable to reduce its toxic action.

Section 3

Recipes for Warming the Channels to Dispel Cold

These recipes are chiefly composed of the drugs for warming the channels to dispel cold and the drugs for nourishing blood and promoting blood circulation, possessing the therapeutic effect of warming the channels to dispel cold. They are indicated for the arthralgia-syndrome marked by insufficiency of *yang-qi*, internal insufficiency of *ying*-blood, and stagnated cold pathogens in the channels.

Chinese Angelica Decoction for Restoring *Yang*

(Danggui Sini Tang)

SOURCE: ***Treatise on Febrile Diseases***

善机能、抗休克等作用。

【使用注意】

1. 本方以治阳虚寒厥为主，若属热厥证者禁用。

2. 若见面红、烦躁属真寒假热者，服用本方时，应以凉服为宜，以避免格拒。

3. 附子宜久煎以减缓毒性。

第三节　温经散寒剂

温经散寒剂主要由温经散寒药和养血通脉药组成，具有温经散寒作用。适用于阳气不足、营血内弱、寒邪凝滞经脉之痹证。

当归四逆汤

【来源】《伤寒论》

INGREDIENTS:

No. 1 Chinese angelica root, *Radix Angelicae Sinensis* 9g
No. 2 Cinnamon twig, *Ramulus Cinnamomi* 9g
No. 3 Peony root, *Radix Paeoniae* 9g
No. 4 Asarum herb, *Herba Asari* 6g
No. 5 Prepared licorice root, *Radix Glycyrrhizae Praeparata* 6g
No. 6 Fiveleaf akebia stem, *Caulis Akebiae* 6g
No. 7 Chinese-dates, *Fructus Ziziphi Jujubae* 8pcs.

DIRECTIONS: All the above drugs are to be decocted in water for oral administration.

FUNCTIONS: Warming the channels to dispel cold, nourishing the blood and promoting blood circulation.

INDICATIONS: Cold limbs due to cold stagnation with insufficiency of blood, marked by cold limbs, thirstlessness, soreness of extremities, or abdominal colic, pale tongue with whitish fur, deep and thready pulse, which is even too thready to be felt

The recipe can be modified to deal with cases such as Raynaud's disease, thrombotic phlebitis, chilblain, chronic rheumatic arthritis, dysmenorrhea, neuralgia, lumbago and gastroduodenal ulcer which pertain to cold stagnation with insufficiency of blood.

INTERPRETATION: The first drug in the recipe, possessing the pungent, bitter and sweet flavor and warm property, acts as a principal and has the functions of enriching and regulating the blood. Used in combination as assistant drugs, No.3 is contributive to nourishing the blood and regulating *ying* and No.2 to warming and promoting blood circulation, both enhancing the effect of the principal drug to warm and nourish the channels. Ingredient No. 4 is able to arouse *yang–qi*, warm the channels exteriorly and warm the viscera interiorly and therefore is administered together with the principal and assistant drugs to eliminate cold pathogens, warm extremities, and relieve arthralgia by removing obstruction in the exterior and

【组成】 当归9克，桂枝9克，芍药9克，细辛6克，甘草(炙)6克，木通6克，大枣8枚。

【用法】 水煎服。

【功用】 温经散寒，养血通脉。

【主治】 血虚寒厥证，表现为四肢厥冷，口不渴，肢体酸痛，或腹中挛急，舌淡苔白，脉沉细，甚则细而欲绝等。

雷诺氏病、血栓性静脉炎、冻疮、慢性风湿性关节炎、痛经、神经痛、腰痛、胃及十二指肠溃疡等证属血虚寒凝者，可用本方加减治疗。

【方解】 方中当归辛苦甘温，补血和血，为主药。芍药养血和营，桂枝温通血脉，以加强当归温养血脉之功，共为辅药。细辛鼓动阳气，外温经脉，内温脏腑，与主辅药合用，通达表里上

interior, superior and inferior of the human body. No. 6 has the abilities of promoting blood circulation and relieving joint trouble, and its cold property can prevent injuring *yin*-blood due to the dry property of No.2 and No.4, playing the role of an adjuvant drug along with No. 4 . Ingredients No. 5 and No.7, as guiding drugs, are used for tonifying and replenishing the spleen and stomach, and tempering the effect of other drugs in the recipe.

Modern researches have ascertained that this recipe possesses the efficacies in improving peripheral circulation, dilating blood vessels, alleviating pain, relieving spasm, promoting digestion and absorption, tonifying the blood and restoring *qi*.

CAUTIONS:

1. The recipe is only indicated for the cold limbs syndrome caused by insufficiency of blood and stagnation of cold. Those related to cold limbs due to excess of heat are prohibited from taking it.

2. The recipe is contraindicated in patients suffering from late-stage chilblain marked by transformation of stagnated cold into heat which is distinct.

下内外，散寒邪，温四末，除痹痛；木通能通血脉，利关节，其寒性能防止桂枝、细辛温燥耗伤阴血，共为佐药。大枣、炙甘草补益脾胃，调和诸药为使药。

现代研究证实，本方具有改善末梢循环、扩张血管、镇痛、解痉、促进消化吸收、养血补虚等作用。

【使用注意】

1. 本方只宜于血虚寒凝所致的厥逆证，若属热厥证禁用。

2. 冻疮后期，寒郁化热，而热较明显者忌用。

Chapter VIII

Mediating Prescriptions

This group of prescriptions may be divided into three types: the recipes for treating *shaoyang* disease by mediation; the recipes for regulating the function of the liver and spleen; and the recipes for regulating the function of the intestine and stomach.

Section 1

Recipes for Treating *Shaoyang* Disease by Mediation

This type of recipes is mainly used to treat *shaoyang* disease, the pathogenic factors of which are neither located in the exterior nor in the interior but in between.

Minor Decoction of Bupleurum

(Xiao Chaihu Tang)

SOURCE: ***Treatise on Febrile Diseases***
INGREDIENTS:
No. 1 Bupleurum root, *Radix Bupleuri* 12g
No. 2 Scutellaria root, *Radix Scutellariae* 9g
No. 3 Pinellia tuber, *Rhizoma Pinelliae* 9g

第八章

和解剂

和解剂可分为和解少阳剂、调和肝脾剂和调和肠胃剂三类。

第一节　和解少阳剂

和解少阳剂主要用于治疗邪在半表半里的少阳病。

小柴胡汤

【来源】《伤寒论》

【组成】 柴胡12克，黄芩9克，半夏9克，生姜9克，人参

No. 4 Fresh ginger, *Rhizoma Zingiberis Recens* 9g
No. 5 Ginseng, *Radix Ginseng* 6g
No. 6 Chinese dates, *Fructus Ziziphi Jujubae* 4 pcs.
No. 7 Prepared licorice root, *Radix Glycyrrhizae Praeparata* 5g

DIRECTIONS: All the drugs listed above are decocted in water for oral administration.

FUNCTIONS: Treating *shaoyang* disease by mediation.

INDICATIONS: *Shaoyang* disease with the pathogenic factors located neither in the exterior nor in the interior but in between marked by alternate attacks of chills and fever, fullness in the chest, hypochondriac discomfort, anorexia, dysphoria, retching, bitterness in the mouth, dry throat, dizziness, thin and white fur of the tongue and stringy pulse, or exogenous febrile diseases occurring in women belonging to invasion of the blood chamber by pathogenic heat.

The common cold, malaria, infection of biliary tract, hepatitis, pleuritis, chronic gastritis, indigestion, mastosis, intercostal neuralgia, neurosis and AIDS marked by the symptoms of *shaoyang* disease can be treated by the modified recipe.

INTERPRETATION: No. 1, as a principal drug, dispels the pathogenic factor located in the half exterior by driving it out. No.2 clears out stagnated heat located in the half interior by clearing away it thoroughly as an assistant drug. The combined use of the two drugs, one for dispelling pathogen, and the other for clearing away stagnated heat, removes pathogenic factors from *shaoyang* channels. No. 3 and No. 4 regulate the function of the stomach and lower the adverse flow of *qi*. No. 5 and No.6 invigorate *qi* and strengthen the middle-warmer. No. 7 coordinates the actions of various drugs in the recipe. The drugs from No. 3 to No. 7 act as adjuvant and guiding drugs.

Modern researches have proved that the recipe has some effects of inhibiting bacteria, viruses and leptospira, relieving the reaction of the human body to the invaded pathogen, and remarkably allaying fever and resisting inflammation. In

6克，大枣4枚，甘草(炙)5克。

【用法】 水煎服。

【功用】 和解少阳。

【主治】 邪在半表半里之少阳病，表现为往来寒热，胸胁苦满，默默不欲饮食，心烦喜呕，口苦咽干，目眩，苔薄白，脉弦，以及妇人伤寒，热入血室等。

感冒、疟疾、胆道感染、肝炎、胸膜炎、慢性胃炎、消化不良、乳房疾病、肋间神经痛、神经官能症以及爱滋病等表现为少阳病者，可用本方加减治疗。

【方解】 方中柴胡疏解半表之邪使之外出，为主药。黄芩清半里之郁热使之内彻，为辅药。二药配伍，一疏一清，共解少阳之邪。半夏、生姜和胃降逆；人参、大枣益气补中，甘草调和诸药，共为佐使药。

现代研究证实，本方对细菌、病毒及钩端螺旋体均有一定的抑制作用，并能缓解机体对入侵病原体产生的反应，有明显的解

addition, the recipe also has the effects of promoting digestion, preventing vomiting, expelling phlegm, relieving cough, protecting the liver, normalizing the functioning of the gallbladder and tranquilizing the mind.

CAUTIONS: Patients with syndromes such as upper excess with lower deficiency, or excess of liver-fire, hyperactivity of the liver-*yang*, haematemesis due to deficiency of *yin* are forbidden to use the recipe.

Supplementary Recipe:

Major Decoction of Bupleurum

(Da Chaihu Tang)

SOURCE: *Synopsis of Prescriptions of the Golden Chamber*

INGREDIENTS:

No. 1 Bupleurum root, *Radix Bupleuri* 15g

No. 2 Scutellaria root, *Radix Scutellariae* 9g

No. 3 White peony root, *Radix Paeoniae Alba* 9g

No. 4 Pinellia tuber, *Rhizoma Pinelliae* 9g

No. 5 Prepared fruit of immature citron or trifoliate orange, *Fructus Aurantii Immaturus Praeparata* 9g

No. 6 Rhubarb root, *Radix et Rhizoma Rhei* 6g

No. 7 Fresh ginger, *Rhizoma Zingiberis Recens* 15g

No. 8 Chinese-dates, *Fructus Ziziphi Jujubae* 5 pcs.

DIRECTIONS: All the drugs listed above are to be decocted in water twice, and after the residue is removed, the decoction is to be taken warm in two separate doses.

FUNCTIONS: Treating *shaoyang* disease by mediation and purging away internal stasis of heat.

INDICATIONS: *Shaoyang* and *yangming* diseases complex marked by alternate attacks of chills and fever, fullness and oppression in the chest, hypochondriac discomfort, frequent

热、抗炎作用。此外，本方尚有促进消化、镇吐、祛痰、镇咳、保肝、利胆、镇静等功效。

【使用注意】 凡上盛下虚、肝火偏盛、肝阳上亢、阴虚吐血等不宜服用。

【附方】 大柴胡汤

【来源】 (《金匮要略》)

【组成】 柴胡15克，黄芩 9 克，芍药 9 克，半夏 9 克，枳实(炙) 9 克，大黄 6 克，生姜15克，大枣 5 枚。

【用法】 水煎二次，去滓，分二次温服。

【功用】 和解少阳，内泻热结。

【主治】 少阳、阳明合病，表现为往来寒热，胸胁苦满，呕

vomiting, mental depression and dysphoria, epigastric fullness and pain or epigastric rigidity, constipation or diarrhea due to interior cold and exterior heat, yellow tongue fur, stringy and forceful pulse.

Patients with acute cholecystitis, cholelithiasis, acute pancreatitis and infection of abdominal activity marked by the above-mentioned symptoms can be treated by the modified recipe.

Section 2

Recipes for Regulating the Function of the Liver and the Spleen

This group of recipes is mainly composed of drugs for soothing the liver and those for strengthening the spleen. It can achieve the effect of regulating the function of the liver and spleen and is fit for the treatment of incoordination between the liver and spleen due to stagnation of the liver-*qi* attacking the spleen or caused by disturbance of the liver-*qi* due to the loss of the normal transporting function of the spleen.

Powder for Treating Cold Limbs

(Sini San)

SOURCE: ***Treatise on Febrile Diseases***

INGREDIENTS:

No. 1 Bupleurum root, *Radix Bupleuri* 6 g

No. 2 White peony root, *Radix Paeoniae Alba* 9 g

No. 3 Fruit of immature citron or trifoliate orange, *Fructus Aurantii Immaturus* 6 g

No. 4 Prepared licorice root, *Radix Glycyrrhizae Praeparata* 6 g

不止，郁郁微烦，心下满痛或心下痞硬，大便不解或协热下利，舌苔黄，脉弦有力。

急性胆囊炎、胆石症、急性胰腺炎、腹腔感染等表现为上述症状者可用本方加减治疗。

第二节 调和肝脾剂

调和肝脾剂主要由疏肝药和健脾药组成，具有调和肝脾的作用。适用于肝气郁结，横逆犯脾，或脾虚不运致肝气不疏而出现的肝脾不和证。

四 逆 散

【来源】《伤寒论》

【组成】 柴胡6克，芍药9克，枳实6克，甘草(炙)6克。

DIRECTIONS: All the drugs listed above are to be decocted in water for oral administration.

FUNCTIONS: Dispersing pathogens and alleviating mental depression, soothing the liver and regulating the spleen.

INDICATIONS: Cold limbs due to the internal depressed *yang–qi* which fails to reach the distal parts of limbs, or epigastric distension and distress, diarrhea with tenesmus and abdominal pain caused by stagnation of the liver-*qi* and the accumulation of the spleen-*qi*, white fur of the tongue and stringy pulse.

Patients with chronic hepatitis, cholecystitis, cholelithiasis, pancreatitis, neuralgia intercostalis and gastroneurosis marked by the symptoms of stagnation of the liver-*qi* and the accumulation of the spleen-*qi* can be treated by the modified recipe.

INTERPRETATION: No. 1 soothes the liver, regulates the circulation of *qi* and normalizes the functional activities of *qi* to render pathogenic heat out of the human body. No. 2 nourishes the liver, relieves spasm and replenishes *yin*, so that pathogenic heat is removed from the body without impairing *yin*. No. 3 purges stagnation from the spleen. No. 4 coordinates the effects of all the drugs in the recipe and can relieve spasm and pain in combination with No. 2.

Modern researches have proved that the recipe has the effects of tranquilizing the mind, relieving spasm and pain, allaying fever and resisting bacteria. In addition, it is also very effective in treating hepatic injury.

CAUTIONS: Since it is indicated for cold limbs due to excess of heat which is caused by stagnation of *yang–qi*, the recipe is contraindicated in patients with cold limbs of other types.

Ease Powder

(Xiaoyao San)

SOURCE: ***Prescription of Peaceful Benevolent Dispensary***

【用法】 水煎服。

【功用】 透邪解表，疏肝理脾。

【主治】 阳气内郁不能达于四末之手足逆冷，肝郁脾壅所致的脘腹胀闷，泻利下重，腹痛，苔白，脉弦。

慢性肝炎、胆囊炎、胆石症、胰腺炎、肋间神经痛、胃神经官能症等表现为肝郁脾壅者，可用本方加减治疗。

【方解】 方中柴胡疏肝解郁，调畅气机，使郁热外达。芍药柔肝、缓急、养阴，使邪热外透而不伤阴。枳实泻脾土之壅滞。甘草调和诸药，配芍药又能缓急止痛。

现代研究证实，本方具有镇静、解痉、镇痛、解热、抗菌等作用。此外，其抗肝损伤的作用也十分显著。

【使用注意】 本方所治之四肢逆冷，系指阳气内郁之热厥，其他厥逆勿用。

逍遥散

【来源】《太平惠民和剂局方》

INGREDIENTS:

No. 1 Bupleurum root, *Radix Bupleuri* 15 g

No. 2 Chinese angelica root, *Radix Angelicae Sinensis* 15 g

No. 3 White peony root, *Radix Paeoniae Alba* 15 g

No. 4 Tuckahoe, *Poria* 15 g

No. 5 Bighead atractylodes rhizome, *Rhizoma Atractylodis Macrocephalae* 15 g

No. 6 Roasted ginger, *Rhizoma Zingiberis Recens Praeparata* a little.

No. 7 Peppermint, *Herba Menthae* a little

No. 8 Prepared licorice root, *Radix Glycyrrhizae Praeparata* 6 g

DIRECTIONS: Grind the above drugs except No. 6 and No. 7 into powder, take 6 to 9 grams each time with a decoction in small amount of roasted ginger and peppermint. If used as decoction the dosage can be reduced proportionally according to the original recipe.

FUNCTIONS: Soothing the liver to disperse the depressed *qi*, and invigorating the spleen to nourish the blood.

INDICATIONS: Stagnation of the liver-*qi* with deficiency of the blood marked by hypochondriac pain, headache, dizziness, bitter mouth, dry throat, mental weariness and poor appetite, or alternate attacks of chills and fever, or irregular menstruation, distension in the breast, light redness of the tongue, taut and feeble pulse.

Patients with chronic hepatitis, pleuritis, chronic gastritis, neurosis, irregular menstruation marked by the symptoms of stagnation of the liver-*qi* with deficiency of the blood can be treated by the modified recipe.

INTERPRETATION: No. 1 in the recipe soothes the liver to disperse the depressed *qi*. No. 2 and No. 3 nourish the blood and the liver. The joint use of the three drugs is able to treat the primary cause of stagnation of the liver-*qi* and deficiency of the blood. No.5 and No.4 strengthen the middle-warmer and reinforce the spleen so as to enrich the source of

【组成】 柴胡、当归、白芍、茯苓、白术各15克，煨姜、薄荷少许，甘草(炙)6克。

【用法】 共为散，每次6～9克，以煨姜、薄荷少许煎汤冲服。若作汤剂，其用量可按原方比例酌减。

【功用】 疏肝解郁，健脾养血。

【主治】 肝郁血虚证，表现为两胁作痛，头痛目眩，口苦咽干，神疲食少，或寒热往来，或月经不调，乳房作胀，舌淡红，脉弦虚。

慢性肝炎、胸膜炎、慢性胃炎、神经衰弱、月经不调等表现为肝郁血虚者，可用本方加减治疗。

【方解】 方中柴胡疏肝解郁，当归、白芍养血柔肝，三者合用以治肝郁血虚之本。白术、茯苓补中健脾，以资气血生化之源，

growth and development of the *qi* and blood. No.6 regulates the stomach and warms the middle-warmer. No.7 assists No. 1 in soothing the liver to disperse the depressed *qi*. No.8 can not only assist No. 5 and No. 4 in replenishing *qi* and invigorating the middle-warmer but also coordinate the effects of all the drugs in the recipe.

Modern researches have proved that the recipe has the remarkable effects of nourishing the liver, tranquilizing the mind and relieving spasm. It is also effective in promoting digestion, coordinating uterine function, nourishing blood, strengthening the stomach and so on.

Supplementary Recipe:

Ease Powder Added with Moutan Bark and Capejasmine Fruit (*Danzhi Xiaoyao San*)

INGREDIENTS: This recipe is made up of all the drugs in the recipe of Ease Powder, 3 grams of moutan bark (*Cortex Moutan Radicis*) and capejasmine fruit (*Fructus Gardeniae*) each.

DIRECTIONS: All the drugs listed above are to be decocted in water for oral administration.

FUNCTIONS: Soothing the liver, strengthening the spleen and nourishing menstruation by regulating the flow of blood.

INDICATIONS: Fire-transmission and heat-production due to blood-deficiency of the liver and spleen marked by irritability, or spontaneous perspiration or night sweat or headache and xeroma, or irregular menstruation, pain and distension in the lower abdómen, difficulty and pain in micturition.

煨姜和胃温中。薄荷助柴胡疏肝解郁。炙甘草既可助术、苓益气补中，又能调和诸药。

现代研究证明，本方具有显著的保肝、镇静、解痉作用，并有促进消化、调节子宫机能以及补血、健胃等作用。

【附方】

丹栀逍遥散

【组成】 由逍遥散原方加丹皮、栀子各3克。

【用法】 水煎服。

【功用】 疏肝健脾，和血调经。

【主治】 肝脾血虚，化生火热，表现为烦躁易怒，或自汗盗汗，或头痛目涩，或月经不调，少腹胀痛，小便涩痛。

Section 3

Recipes for Regulating the Intestine and Stomach

The recipe, mainly composed of the pungent drugs with dispersing effect and the bitter drugs with purging effect, has the actions of regulating the functions of the intestine and stomach. It is fit for the treatment of disorder of gastrointestinal function caused by the invasion of pathogenic factors to the intestine and stomach.

Pinellia Decoction for Purging Stomach-fire

(Banxia Xiexin Tang)

SOURCE: ***Treatise on Febrile Diseases***

INGREDIENTS:

No. 1 Pinellia tuber, *Rhizoma Pinelliae* (washed) 9 g

No. 2 Dried ginger, *Rhizoma Zingiberis* 6 g

No. 3 Scutellaria root, *Radix Scutellariae* 6 g

No. 4 Chinese goldthread root, *Rhizoma Coptidis* 3 g

No. 5 Ginseng root, *Radix Ginseng* 6 g

No. 6 Prepared licorice root, *Radix Glycyrrhizae praeparata* 6 g

No. 7 Chinese-dates, *Fructus Ziziphi Jujubae* 4 pcs.

DIRECTIONS: All the drugs listed above are to be decocted in water for oral administration.

FUNCTIONS: Regulating the stomach and purging the adverse flow of *qi*, and relieving stagnation and flatulence.

INDICATIONS: Disorder of the stomach due to stagnation of *qi* marked by loss of appetite, epigastric fullness sensation without pain, retching or vomiting, excited intestinal gurgling

第三节　调和肠胃剂

调和肠胃剂主要由辛开苦降药物组成，具有调和肠胃的作用，适用于邪犯肠胃所致的肠胃功能失调证。

半夏泻心汤

【来源】 《伤寒论》

【组成】 半夏(洗) 9 克，干姜 6 克，黄芩 6 克，黄连 3 克，人参 6 克，甘草(炙) 6 克，大枣 4 枚。

【用法】 水煎服。

【功用】 和胃降逆，开结除痞。

【主治】 胃呆气滞，表现为纳呆，心下痞满不痛，干呕或呕

sound and diarrhea, yellow and greasy fur of the tongue and taut and rapid pulse.

Acute gastroenteritis, chronic gastritis, gastroduodenal ulcer, indigestion, gastrointestinal neurosis, vomiting of pregnancy and others marked by the symptoms of disorder of the stomach due to stagnation of *qi* can be treated by the modified recipe.

INTERPRETATION: No. 1 and No. 2, with a pungent flavor and dispersing effect, can relieve flatulence as principal drugs. No. 3 and No. 4, bitter in taste, can purge accumulation of pathogenic heat. The joint use of the four drugs, with the pungent drugs for dispersion and the bitter drugs for purgation, can treat flatulence due to stomach disorder caused by stagnation of *qi*. No. 5, No. 6 and No. 7 supplement *qi* and strengthen the middle-warmer. The combination of the seven drugs in the recipe can cure flatulence, fullness, vomiting and diarrhea.

Modern researches have proved that the recipe has the effects of relieving inflammation, tranquilizing the mind, arresting vomiting and diarrhea, strengthening the stomach and regulating the function of the intestinal tract.

CAUTIONS: Since most drugs in the recipe are dry and drastic in nature, so the recipe is contraindicated in patients with nausea and retching due to deficiency of the stomach-*yin*.

吐，肠鸣下利，舌苔黄而腻，脉弦数等。

急性胃肠炎、慢性胃炎、胃及十二指肠溃疡、消化不良、胃肠神经官能症、妊娠呕吐等表现为胃呆气滞者可用本方加减治疗。

【方解】 方中半夏、干姜辛开消痞，为主药。黄芩、黄连苦降热结，为辅药。四药相配，辛开苦降以治胃呆气滞之痞。人参、甘草、大枣益气补中。七味相配，共治痞、满、吐、利诸证。

现代研究证实，本方具有消炎、镇静、制吐、止泻、健胃、调整胃肠道机能等作用。

【使用注意】 本方药物性多燥烈，胃阴虚恶心、干呕者禁用。

Chapter IX

Prescriptions for Regulating the Flow of *Qi*

This group of prescriptions is mainly composed of drugs for regulating the flow of *qi*, having the effects of promoting the circulation of *qi*, sending down its upward adverse flow. It can be used to treat the stagnation and the reversed flow of *qi*. This type of prescriptions is divided into two kinds: the recipes for promoting the circulation of *qi* and the recipes for sending down the abnormally-ascending *qi*.

Section 1

Recipes for Promoting the Circulation of *Qi*

Qi-promoting recipes with the effects of promoting the functional activities of *qi* is fit for the treatment of disturbance of the visceral function.

Pill for Relieving Stagnancy

(Yueju Wan)

SOURCE: ***Danxi's Experiential Therapy***

INGREDIENTS:

No. 1 Nutgrass flatsedge rhizome, *Rhizoma Cyperi*

No. 2 Chuanxiong rhizome, *Rhizoma Ligustici Chuanxiong*

No. 3 Atractylodes rhizome, *Rhizoma Atractylodis*

No. 4 Capejasmine fruit, *Fuctus Gardeniae*

No. 5 Medicated leaven, *Massa Fermentata Medicinalis*

The dose of all the ingredients is equal in amount.

DIRECTIONS: Grind the above-mentioned ingredients

第九章

理气剂

理气剂以理气药为主组成，具有行气或降气的作用，用于治疗气滞、气逆等病证。本章方剂分为行气剂和降气剂两类。

第一节 行气剂

行气剂具有疏畅气机的作用，适用于气机郁滞证。

越鞠丸（又名芎术丸）

【来源】 《丹溪心法》

【组成】 香附、川芎、苍术、栀子、神曲各等分。

【用法】 上药研末，水泛为小丸，每服6～9克。亦可按原

into fine powder first, and then make pills with water. Take 6 to 9 grams each time. It can also be decocted in water for oral administration with the dosage modified proportionally according to the original recipe.

FUNCTIONS: Promoting the circulation of *qi* to relieve the stagnation.

INDICATIONS: Syndrome of six kinds of stagnations marked by oppressed sensation and feeling of stuffiness in the chest, epigastric distension and pain, gastric discomfort with acid regurgitation, indigestion, eructation, vomiting and nausea, white and greasy fur of the tongue, taut pulse.

Gastrointestinal neurosis, gastroduodenal ulcer, chronic gastritis, infectious hepatitis, cholecystitis, cholelithiasis, intercostal neuralgia, dysmenorrhea and others marked by symptoms of six kinds of stagnations can be treated by the modified recipe.

INTERPRETATION: No. 1 in the recipe is used as a principal drug to deal with stagnancy of *qi* by promoting the circulation of *qi*. No. 2 promotes the circulation of *qi* and blood to treat stagnancy of blood. No.3 can treat stagnancy of dampness by reinforcing the spleen. No. 4 can treat stagnancy of fire by clearing away pathogenic heat and purging pathogenic fire. No. 5 can treat stagnancy of food by promoting digestion and normalizing the function of the stomach. All the abovementioned drugs are used as assistant drugs. As the stagnancy of phlegm is mainly caused by spleen-dampness and associated with stagnancy of *qi*, fire and food, and it can be cleared away when the other various stagnancies are removed.

Modern studies have proved that this recipe has the effects of tranquilizing the mind, alleviating pain, promoting digestion, and relieving spasm of uterine smooth muscle.

CAUTIONS: This recipe is indicated only for the stagnancies belonging to excess syndromes. Stagnancies associated with deficiency type should not be treated only with this recipe.

方比例酌情增减用量，水煎服。

【功用】 行气解郁。

【主治】 六郁证，表现为胸膈痞闷，脘腹胀痛，嘈杂吞酸，饮食不化，嗳气呕恶，苔白腻，脉弦。

胃肠神经官能症、胃及十二指肠溃疡、慢性胃炎、传染性肝炎、胆囊炎、胆石症、肋间神经痛、痛经等表现为六郁证者，可用本方加减治疗。

【方解】 方中香附行气开郁以治气郁，为主药。川芎行气活血以治血郁；苍术燥湿健脾以治湿郁；栀子清热泻火以治火郁；神曲消食和胃以治食郁，均为辅药。由于痰郁多由脾湿引起，且与气、火、食郁有关，诸郁得解，痰郁亦可消除。

现代研究证实，本方具有镇静、镇痛、促进消化及缓解子宫平滑肌痉挛等作用。

【使用注意】 本方所治诸郁均属实证，虚证郁滞不宜单独使

Decoction of Pinellia and Magnolia Bark

(Banxia Houpo Tang)

SOURCE: *Synopsis of Prescriptions of the Golden Chamber*

INGREDIENTS:

No. 1 Pinellia tuber, *Rhizoma Pinelliae* 12 g

No. 2 Magnolia bark, *Cortex Magnoliae Officinalis* 9 g

No. 3 Poria, *Poria* 12 g

No. 4 Fresh ginger, *Rhizoma Zingiberis Recens* 9 g

No. 5 Perilla leaf, *Folium Perillae* 6g

DIRECTIONS: All the drugs listed above are to be decocted in water for oral administration.

FUNCTIONS: Promoting the circulation of *qi* to alleviate mental depression, lowering the adverse flow of *qi* and resolving phlegm.

INDICATIONS: Globus hystericus marked by a subjective sensation as if a plum pit is stuck in the throat which can neither be thrown up nor swallowed down, or accompanied by fullness and distress in the chest and hypochondrium, or cough or vomiting, white, moist or greasy fur of the tongue, and slippery or taut pulse.

Pharyngoneurosis, pharyngitis, edema of plica vocalis, bronchitis, bronchial asthma, neurogenic vomiting, gastirc neurosis and vomiting of pregnancy marked by stagnancy of phlegm and *qi* or reversed flow of *qi* can be treated by the modified recipe.

INTERPRETATION: No.1 in the recipe, with a pungent flavor and warm nature, is used as a principal drug to resolve phlegm, disperse stagnancy and regulate the stomach and lower the adverse flow of *qi*. No. 2 ,pungent in flavor, bitter in taste and warm in nature, can achieve the effects of sending down the ascending *qi*, relieving the sensation of fullness and assisting No. 1 in dispersing stagnation and lowering the ad-

用。

半夏厚朴汤

【来源】 《金匮要略》

【组成】 半夏12克，厚朴9克，茯苓12克，生姜9克，苏叶6克。

【用法】 水煎温服。

【功用】 行气解郁，降逆化痰。

【主治】 梅核气，表现为咽中如有物阻，吐之不出、咽之不下，胸胁满闷，或咳或吐，舌苔白润或滑腻，脉滑或弦等。

咽部神经官能症、咽炎、声带水肿、支气管炎、支气管哮喘、神经性呕吐、胃神经官能症、妊娠呕吐等表现为痰气郁结或气逆者，可用本方加减治疗。

【方解】 方中半夏辛温化痰开结，和胃降逆，为主药。厚朴辛苦温，下气除满，助半夏散结降逆；茯苓甘淡渗利，助半夏化

verse flow of *qi*. No. 3, sweet and bland in taste, can be used to induce diuresis and assist No. 1 in resolving phlegm. The two drugs are regarded as assistant drugs. No. 4, pungent in flavor and warm in nature, can be used to disperse stagnation, regulate the stomach and relieve vomiting. No. 5 promotes the circulation of *qi*, soothes the liver and regulates the spleen by means of its aroma. The two drugs are used as adjuvant drugs.

Modern researches have proved that the recipe has the effects of expelling phlegm, arresting cough, relieving spasm of smooth muscles of bronchus and regulating the function of autonomic nerve and removing edema.

CAUTIONS: The recipe is mainly composed of drugs bitter and pungent in taste, warm and dry in nature, so it is only indicated for stagnation of phlegm and *qi*, partially for the phlegm-dampness. It is contraindicated in patients with deficiency of *yin*-fluid or hyperactivity of pathogenic fire due to *yin* deficiency.

Decoction of Trichosanthes and Macrostem with Liquor

(Gualou Xiebai Baijiu Tang)

SOURCE: *Synopsis of Prescriptions of the Golden Chamber*

INGREDIENTS:

No. 1 Trichosanthes fruit, *Fructus Trichosanthis* 12 g

No. 2 Macrostem onion, *Bulbus Allii Macrostemi* 9 g

No. 3 Liquor, proper amount (or 30 to 60 ml)

DIRECTIONS: All the above are to be decocted in water for oral administration.

FUNCTIONS: Dispersing obstruction of chest-*yang*, promoting the circulation of *qi* to expel phlegm.

INDICATIONS: Obstruction of *qi* in the chest marked by cheking pain in the chest, even radiating to the back, usually accompanied by dyspnea, cough, shortness of breath, white and

痰，共为辅药。生姜辛温散结，和胃止呕；苏叶芳香行气，疏肝理脾，共为佐使药。

现代研究证实，本方具有祛痰、镇咳、缓解支气管平滑肌痉挛、调整植物神经、消除水肿等作用。

【使用注意】 本方药物多苦温性燥，仅适宜于气郁痰结、偏于痰湿者，若属阴亏津少或阴虚火盛者禁用。

瓜蒌薤白白酒汤

【来源】 《金匮要略》

【组成】 瓜蒌12克，薤白 9 克，白酒适量(约 30 ～60 毫升)。

【用法】 水煎服。

【功用】 宣通胸阳，行气祛痰。

【主治】 胸痹，表现为胸部闷痛，甚则胸痛彻背，喘息咳唾，

greasy fur of the tongue, taut and deep pulse or tense pulse.

Patients with angina pectoris of coronary heart disease, intercostal neuralgia, non-suppurative costochondritis, chronic bronchitis marked by the syndrome of obstruction of *qi* in the chest can be treated by the modified recipe.

INTERPRETATION: No. 1, as a principal drug, disperses obstruction of the chest-*yang*, resolves phlegm and expels stagnation. No.2, as an assistant drug, activates *yang* and disperses the obstruction and promotes the circulation of *qi* to relieve pain. The two drugs, one for expelling the stagnancy of phlegm and the other for promoting the functional activities of *qi*, supplement each other in the combined use and are important in treating obstruction of *qi* in the chest. No. 3, with lifting and warming effects, strengthens the effects of the above-mentioned two drugs in promoting the circulation of *qi* and activating *yang* as adjuvant and guiding drugs.

Modern researches have proved that the recipe has the effects of dilating coronary artery, and relieving inflammation and pain.

CAUTIONS:

1. The amount of liquor can be reduced at discretion in treating patients who are not good at drinking it.

2. When the recipe is used to treat angina pectoris due to blood stasis, drugs for activating blood flow can be added to the recipe, such as peach kernel, safflower, red sage root, Chinese angelica root, chuanxiong rhizome, red peony and so on.

Section 2

Prescriptions for Lowering the Adverse Flow of *Qi*

This group of prescriptions is mainly composed of the drugs

短气，苔白腻，脉沉弦或紧。

冠心病心绞痛、肋间神经痛、非化脓性肋软骨炎、慢性支气管炎等表现为胸痹证者，可用本方加减治疗。

【方解】 方中瓜蒌宣通胸阳，祛痰散结，为主药。薤白通阳散结，行气止痛，为辅药。两药合用，一除痰结，一通气机，相辅相成，为治胸痹要药。再借白酒温升之力，增强两药行气通阳之功，为佐使之用。

现代研究证实，本方具有扩张冠状动脉、抗炎、镇痛等作用。

【使用注意】

1．若患者不善饮酒，方中白酒用量可酌减。

2．治疗血瘀型心绞痛，常加用桃仁、红花、丹参、当归、川芎、赤芍等活血药。

第二节 降 气 剂

降气剂主要由降逆止呕或降气平喘药物组成，具有降气平喘、

for lowering the adverse flow of the stomach-*qi* to arrest vomiting, or the drugs for checking the upward adverse flow of the lung-*qi* to relieve asthma. It has the effects of relieving asthma, preventing vomiting and relieving hiccup, and is fit for treating syndrome of reversed flow of the lung-*qi* or stomach-*qi*.

Decoction of Perilla Seed for Descending *Qi*

(Suzi Jiangqi Tang)

SOURCE: ***Prescription of Peaceful Benevolent Dispensary***

INGREDIENTS:

No. 1 Perilla fruit, *Fructus Perillae* 9g

No. 2 Pinellia tuber, *Rhizoma Pinelliae* 9 g

No. 3 Magnolia bark, *Cortex Magnoliae officinalis* 6 g

No. 4 Root of purple-flowered peucedanum, *Radix Peucedani* 6 g

No. 5 Bark of Chinese cassia tree, *Cortex Cinnamomi* 3 g

No. 6 Chinese angelica root, *Radix Angelicae Sinensis* 6 g

No. 7 Fresh ginger, *Rhizoma Zingiberis Recens* 3 g

No. 8 Perilla leaf, *Folium Perillae* 2 g

No. 9 Licorice root, *Radix Glycyrrhizae* 6 g

No.10 Chinese-dates, *Fructus Ziziphi Jujubae* 3 pcs.

DIRECTIONS: All the drugs listed above are to be decocted in water for oral administration.

FUNCTIONS: Lowering the abnormally ascending *qi* to relieve asthma and expelling phlegm to arrest cough.

INDICATIONS: Abundant expectoration due to excess in the upper part and deficiency in the lower part marked by cough with dyspnea, shortness of breath, fullness sensation and choking sensation in the chest and hypochondrium, chest pain, weakness of feet, fatigue of the limbs, white and smooth fur or white, greasy fur of the tongue.

Cough and asthma due to chronic bronchitis, bronchial

止呕、止呃等作用，适用于肺胃气逆证。

苏子降气汤

【来源】《太平惠民和剂局方》

【组成】苏子、半夏各9克，厚朴、前胡各6克，肉桂3克，当归6克，生姜3克，苏叶2克，甘草6克，大枣3枚。

【用法】水煎服。

【功用】降气平喘，祛痰止咳。

【主治】上实下虚之痰涎壅盛证，表现为喘咳短气，胸膈满闷，胸痛脚软，肢体倦怠，苔白滑或白腻等。

慢性支气管炎、支气管哮喘、肺气肿、肺心病之咳嗽、气喘

asthma, pulmonary emphysema and pulmonary heart disease marked by the symptoms of abundant expectoration due to excess in the upper part and deficiency in the lower part in the body can be treated by the modified recipe.

INTERPRETATION: No. 1 produces the effects of lowering the abnormally ascending *qi* to relieve asthma, arresting cough and expelling phlegm. No. 2, No. 3 and No. 4 expel phlegm to relieve cough and asthma due to abundant expectoration. No. 5 has the effect of warming the kidney to expel cold and improve inspiration to relieve asthma. No. 6 functions in nourishing the blood and regulating the blood flow. When combined, the two drugs not only warm and restore *qi* in the lower but also treat cough and dyspnea. No.7 and No.8 expel pathogenic cold and promote the dispersing function of the lung. No.9 and No.10 coordinate the effects of all the other drugs in the recipe and normalize the functions of the stomach and spleen.

Modern researches have proved that this recipe has a stronger phlegm-expelling effect as well as better cough-arresting and asthma-relieving effects. In addition, it can improve the pituitary-adrenal function, promote blood circulation and strengthen the cold-resisting ability of the body.

CAUTIONS: The recipe is mainly aimed at eliminating the pathogenic factor and treating the excess in the upper and the ingredients in it tend to be warm and dry in nature, so it should not be used to treat cough and asthma due to deficiency of both the lung and kidney or phlegm-dyspnea due to lung-heat.

Asthma-relieving Decoction

(Dingchuan Tang)

SOURCE: ***Effective Prescriptions for Health Conservation***

INGREDIENTS:

等证属上实下虚、痰涎壅盛者，可用本方加减治疗。

【方解】 方中苏子降气平喘、止咳祛痰，半夏、厚朴、前胡祛痰、止咳、平喘，共治痰壅咳喘。肉桂温肾散寒、纳气平喘，当归养血和血，两者既能温补下虚，又治咳逆上气。生姜、苏叶散寒宣肺，甘草、大枣调药和中。

现代研究证实，本方具有较强的祛痰作用，镇咳、平喘效果也较好。此外，尚有改善垂体-肾上腺功能、增加血液循环、提高机体抗寒能力的功效。

【使用注意】 本方以祛邪治上实为主，其药偏于温燥，故肺肾两虚型喘咳或肺热痰喘均不宜使用。

定喘汤

【来源】《摄生众妙方》

No. 1 Ephedra, *Herba Ephedrae* 9 g
No. 2 Gingko-nut, *Semen Ginkgo* 9 g
No. 3 Perilla fruit, *Fructus Perillae* 6g
No. 4 Bitter apricot kernel, *Semen Armeniacae Amarum* 9g
No. 5 Pinellia tuber, *Rhizoma Pinelliae* 9g
No. 6 Coltsfoot flower, *Flos Farfarae* 9 g
No. 7 Mulberry bark, *Cortex Mori Radicis* 9 g
No. 8 Baikal Skullcap root, *Radix Scutellariae* 6 g
No. 9 Licorice root, *Radix Glycyrrhizae* 3 g

DIRECTIONS: All the drugs listed above are to be decocted in water for oral administration.

FUNCTIONS: Facilitating the flow of the lung-*qi* and removing heat-phlegm to relieve asthma.

INDICATIONS: Accumulation of phlegm and heat in the lung with the attack of wind cold on the body surface marked by cough, dyspnea, profuse yellowish and viscid sputa, or accompanied by aversion to cold, fever, yellowish, greasy fur of the tongue, slippery rapid pulse.

Chronic bronchitis, bronchial asthma marked by the abovementioned symptoms can be treated by the modified recipe.

INTERPRETATION: No.1 facilitates the flow of the lung-*qi* and disperses pathogenic factors to relieve asthma, while No.2 astringes the lung and removes phlegm to relieve asthma. The two ingredients, one with astringing effect, and the other with the effect of dispersion, are combined to reinforce the asthma-relieving effect as well as to prevent No.1 from consuming the lung-*qi*. No.3, No.4, No.5, and No.6 lower the adverse flow of *qi* and remove phlegm to relieve asthma and cough. No. 7 and No. 8 clear away lung-heat to relieve cough and asthma. No. 9 coordinates the effects of all the other ingredients in the recipe. These drugs are combined to get the lung-*qi* facilitated, phlegm-heat cleared away, wind-cold pathogens expelled so that all the symptoms will disappear.

Modern researches have proved that the recipe can

【组成】 麻黄9克，白果9克，苏子6克，杏仁9克，半夏9克，款冬花9克，桑白皮9克，黄芩6克，甘草3克。

【用法】 水煎服。

【功用】 宣肺平喘，清热化痰。

【主治】 痰热阻肺，风寒外束，表现为咳嗽气喘，痰多黄稠，或伴有恶寒发热，苔黄腻，脉滑数。

慢性支气管炎、支气管哮喘有上述证候者，可用本方加减治疗。

【方解】 方中麻黄宣肺散邪以平喘，白果敛肺祛痰而定喘，二者一散一收，既可加强平喘之功，又防麻黄耗散肺气。苏子、杏仁、半夏、款冬花降气平喘，祛痰止咳。桑白皮、黄芩清泻肺热，止咳平喘。甘草调和诸药。诸药合用，使肺气得宣，痰热得清，风寒得解而诸症自除。

现代研究证实，本方具有解除支气管平滑肌痉挛、祛痰、镇

achieve the effects of relieving spasm of bronchial smooth muscle, expelling phlegm, arresting cough, inducing sweet and allaying fever.

CAUTIONS:

1. The recipe is contraindicated in patients with recent attack of wind-cold on the body surface without interior phelgm-heat marked by absence of sweating but asthma.

2. It is also contraindicated in patients with persistent asthma due to deficiency of *qi* marked by feeble pulse.

Decoction of Inula and Red Ochre

(Xuanfu Daizhe Tang)

SOURCE: ***Treatise on Febrile Disease***

INGREDIENTS:

No. 1 Inula flower, *Flos Inulae* 9 g (Wrapped with a piece of cloth when the decoction is being made) 9 g

No. 2 Red ochre, *Ochra Haematitum* 15 g

No. 3 Pinellia tuber, *Rhizoma Pinelliae* 9 g

No. 4 Fresh ginger, *Rhizoma Zingiberis Recens* 9 g

No. 5 Ginseng, *Radix Ginseng* 6 g

No. 6 Chinese-dates, *Fructus Ziziphi Jujubae* 4 pcs.

No. 7 Prepared licorice root, *Radix Glycyrrhizae praeparata* 6 g

DIRECTIONS: All the drugs listed above are to be decocted in water for oral administration.

FUNCTIONS: Lowering the adverse flow of *qi* and resolving phlegm, invigorating *qi* and regulating the function of the stomach.

INDICATIONS: Syndrome of the deficient stomach-*qi* with reversed flow of *qi* marked by epigastric fullness and rigidity, frequent eructation, vomiting, salivation, white smooth fur of the tongue, taut and feeble pulse.

Chronic gastritis, gastroptosis, gastric dilatation, ulcerous pylorospasm or incomplete pylorochesis, neurogenic hiccup or

咳等作用，并可发汗解热。

【使用注意】

1. 新感风寒，无汗而喘，内无痰热者忌用。

2. 哮喘日久，气虚脉弱者禁用。

旋覆代赭汤

【来源】《伤寒论》

【组成】旋覆花9克(布包煎)，代赭石15克，半夏9克，生姜9克，人参6克，大枣4枚，甘草(炙)6克。

【用法】水煎服。

【功用】降逆化痰，益气和胃。

【主治】胃虚气逆证，症见心下痞硬，噫气不除，反胃呕吐，吐涎沫，苔白滑，脉弦而虚。

慢性胃炎、胃下垂、胃扩张、溃疡病幽门痉挛或不完全性梗

vomiting, Meniere's disease and others marked by the symptoms of deficient stomach-*qi* with reversed flow of *qi* can be treated by the modified recipe.

INTERPRETATION: No. 1 in the recipe lowers the adverse flow of *qi* and expels phlegm, softens hard mass in the abdomen and relieves flatulence, and No.2, being a heavy material, functions in lowering the adverse flow of *qi* and promoting expectoration. The two drugs mentioned above act as principal drugs. No. 3 and No. 4, as assistant drugs, expel phlegm, lower the adverse flow of *qi*, relieve flatulence and resolve mass. No. 5, No. 6 and No. 7 invigorate *qi*, regulate the function of stomach, coordinate the effects of all the other ingredients and act as adjuvant and guiding drugs.

Modern researches have proved that the recipe can produce the effects of tranquilizing the mind, relieving cough, expelling phlegm, arresting vomiting, relieving spasm of bronchial smooth muscle, protecting gastric mucosa and promoting the reproduction of the red blood cells and hemoglobin.

Tangerine Peel and Bamboo Shavings Decoction

(Jupi Zhuru Tang)

SOUCE: ***Synopsis of Prescriptions of the Golden Chamber***
INGREDIENTS:

No. 1 Tangerine peel, *Pericarpium Citri Reticulatae* 9 g
No. 2 Bamboo shavings, *Caulis Bambusae in Taenis* 9 g
No. 3 Fresh ginger, *Rhizoma Zingiberis Recens* 9 g
No. 4 Ginseng, *Radix Ginseng* 3 g
No. 5 Licorice root, *Radix Glycyrrhizae* 6 g
No. 6 Chinese-dates, *Fructus Ziziphi Jujubae* 5 pcs.

DIRECTIONS: All the drugs prescribed above are to be decocted in water for oral administration.

阻、神经性呃逆或呕吐、美尼尔氏综合征等，表现为胃虚气逆者，可用本方加减治疗。

【方解】 方中旋覆花降逆祛痰，软坚消痞；代赭石质重降逆坠痰，共为主药。半夏、生姜祛痰降逆，消痞散结，为辅药。人参、甘草、大枣益气和胃，调和诸药，为佐使之品。

现代研究证实，本方具有镇静、镇咳、祛痰、镇吐、缓解支气管平滑肌痉挛、保护胃粘膜以及促进红细胞再生、增加血红蛋白等多种作用。

橘皮竹茹汤

【来源】 《金匮要略》

【组成】 橘皮9克，竹茹9克，生姜9克，人参3克，甘草6克，大枣5枚。

【用法】 水煎服。

FUNCTIONS: Lowering the adverse flow of *qi* to relieve vomiting, invigorating *qi* and clearing away heat.

INDICATIONS: Reversed flow of *qi* due to weak stomach with heat marked by hiccup, vomiting, anorexia, reddish tongue, feeble and rapid pulse.

Vomiting of pregnancy, incomplete pylorochesis, gastritic vomiting, neurogenic vomiting, ceaseless hiccup after abdominal operation and others marked by the symptoms of reversed flow of *qi* due to weak stomach with heat can be treated by the modified recipe.

INTERPRETATION: No. 1 regulates the flow of *qi*, strengthens and normalizes the functions of the stomach and spleen to relieve vomiting. No.2 clears away stomach-heat to relieve hiccup. The combined use of the two drugs can clear away stomach-heat as well as lower the adverse flow of *qi* to relieve vomiting. They are both used as principal drugs. No.3 is used to assist the principal drugs in regulating the stomach to arrest vomiting, and combined with No.2, achieves the effects of both clearing and warming so as to prevent the impairment of middle-warmer due to excessive administration of the drugs cold in nature, so they are considered as assistant drugs. No.4, No.5 and No.6, as adjuvant and guiding drugs, invigorate *qi*, supplement the spleen, regulate the stomach and coordinate the effects of all the other ingredients in the recipe.

Modern studies have proved that the recipe can produce the effects of tranquilizing the mind, relieving inflammation, preventing vomiting and relieving phrenospasm, etc.

CAUTIONS: Hiccup due to heat of excess type or cold of insufficiency type should not be treated with the recipe.

【功用】 降逆止呕，益气清热。

【主治】 胃虚气逆偏热证，表现为呃逆或呕吐，不思饮食，舌嫩红，脉虚数。

妊娠呕吐、幽门不完全性梗阻、胃炎呕吐、神经性呕吐和腹部手术后呃逆不止表现为胃虚气逆偏热者，可用本方加减治疗。

【方解】 方中橘皮理气健胃，和中止呕；竹茹清胃热，止呃逆。两药合用，既能降逆止呕，又能清泻胃热，共为主药。生姜助主药和胃止呕，与竹茹配用，清中有温，以防过寒伤中，为辅药。人参、甘草、大枣益气、补脾、和胃，并调和诸药，为佐使之品。

现代研究证实，本方具有镇静、消炎、镇吐、缓解膈肌痉挛等作用。

【使用注意】 呃逆属于实热或虚寒者，不宜用本方治疗。

Chapter X

Prescriptions for Treating Blood Disorders

This kind of prescriptions is composed of drugs for treating blood troubles and has the effect of regulating *qi* and blood to treat blood disorders.

Blood disorder is wide in scope and complex in therapy. Usually the methods of treating blood disorder include enriching the blood, arresting bleeding and promoting blood circulation to remove blood stasis. The method of enriching blood belongs to the section of the recipes for enriching blood. Here are only introduced the recipes for promoting blood circulation to remove blood stasis and those for arresting bleeding.

Section 1

Recipes for Promoting Blood Circulation To Remove Blood Stasis

This group of recipes is mainly composed of drugs used to promote blood circulation and remove blood stasis, fit for the treatment of syndrome of blood retention and syndrome of blood stasis.

Decoction for Removing Blood Stasis in the Chest

(Xuefu Zhuyu Tang)

SOURCE: *Corrections on the Errors of Medical Works*

第十章

理血剂

凡主要由理血药物组成，具有调理气血的作用，治疗血病的方剂，称为理血剂。

血病所包括的范围较广，其治疗方法亦较复杂，一般可概括为补血、止血、活血祛瘀三个方面。补血法已归入补血剂。这里仅介绍活血祛瘀剂和止血剂两类。

第一节　活血祛瘀剂

活血祛瘀剂常以活血祛瘀药为主组成，适用于蓄血及瘀血证。

血府逐瘀汤

【来源】《医林改错》

INGREDIENTS:

No. 1 Chinese angelica root, *Radix Angelicae Sinensis* 9 g
No. 2 Chuanxiong rhizome, *Rhizoma Ligustici Chuanxiong* 5 g
No. 3 Red peony root, *Radix Paeoniae Rubra* 9 g
No. 4 Peach kernel, *Semen Persicae* 12 g
No. 5 Safflower, *Flos Carthami* 9 g
No. 6 Achyranthes root, *Radix Achyranthis Bidentatae* 9 g
No. 7 Bupleurum root, *Radix Bupleuri* 3 g
No. 8 Balloonflower root, *Radix Platycodi* 5 g
No. 9 Fruit of citron or trifoliate orange, *Fructus Aurantii* 6 g
No.10 Dried root of rehmannia, *Radix Rehmanniae* 9 g
No.11 Licorice root, *Radix Glycyrrhizae* 3 g

DIRECTIONS: All the drugs listed above are to be decocted in water for oral administration.

FUNCTIONS: Promoting blood circulation to remove blood stasis and promoting circulation of *qi* to relieve pain.

INDICATIONS: Syndrome of blood stasis in the chest marked by long-standing prickly chest pain and headache which exist in a certain region, or endless hiccup, dysphoria due to interior heat, palpitation, insomnia, irritability and liability to a fit of temper, running a fever gradually at dusk, deep-red tongue with ecchymoses, dark-purple lips or dark eyes, uneven pulse or taut and tense pulse.

Coronary heart disease, cerebral thrombosis, thromboangiitis obliterans, hypertension, cirrhosis of liver, dysmenorrhea, amenia, postabortal retention of placenta, headache, chest pain and hypochondriac pain marked by stagnancy of *qi* and blood stasis can be treated by the modified recipe.

INTERPRETATION: The leading ingredients in the recipe are No. 1, No. 2, No. 3, No. 4, No. 5 and No. 6 which promote blood circulation to remove blood stasis. Among them, No.6 also ensures proper downward flow of the blood. No.7 soothes the liver and regulates the circulation of *qi*. No. 8 and No. 9 relieve the oppressed feeling in the chest, promote

【组成】 当归9克，川芎5克，赤芍9克，桃仁12克，红花9克，牛膝9克，柴胡3克，桔梗5克，枳壳6克，生地9克，甘草3克。

【用法】 水煎服。

【功用】 活血祛瘀，行气止痛。

【主治】 胸中瘀血证。表现为胸痛、头痛，日久不愈，痛如针刺而有定处，或呃逆不止，或内热烦闷，心悸失眠，急躁善怒，入暮渐热，舌质暗红或有瘀斑、瘀点，唇暗或两目暗黑，脉涩或弦紧。

冠心病、脑血栓形成、血栓闭塞性脉管炎、高血压病、肝硬化、痛经、闭经、流产后胎盘滞留，以及头、胸、胁等疼痛表现为气滞血瘀者可用本方加减治疗。

【方解】 方中当归、川芎、赤芍、桃仁、红花活血祛瘀；牛膝通血脉、祛瘀血并引血下行，为方中主要组成部分。柴胡疏肝

the circulation of *qi* to render blood circulation normal. No. 10 removes heat from the blood and combines No. 1 to enrich the blood and moisten dryness so as to remove blood stasis without impairment of *yin*. No. 11 coordinates the effects of all the other ingredients in the recipe.

Modern researches have proved that this recipe is especially effective in anti-coagulation and antispasm. Besides, it has some effect on uterine contraction.

CAUTIONS:

1. Since this recipe is mainly composed of drugs for removing blood stasis, it should not be used to treat the syndrome without distinct stasis.

2. It is contraindicated in pregnancy.

Supplementary Recipe:

1. Decoction for Dissipating Blood Stasis under Diaphram (*Gexia Zhuyu Tang*)

SOURCE: ***Corrections on the Errors of Medical Works***

INGREDIENTS:

No. 1 Trogopterus dung, *Faeces Trogopterorum* 9 g
No. 2 Chinese angelica root, *Radix Angelicae Sinensis* 9g
No. 3 Chuanxiong rhizome, *Rhizoma Ligustici Chuanxiong* 6g
No. 4 Peach kernel, *Semen Persicae* 9 g
No. 5 Moutan bark, *Cortex Moutan Radicis* 6 g
No. 6 Red peony root, *Radix Paeoniae Rubra* 6 g
No. 7 Spicebush root, *Radix Linderae* 6 g
No. 8 Corydalis tuber, *Rhizoma Corydalis* 3 g
No. 9 Licorice root, *Radix Glycyrrhizae* 9 g
No.10 Nutgrass flatsedge rhizome, *Rhizoma Cyperi* 3 g
No.11 Safflower, *Flos Carthami* 9 g
No.12 Fruit of citron or trifoliate orange, *Fructus Aurantii* 5g

DIRECTIONS: All the above drugs are to be decocted in water for oral administration.

FUNCTIONS: Promoting blood circulation to remove blood stasis, and promoting circulation of *qi* to relieve pain.

理气，桔梗、枳壳开胸行气，使气行则血行。生地凉血清热，配当归又能养血润燥，使瘀祛而不伤阴血。甘草调和诸药。

现代研究证实，本方抗凝血与扩张血管的作用尤为突出，镇静和解痉作用也较明显。此外，尚有收缩子宫的作用。

【使用注意】

1. 本方祛瘀药较多，非确有“血瘀”之证不宜使用。

2. 孕妇忌服。

【附方】

1. 膈下逐瘀汤(《医林改错》)

【组成】 五灵脂9克，当归9克，川芎6克，桃仁9克，丹皮6克，赤芍6克，乌药6克，延胡索3克，甘草9克，香附3克，红花9克，枳壳5克。

【用法】 水煎服。

【功用】 活血祛瘀，行气止痛。

INDICATIONS: Mass under the diaphram caused by blood stasis, infantile mass in the abdomen, abdominal pain with a fixed region or a feeling of abdominal falling as if there were something heavy in it.

2. Decoction for Removing Blood Stagnation in the Lower Abdomen (*Shaofu Zhuyu Tang*)

SOURCE: ***Corrections on Errors of Medical Works***

INGREDIENTS:

No. 1 Common fennel fruit, *Fructus Foenicuii* 1.5g
No. 2 Dried ginger, *Rhizoma Zingiberis* 3 g
No. 3 Corydalis tuber, *Rhizoma Corydalis* 3 g
No. 4 Chinese angelica root, *Radix Angelicae Sinensis* 9 g
No. 5 Chuanxiong rhizome, *Rhizoma Ligustici Chuanxiong* 3 g
No. 6 Bark of Chinese cassia tree, *Cortex Cinnamomi* 3 g
No. 7 Red peony root, *Radix Paeoniae Rubra* 6 g
No. 8 Cat-tail pollen, *Pollen Typhae* 9 g
No. 9 Trogopterus dung, *Faeces Trogopterorum* 6 g

DIRECTIONS: All the above drugs are to be decocted in water for oral administration.

FUNCTIONS: Promoting blood circulation to remove blood stasis, and warming the channels to relieve pain.

INDICATIONS: Mass in the lower abdomen caused by blood stasis with or without pain, or pain in the lower abdomen without mass, or distension in the lowr abdomen, or soreness of waist and abdominal distension during menstruation of women, or menorrhagia with dark color and mass, or metrorrhagia and metrostaxis with pain in the lower abdomen.

3. Decoction for Relieving Pantalgia due to Blood Stagnation (*Shentong Zhuyu Tang*)

SOURCE: ***Corrections on Errors of Medical Works***

INGREDIENTS:

No. 1 Root of large-leaf gentian, *Radix Gentianae Macrophyllae* 3 g
No. 2 Chuanxiong rhizome, *Rhizoma Ligustici Chuanxiong* 6 g

【主治】 瘀在膈下，形成积块；或小儿痞块；或肚腹疼痛，痛处不移；或腹坠似有物者。

2. 少腹逐瘀汤(《医林改错》)

【组成】 小茴香1.5克，干姜3克，延胡索3克，当归9克，川芎3克，官桂3克，赤芍6克，蒲黄9克，五灵脂6克。

【用法】 水煎服。

【功用】 活血祛瘀，温经止痛。

【主治】 少腹瘀血积块，疼痛或不痛；或痛而无积块；或少腹胀满；或妇女经期腰酸腹胀；或月经量多色黑有块；或崩漏兼少腹疼痛等症。

3. 身痛逐瘀汤(《医林改错》)

【组成】 秦艽3克，川芎6克，桃仁9克，红花9克，甘草

No. 3 Peach kernel, *Seman Persicae* 9 g
No. 4 Safflower, *Flos Carthami* 9 g
No. 5 Licorice root, *Radix Glycyrrhizae* 6 g
No. 6 Notopterygium root, *Rhizoma seu Radix Notopterygii* 3 g
No. 7 Myrrh, *Myrrha* 6 g
No. 8 Chinese angelica root, *Radix Angelicae Sinensis* 9 g
No. 9 Trogopterus dung, *Faeces Trogopterorum* 6 g
No.10 Nutgrass flatsedge rhizome, *Rhizoma Cyperi* 3 g
No.11 Achyranthes root, *Radix Achyranthis Bidentatae* 9 g
No.12 Earth worm, *Lumbricus* 6 g

DIRECTIONS: All the above drugs are to be decocted in water for oral administration.

FUNCTIONS: Promoting circulation of blood and *qi* to remove blood stasis from the channels, and treating arthralgia-syndrome and relieving other pain.

INDICATIONS: Symptoms caused by the obstruction of *qi* and blood in the channels marked by long-standing omalgia, brachialgia, lumbago, pain in legs or pantalgia.

Decoction for Recovery and Activating Blood Circulation

(Fuyuan Huoxue Tang)

SOURCE: ***Invention of Medicine***

No. 1 Rhubarb, *Radix et Rhizoma Rhei* (soaked in wine) 12 g
No. 2 Bupleurum root, *Radix Bupleuri* 15 g
No. 3 Chinese angelica root, *Radix Angelicae Sinensis* 9 g
No. 4 Peach kernel, *Semen Persicae* (soaked in wine, peeled and ground into paste) 9 g
No. 5 Safflower, *Flos Carthami* 6 g
No. 6 Pangolin scales, *Squama Manitis* (roasted) 6 g
No. 7 Snakegourd root, *Radix Trichosanthis* 9 g

6克，羌活3克，没药6克，当归9克，五灵脂6克，香附3克牛膝9克，地龙6克。

【用法】 水煎服。

【功用】 活血行气，祛瘀通络，通痹止痛。

【主治】 气血痹阻经络所致的肩痛、臂痛、腰痛、腿痛或周身疼痛，经久不愈。

复元活血汤

【来源】《医学发明》

【组成】 大黄(酒浸)12克，柴胡15克，当归9克，桃仁（酒浸，去皮尖，研如泥）9克，红花6克，穿山甲(炮) 6克，瓜蒌

No. 8 Licorice root, *Radix Glycyrrhizae* 6 g

DIRECTIONS: All the above drugs are to be decocted in water for oral administration.

FUNCTIONS: Promoting blood circulation to remove blood stasis, soothing the liver and removing the obstruction in the channels.

INDICATIONS: Blood stasis in the hypochondriac region due to traumatic injury characterized by hypochondriac pain.

Traumatic swelling pain, intercostal neuralgia, costal chrondritis marked by accumulation of blood stasis can be treated by the modified recipe.

INTERPRETATION: No. 1 is used in large dosage to remove blood stasis, while No.2 is used to soothe the liver and regulate the flow of *qi*. The two ingredients are used as principal drugs to remove blood stasis in the hypochondriac region. No.3, No. 4 and No. 5 promote blood circulation to remove blood stasis, relieve swelling and pain as assistant drugs. No. 6 removes blood stasis in the channels and No. 7 clears away pathogenic heat to subdue swelling, promotes reunion of fractured bones and the healing of traumatic injuries. The two drugs mentioned above act as adjuvant drugs. No. 8 regulates the stomach, relieves spasm and pain and coordinates the effects of all the other drugs in the recipe.

Modern researches have proved that the recipe has the effects of promoting blood circulation to expel blood stasis, relieving inflammation and swelling, tranquilizing the mind, alleviating pain and regulating the function of autonomic nerve.

CAUTIONS: Patients who are very weak physically should be treated with the recipe very carefully; it is contraindicated in pregnancy.

根9克，甘草6克。

【用法】 水煎服。

【功用】 活血祛瘀，疏肝通络。

【主治】 跌打损伤，瘀血留于胁下，痛不可忍者。

外伤性肿胀疼痛、肋间神经痛、肋软骨炎，表现为瘀血停滞者，可用本方加减治疗。

【方解】 方中重用大黄荡涤留瘀败血；柴胡疏肝调气。两药合用，以散胁下瘀滞，共为主药。当归、桃仁、红花活血祛瘀，消肿止痛，共为辅药。穿山甲破瘀通络；瓜蒌根清热消肿，续骨伤，消仆损，均为佐药。甘草和中、缓急止痛，调和诸药，为使药。

现代研究证实，本方具有活血化瘀、消炎、消肿、镇静、镇痛、调整植物神经等作用。

【使用注意】 虚人慎用，孕妇忌用。

Decoction Invigorating *Yang* for Recuperation

(Buyang Huanwu Tang)

SOURCE: *Corrections on Errors of Medical Works*

INGREDIENTS:

No. 1 Astragalus root, *Radix Astragali seu Hedysari* 120 g
No. 2 Chinese angelica root, *Radix Angelicae Sinensis* 6 g
No. 3 Chuanxiong rhizome, *Rhizoma Ligustici Chuanxiong* 3 g
No. 4 Red peony root, *Radix Paeoniae Rubra* 6 g
No. 5 Peach kernel, *Semen Persicae* 3 g
No. 6 Safflower, *Flcs Carthami* 3 g
No. 7 Earth-worm, *Lumbricus* 3 g

DIRECTIONS: All the above drugs are to be decocted in water for oral administration.

FUNCTIONS: Invigorating *qi*, and promoting blood circulation to remove blood stasis from the channels.

INDICATIONS: Hemiplegia of sequelae of apoplexy, deviation of the eye and mouth, intricate and obscure speech, involuntary drooling, atrophy and disability of lower limbs, frequent urination or involuntary enuresis, white tongue fur and slow pulse.

Sequelae of cerebrovascular accident, sequelae of infantile paralysis or disturbance of extremity movement due to other diseases marked by the syndrome of blood stasis due to deficiency of *qi* can be treated by the modified recipe.

INTERPRETATION: The recipe is aimed at the treatment of hemiplegia after apoplexy, the cause of which is deficiency of *qi* and the manifestation of which is blood stasis, therefore, No.1, acting as a principal drug, is used in large dosage to invigorate primordial *qi* so as to promote blood circulation and remove blood stasis whithout impairing the vital *qi*. No.2 also promotes blood circulation and expels blood stasis without

补阳还五汤

【来源】《医林改错》

【组成】 生黄芪120克，当归尾6克，川芎3克，赤芍6克，桃仁3克，红花3克，地龙3克。

【用法】 水煎服。

【功用】 补气，活血，通络。

【主治】 中风后遗症之半身不遂，口眼歪斜，语言蹇涩，口角流涎，下肢萎废，小便频数或遗尿不禁，苔白，脉缓。

脑血管意外后遗症、小儿麻痹后遗症及其他原因引起的肢体活动障碍证属气虚血瘀者，可用本方加减治疗。

【方解】 本方是为中风后半身不遂而设，此证气虚为本，血瘀为标。故方中重用生黄芪大补元气，使气旺血行，祛瘀而不伤正，为主药。当归尾活血祛瘀而不伤阴血，为辅药。川芎、赤芍、

impairing *yin* and blood as an assistant drug. The following drugs are adjuvant and guiding drugs. Among them, No. 3, No. 4, No. 5 and No. 6 promote blood circulation to remove blood stasis, No. 7 clears and activates the channels and collaterals. The combination of the above drugs in the recipe gets *qi* activated and blood circulated normally, stasis removed and the channels and collaterals cleared, thus bring about the recovery.

Modern researches have proved that the recipe has the effects of dilating the blood vessels of brain, promoting blood circulation, removing stagnated blood, relieving the state of insufficiency of blood supply, strengthening fibrinolytic activity, checking platelet aggregation, retarding thrombosis and promoting absorption of extravascular auto-blood and clot.

CAUTIONS:

1. The recipe can only be used to treat the conscious patients with normal body temperature and arrested bleeding. It is contraindicated in the patients with syndromes such as upstirring of liver-wind, stagnation of phlegm in the channels, blood heat due to deficiency of *yin*.

2. The dosage of No.1 usually begins with 30 to 60 grams and then is increased gradually to 120 grams. The patient must continue to take the decoction after recovery for a certain period to prevent relapse.

Decoction for Warming Channels

(Wenjing Tang)

SOURCE: ***Synopsis of Prescriptions of the Golden Chamber***

INGREDIENTS:

No. 1 Evodia fruit, *Fructus Evodiae* 9 g

No. 2 Cinnamon twig, *Ramulus Cinnamomi* 6 g

No. 3 Chinese angelica root, *Radix Angelicae Sinensis* 9 g

桃仁、红花活血化瘀，地龙通经活络，均为佐使药。诸药合用，使气旺血行，瘀祛络通，诸症可愈。

现代研究证实，本方具有扩张脑血管、改善血液循环、解除郁血或供血不足的状态、增强纤维蛋白溶解活性、抑制血小板聚集、减缓血栓形成、促进血管外的自体血液及血块的吸收等作用。

【使用注意】

1. 使用本方应以病人清醒、体温正常、出血停止者为宜。凡肝风内动、痰阻经络、阴虚血热者均忌服。

2. 本方黄芪用量一般从30～60克开始，逐渐加大至120克，且愈后仍须继续服用，以防复发。

温经汤

【来源】《金匮要略》

【组成】 吴茱萸9克．桂枝6克，当归9克，川芎6克，芍

No. 4 Chuanxiong rhizome, *Rhizoma Ligustici Chuanxiong* 6 g
No. 5 Peony root, *Radix Paeoniae* 9 g
No. 6 Donkey-hide gelatin, *Colla Corii Asini* 6 g
No. 7 Lilyturf root, *Radix Ophiopogonis* 9 g
No. 8 Moutan bark, *Cortex Moutan Radicis* 6 g
No. 9 Ginseng, *Radix Ginseng* 6 g
No.10 Licorice root, *Radix Glycyrrhizae* 6 g
No.11 Pinellia tuber, *Rhizoma Pinelliae* 9 g
No.12 Fresh ginger, *Rhizoma Zingiberis Recens* 6 g

DIRECTIONS: All the above drugs are to be decocted in water for oral administration.

FUNCTIONS: Warming the channels and expelling cold, nourishing the blood and dispelling blood stasis.

INDICATIONS: Irregular menstruation due to the deficiency-cold in the *chong* and *ren* channels and accumulation of stagnant blood, marked by preceded or delayed menstrual cycle, or overdue or persistent menstrual duration, or occurence of menstruation twice or more in one month, or nightfall fever, feverish sensation in the palms, parched lips and dry mouth, pain and cold in the lower abdomen, failure to conceive for a long time.

Dysfunctional uterine bleeding, chronic pelvic inflammation and hysteromyoma marked by the above-mentioned symptoms can be treated by the modified recipe.

INTERPRETATION: No. 1 and No. 2 warm the channels and dispel cold to promote blood circulation as principal drugs. No. 3, No. 4 and No. 5 activate the blood, eliminate blood stasis and nourish the blood to regulate menstruation and keep it normal. No. 6, No. 7 and No. 8 nourish the blood and *yin*, regulate the liver to get the stagnant blood dispelled and fresh blood reproduced, remove the blood stasis without impairing the vital *qi*. All the drugs mentioned above are assistant drugs. No. 9 and No. 10 tonify the middle-warmer and strengthen the spleen to enrich the source of *qi* and blood, assisting No.3 and No.6

药9克，阿胶6克，麦冬9克，丹皮6克，人参6克，甘草6克，半夏9克，生姜6克。

【用法】 水煎服。

【功用】 温经散寒，养血祛瘀。

【主治】 冲任虚寒、瘀血阻滞所致的月经不调，或前或后，或逾期不止，或一月再行，或傍晚发热，手心烦热，唇干口燥，或小腹冷痛，久不受孕。

功能性子宫出血、慢性盆腔炎、子宫肌瘤等表现为上述症状者，可用本方加减治疗。

【方解】 方中吴茱萸、桂枝温经散寒，通利血脉，为主药。当归、川芎、芍药活血祛瘀，养血调经，以畅血行；阿胶、麦冬、丹皮养血益阴调肝，使瘀血祛、新血生，瘀祛而不伤正，共为辅药。人参、甘草补中健脾以资气血生化之源，以助归、胶益阴养血；

to tonify *yin* and nourish the blood; No. 11 regulates and sends down the abnormally ascending stomach-*qi* to disperse accumulation of *qi*, helpful in removing blood stasis and regulating menstruation; No. 12 warms the stomach to promote the production of blood and *qi*. The above drugs act together as adjuvant drugs. In addition, No. 10, as a guiding drug, can coordinate the actions of the drugs in the recipe.

Modern researches have proved that the recipe has the effects of regulating the functions of uterus, relieving spasm and arresting pain, tranquilizing the mind and relieving inflammation.

Decoction for Postpartum Troubles

(Shenghua Tang)

SOURCE: ***Fu Qingzhu's Obstetrics and Gynecology***

INGREDIENTS:

No. 1 Chinese angelica root, *Radix Angelicae Sinensis* 24 g

No. 2 Chuanxiong rhizome, *Rhizoma Ligustici Chuanxiong* 9 g

No. 3 Peach kernel, *Semen Persicae* (peeled) 6 g

No. 4 Baked ginger, *Rhizoma Zingiberis* 2 g

No. 5 Prepared licorice root, *Radix Glycyrrhizae Praeparata* 2 g

DIRECTIONS: All the above drugs are to be decocted in water or added with some yellow rice wine for oral administration.

FUNCTIONS: Promoting blood circulation to remove blood stasis and warming the channels to relieve pain.

INDICATIONS: Retention of lochia after childbirth or scanty amount of discharge of lochia, pain in the lower abdomen with tenderness or with some mass in the sore region, dark-purplish margin of the tongue and deep and uneven pulse.

Lochiostasis, hysteromyoma, blood stasis of the pelvis and others marked by blood stasis with coldness can be treated by the modified recipe.

INTERPRETATION: No. 1, used in large dosage as

半夏通降胃气而散结，有助于祛瘀调经；生姜温胃以助运化，共为佐药。甘草又可调和诸药，为使药。

现代研究证实，本方具有调节子宫机能、解痉、镇痛、镇静、消炎等作用。

生 化 汤

【来源】《傅青主女科》

【组成】 全当归24克，川芎 9 克，桃仁（去皮尖）6 克，干姜（炮黑）2 克，甘草（炙）2 克。

【用法】 水煎服，或酌加黄酒同煎。

【功用】 活血化瘀，温经止痛。

【主治】 产后恶露不下，或下亦甚少，小腹疼痛拒按，痛处有块，舌边黯紫，脉沉涩。

产后恶露停滞、子宫肌瘤、盆腔瘀血症等属血瘀兼寒者，可用本方加减治疗。

【方解】 方中重用当归补血活血，化瘀生新，为主药。川芎

a principal drug, has the functions of promoting blood circulation and removing blood stasis to promote the regeneration of blood. No. 2, susceptible to run in the channels of the human body, promotes the circulation of blood and *qi*. No. 3 removes blood stasis with drastic effect. The above two drugs are assistant drugs. The following are adjuvant drugs: No. 4 goes into the blood to expel cold and warms the channels to relieve pain; yellow rice wine with warm nature and expelling effect, reinforces potency of the other drugs in the recipe; No. 5 relieves spasm and arrests pain, coordinating the effects of other drugs as a guiding drug.

Modern researches have proved that the recipe has the effects of contracting uterus, regulating the functions of the uterus, dilating blood vessels, promoting blood circulation, absorbing internal hemorrhage and promoting secretion of mammary gland.

CAUTIONS: The recipe is fit for the treatment of postpartum pain in the lower abdomen with blood stasis. However, the patient who has the syndrome of blood heat with blood stasis is forbidden to use it.

Prescription for Extrauterine Pregnancy

(Gongwaiyun Fang)

SOURCE: Shanxi Medical College

INGREDIENTS:

Recipe I

No. 1 Red sage root, *Radix Salviae Miltirorrhizae* 15 g

No. 2 Red peony root, *Radix Paeoniae Rubra* 9 g

No. 3 Peach kernel, *Semen Persicae* 9 g

No. 4 Olibanum, *Resina Olibani* 9 g

No. 5 Myrrh, *Myrrha* 9 g

Recipe II

Adding the following drugs to Recipe I.

善走，活血行气；桃仁善破，活血祛瘀，共为辅药。炮姜入血散寒，温经止痛；黄酒温散以助药力，均为佐药。甘草缓急止痛，调和诸药，为使药。

现代研究证实，本方具有收缩子宫、调整子宫机能、扩张血管、促进血液循环、吸收内出血、促进乳汁分泌等作用。

【使用注意】 本方以产后少腹痛而挟瘀者为宜，血热而有瘀滞者忌用。

宫外孕方

【来源】 山西医学院

【组成】 Ⅰ号方：丹参15克，赤芍9克，桃仁9克，乳香9克，没药9克。

Ⅱ号方：Ⅰ号方加三棱6克，莪术6克。

No. 6 Burreed tuber, *Rhizoma Sparganii* 6 g
No. 7 Zedoary, *Rhizoma Zedoariae* 6 g

DIRECTIONS: All the above drugs are to be decocted in water for oral administration.

FUNCTIONS: Promoting blood circulation to remove blood stasis and abdominal mass and relieving pain.

INDICATIONS: Rupture of extra-uterine pregnancy marked by sudden attack of pain in the lower abdomen after amenorrhea, colporrhagia, blood dark in colour or mixed up with mucous-like substance and severe tenderness in the lower abdomen.

INTERPRETATION: No. 1 and No. 2 ,bitter in taste and slight cold in nature, go into the blood system to promote blood circulation, remove blood stasis, cool the blood and relieve pain. No. 3 ,bitter but slightly sweet in taste and neutral in nature, removes blood stasis to promote blood circulation, effective in the treatment of abdominal pain due to postpartum blood stasis. No. 4 and No. 5 activate the flow of blood and *qi* and expel blood stasis by means of aromatics, acting as specific drugs for removing blood stasis and relieving pain. No. 6 and No. 7 remove blood stasis and promote the flow of *qi* to resolve mass and relieve pain. But No. 6, bitter in taste and neutral in nature without fragrant smell, tends to remove the *qi*-stagnation in the blood to promote menstrual flow, while No.7, bitter in taste, pungent in flavor, warm in nature and fragrant in smell, tends to remove the blood stasis in *qi* to dispel stagnation. The combined use of the two drugs can produce the effects of resolving hard mass and expelling accumulation.

Modern researches have proved that the recipe has the effects of dilating blood vessels, increasing the volume of blood flow, absorbing retained blood or hematoma, increasing capillary permeability, raising phagocytic power of the phagocyte, promoting the activity of fibrinolytic system and so on.

CAUTIONS: The recipe is contraindicated in patients

【用法】 水煎服。

【功用】 活血祛瘀，消癥止痛。

【主治】 子宫外妊娠破裂，表现为闭经后突然发生小腹疼痛，阴道下血，色暗或夹杂有粘膜样物，下腹部有强烈压痛。

【方解】 方中丹参、赤芍苦微寒，入血分活血祛瘀，凉血止痛；桃仁苦甘性平，破瘀行血，善治产后瘀阻之腹痛；乳香、没药气香走窜而善行，能活血散瘀，利气通络，血行气利则疼痛自止，为散瘀止痛之专药。三棱、莪术破血行气，消积止痛。但三棱苦平不香，长于破血中之气而通经，而莪术苦辛温香，偏于破气中之血而消积，两药合用，具有攻坚消积之功。

研究证实，本方具有扩张血管、增加血流量、吸收滞留的血液或血肿、增加血管通透性、提高吞噬细胞的吞噬能力、促进纤维蛋白溶解系统的活性等作用。

【使用注意】 对子宫外妊娠破裂所致的大量出血或休克者，

with hematorrhea or shock due to rupture of extra-uterine pregnancy. In this case emergency treatment must be taken and operation must be performed promptly.

Recipe No.II for Coronary Heart Disease

(Guanxin Er Hao Fang)

SOURCE: China Academy of Traditional Chinese Medicine

INGREDIENTS:

No. 1 Chuanxiong rhizome, *Rhizoma Ligustici Chuanxiong* 15 g
No. 2 Red sage root, *Radix Salviae Miltiorrhizae* 24 g
No. 3 Safflower, *Flos Carthami* 12 g
No. 4 Red peony root, *Radix Paeoniae Rubra* 15g
No. 5 Dalbergia wood, *Lignum Dalbergiae Odoriferae* 12 g

DIRECTIONS: All the drug listed above are to be decocted in water for oral administration.

FUNCTIONS: Promoting blood circulation and removing blood stasis to relieve pain.

INDICATIONS: Angina pectoris due to blood stasis marked by precordial fixed pain or megalgia radiating to the left shoulder or left back, chest distress or oppressed sensation in the sternal part, dark-red or purplish tongue or with ecchymosis, uneven and slow pulse or knotted and intermittent pulse.

Coronary heart disease, angina pectoris, cardiac infarction or cerebral thrombosis or cerebral embolism in their initial stages can be treated by the modified recipe.

INTERPRETATION: No. 1, pungent in flavor, warm in nature, fragrant in smell and active in nature, promotes the flow of *qi* and blood circulation. No. 2 bitter in taste and slight cold in nature and No. 3 with a pungent flavor for dispersion and a warm nature for promotion of circulation, are both able to promote blood circulation and remove blood stasis from the channels to relieve pain. No. 4, bitter in taste and slight cold in

必须采用急救措施和手术，忌用本方。

冠心II号方

【来源】 中国中医研究院

【组成】 川芎15克，丹参24克，红花12克，赤芍15克，降香12克。

【用法】 水煎服。

【功用】 活血化瘀止痛。

【主治】 血瘀型心绞痛，表现为心前区固定性疼痛或剧痛，放射到左肩背，胸闷或有胸骨部压迫感，舌暗红或紫，或有瘀点，脉涩而迟或结代。

冠心病、心绞痛、心肌梗塞初期、脑血栓或脑栓塞初期等，可用本方加减治疗。

【方解】 方中川芎辛温香窜，走而不守，为血中之气药，能活血行气止痛；丹参苦微寒，红花辛散温通，二药均能活血祛瘀，

nature, can cool and activate the blood flow and remove blood stasis to arrest pain. No. 5 removes obstruction by its pungent flavor and warm nature, and relieve pain by removing blood stasis. The five drugs produce jointly the effects of promoting blood circulation and removing blood stasis to arrest pain.

Modern researches have proved that the recipe has remarkable effects in dilating coronary artery, increasing the volume of blood flow of coronary artery, raising the hypoxia toleration of cardiac muscle, inhibiting thrombosis, promoting the activity of fibrinolytic system, inhibiting platelet aggregation and promoting the restoration of necrotic cardiac muscle.

CAUTIONS: Patients with menorrhagia and the deficiency of blood but without blood stasis should not be treated with this recipe. Pregnant women are especially forbidden to use the recipe in case abortion occurs.

Section 2

Hemostatic Recipes

This group of recipes, mainly composed of hemostatic drugs and effective in stopping bleeding ,is used to treat various hemorrhagic syndromes.

Small Thistle Decoction

(Xiaoji Yinzi)

SOURCE: ***Prescriptions for Succouring the Sick***

INGREDIENTS:

No. 1 Field thistle, *Herba Cephalanoploris* 15 g
No. 2 Node of lotus rhizome, *Nodus Nelumbinis Rhizomatis* 9 g
No. 3 Cat-tail pollen, *Pollen Typhae* (parched) 9 g
No. 4 Dried rehmannia root, *Radix Rehmanniae* 30 g

通经止痛；赤芍苦微寒，凉血活血，祛瘀止痛；降香辛散温通，行瘀止血定痛。五药合用，共奏活血祛瘀止痛之效。

现代研究证实，本方具有明显的扩张冠状动脉、增加冠状动脉血流量、提高心肌对缺氧的耐受性、抑制血栓形成、提高纤维蛋白溶解系统活性、抑制血液凝集、促进坏死心肌的修复等作用。

【使用注意】 凡月经过多或血虚无瘀滞者不宜应用。孕妇尤当禁用，以免引起流产。

第二节 止 血 剂

止血剂主要由止血药组成，具有止血作用，用于治疗各种出血证。

小蓟饮子

【来源】《济生方》

【组成】 小蓟15克，藕节9克，蒲黄（炒）9克，生地黄30克，

No. 5 Capejasmine fruit, *Fructus Gardeniae* 9 g
No. 6 Fiveleaf akebia (stem), *Caulis Akebiae* 9 g
No. 7 Lophatherum, *Herba Lophatheri* 9 g
No. 8 Talcum powder, *Talcum Pulveratum* 12 g
No. 9 Chinese angelica root, *Radix Angelicae Sinensis* (washed with wine) 9 g
No.10 Prepared licorice root, *Radix Glycyrrhizae Praeparata* 6 g

DIRECTIONS: All the above drugs are to be decocted in water for oral use.

FUNCTIONS: Removing heat from the blood to stop bleeding and inducing diuresis to treat stranguria.

INDICATIONS: Stranguria with hematuria due to accumulation of pathogenic heat characterized by frequent, painful and dribbling urination, red tongue with thin and white fur and rapid pulse.

Patients with urinary tract infection, lithangiuria, acute glomerulonephritis and renal tuberculosis marked by stranguria with hematuria due to accumulation of pathogenic heat can be treated by the modified recipe.

INTERPRETATION: No. 1 removes heat from the blood to stop bleeding as a principal drug. No. 2 and No. 3 can be used to assist No. 1 in cooling the blood to stop bleeding and remove blood stasis to make the bleeding stop without any blood stasis left. No. 4 and No. 5 remove heat from the blood to stop bleeding and eliminate pathogenic heat by inducing diuresis. No. 6, No. 7 and No.8 remove heat, induce diuresis to treat stranguria. No. 9, warm in nature, regulates and nourishes the blood, not only preventing the excessive cold of various drugs in the recipe but also guiding the blood back to circulate in the vessels to arrest bleeding. The above-mentioned drugs are used as assistant and adjuvant drugs. No. 10, as a guiding drug, relieves spasm and pain and coordinates the actions of the other drugs in the recipe.

Modern researches have proved that the recipe has remark-

栀子 9 克，木通 9 克，淡竹叶 9 克，滑石12克，当归(酒洗) 9 克，甘草(炙) 6 克。

【用法】 水煎服。

【功用】 凉血止血，利尿通淋。

【主治】 热结血淋，小便频数，赤涩热痛，舌质红，苔薄白，脉数。

急性泌尿道感染、尿路结石、急性肾小球肾炎、肾结核等表现为热结血淋证者可用本方加减治疗。

【方解】 方中小蓟凉血止血，为主药。辅以藕节、蒲黄助主药凉血止血，并能化瘀，使血止而不留瘀。生地、栀子清热、凉血、止血，凉而导之，以竭其热。木通、竹叶、滑石清热、利尿通淋，淡而渗之，使邪热从下窍而出。当归性温，和血养血，既防诸药寒凉太过，又能引血归经。以上皆为辅佐药。甘草缓急止痛，调和诸药，为使药。

现代研究证实，本方止血作用显著，利尿作用亦较明显，并

able bleeding-stopping and better diuresis-inducing effects. It also has the functions of allaying fever, resisting-bacteria and relieving inflammation, etc.

CAUTIONS:

1. Most of the drugs in the recipe are cold-natured drugs and diuretics, therefore, patients suffering from stranguria with hematuria for a long time and patients with weakened body resistance should not be treated with this recipe.

2. The recipe is mainly indicated for symptoms such as more erythrocytes or macroscopic hematuria.

Sophora Powder

(Huaihua San)

SOURCE: ***Effective Prescriptions for Universal Relief***

INGREDIENTS:

No. 1 Sophora flower, *Flos Sophorae* (parched) 12g

No. 2 Biota tops, *Cacumen Biotae* 12 g

No. 3 Schizonepeta spike, *Spica Schizonepetae* 6 g

No. 4 Fruit of citron or trifoliate orange, *Fructus Aurantikii* (parched with bran) 6 g

DIRECTIONS: All the above drugs are to be decocted in water for oral administration.

FUNCTIONS: Clearing the bowels to stop bleeding, dispelling pathogenic wind to keep the adverse *qi* flowing downward.

INDICATIONS: Hematochezia due to pathogenic wind accumulated in the large intestine marked by bleeding before or after passing stools, or fresh blood in the stools, or dull purplish bloody stools caused by toxic heat in the stomach and large intestine as well as hemorrhoidal bleeding.

Patients with hemorrhoid, colitis and proctopolypus marked by hematochezia caused by pathogenic wind accumulated in the intestine can be treated by the modified recipe.

INTERPRETATION: No. 1, as a principal drug, clears

有解热、抗菌、消炎等作用。

【使用注意】

1. 本方药物多为性寒通利之品，血淋日久正虚者则非其所宜。

2. 使用本方以尿检红细胞较多或肉眼血尿为主要指征。

槐 花 散

【来源】《本事方》

【组成】 槐花(炒)12克，侧柏叶12克，荆芥穗6克，枳壳(麸炒)6克。

【用法】 水煎服。

【功用】 清肠止血，疏风下气。

【主治】 肠风下血，表现为便前或便后出血，或粪中带血，血色鲜红，或脏毒便血，血色紫暗，以及痔疮出血等。

痔核、结肠炎、直肠息肉等证属肠风下血者，可用本方加减治疗。

away heat and toxins, cools the blood and removes damp-heat from the large intestine to stop hematochezia. No. 2 removes heat from the blood, eliminates dampness from the large intestine and assists No. 1 in stopping bleeding; No. 3 dispels pathogenic wind and stops bleeding. The two drugs mentioned above are assistant drugs. No. 4, as an adjuvant and guiding drug, soothes the large intestine to keep the adverse *qi* flowing downward.

Modern researches have proved that the recipe has the effects of stopping bleeding, relieving inflammation and resisting bacteria.

CAUTIONS: Drugs in the recipe with cold or cool nature can not be taken for a long time. Patients passing bloody stools without damp-heat are forbidden to use the recipe.

Decoction of Baked Yellow Earth

(Huangtu Tang)

SOURCE: *Synopsis of Precriptions of the Golden Chamber*

INGREDIENTS:

No. 1 Baked yellow earth, *Terra Flava Vsta* 30 g

No. 2 Large-headed atractylodes rhizome, *Rhizoma Atractylodis Macrocephalae* 9 g

No. 3 Prepared aconite root, *Radix Aconite Praeparata* 9 g

No. 4 Dried rehmannia root, *Radix Rehmanniae* 9 g

No. 5 Donkey-hide gelatin, *Colla Corii Asini* 9 g

No. 6 Scutellaria root, *Radix Scutellariae* 9 g

No. 7 Licorice root, *Radix Glycyrrhizae* 9 g

DIRECTIONS: Decoct the baked yellow earth in water to get its decoction and then decoct the other drugs in the decoction for oral administration.

FUNCTIONS: Warming *yang*, strengthening the spleen, nourishing the blood and stopping bleeding.

INDICATIONS: Hemorrhage which belongs to cold

【方解】 方中槐花清热解毒，凉血止血，善清大肠之湿热，凉大肠而止便血，为主药。侧柏叶苦涩微寒，入血分以清血热，燥湿、凉血而收敛，助槐花以止血；荆芥穗疏风止血，举清气，又能入血分以搜血分之风，共为辅药。枳壳宽肠下气，为佐使药。

现代研究证实，本方具有止血、消炎和抗菌作用。

【使用注意】 药性寒凉，不宜久服。便血无湿热者忌用。

黄土汤

【来源】 《金匮要略》

【组成】 灶心黄土30克，白术、附子、干地黄、阿胶、黄芩、甘草各9克。

【用法】 先将灶心土水煎取汤，再煎余药。

【功用】 温阳健脾，养血止血。

【主治】 虚寒失血证，表现为吐血，衄血，便血，妇人血崩，

syndrome of insufficiency type manifested by hematemesis, epistaxis, hematochezia and metrorrhagia characterized by dark-red blood, cold limbs, sallow complexion, pale tongue with white fur, and deep thready and feeble pulse.

Patients with chronic hemorrhage of gastrointestinal tract and chronic dysfunctional uterine bleeding, marked by the symptoms of cold syndrome of insufficiency type can be treated by the modified recipe.

INTERPRETATION: No. 1, as a principal drug in the recipe, warms the middle-warmer to stop bleeding. No. 2 and No. 3 warm *yang* and strengthen the spleen to restore its function of keeping the blood flowing in the vessels and plays the role of assistant drugs. No. 4 and No. 5 nourish *yin*, supplement the blood and stop bleeding, thus not only helping No. 1 in stopping bleeding but also compensating for the loss of *yin*-blood. No. 6, bitter in taste and cold in nature, can be used together with No. 4 and No. 5 to restrict the pungent, warm, dry and drastic nature of No. 2 and No. 3 to prevent wasting the blood. The drugs from No. 4 to No. 6 are adjuvant drugs. No. 7, as a guiding drug, coordinates the actions of the other drugs in the recipe and regulates the middle-warmer.

Modern researches have proved that the recipe can produce the effects of protecting the gastrointestinal mucous membrane, promoting the healing of ulcers, shortening the clotting time, promoting the regeneration of red blood cells and increasing hemoglobin.

CAUTIONS: Patients with symptoms due to exogenous pathogenic factors should not be treated by this recipe.

Ass-hide Glue and Argyi Leaf Decoction

(Jiao Ai Tang)

SOURCE: *Synopsis of Prescription of the Golden Chamber*

血色暗淡，四肢不温，面色萎黄，舌淡，苔白，脉沉细无力。

慢性胃肠道出血及慢性功能性子宫出血，证属虚寒失血者，可用本方加减治疗。

【方解】 方中灶心土温中止血，为主药。白术、附子温阳健脾，以复其统血之权，为辅药。生地、阿胶滋阴、养血、止血，既助灶心土止血，又可填充已失之阴血；黄芩苦寒，与生地、阿胶同用制约术、附辛温燥烈之性，防其耗血动血，同为佐药。甘草调药和中，为使药。

现代研究证实，本方具有保护胃肠粘膜、促进溃疡面愈合、缩短凝血时间、促进红细胞再生、增加血红蛋白等作用。

【使用注意】

有外邪者不宜用。

胶 艾 汤

【来源】 《金匮要略》

INGREDIENTS:

No. 1 Donkey-hide gelatin, *Colla Corii Asini* 6 g
No. 2 Chinese mugwort leaf, *Folium Artemisiae Argyi* 9 g
No. 3 Chinese angelica root, *Radix Angelicae Sinensis* 9 g
No. 4 Peony root, *Radix Paeoniae* 12 g
No. 5 Dried root of rehmannia, *Radix Rehmanniae* 12g
No. 6 Chuanxiong rhizome, *Rhizoma Ligustici Chuanxiong* 12 g
No. 7 Licorice root, *Radix Glycyrrhizae* 6 g

DIRECTIONS: Decoct the drugs except No. 1 in water. Remove the residue to get the decoction or add in an appropriate amount of wine, then put No. 1 in the decoction. Get it melted and take it warm.

FUNCTIONS: Nourishing the blood and stopping bleeding, regulating menstruation and preventing abortion.

INDICATIONS: Metrorrhagia and metrostaxis due to deficiency and impairment of the *chong* and *ren* channels marked by menorrhagia without stopping, or ceaseless bleeding due to miscarriage; vaginal bleeding occurring during pregnancy with abdominal pain.

Patients with threatened abortion, habitual abortion, dysfunctional uterine bleeding, ceaseless bleeding due to subinvolution of uterus marked by syndrome of deficiency and impairment of the *chong* and *ren* channels can be treated by the modified recipe.

INTERPRETATION: No. 1 nourishes the blood and stops bleeding while No. 2 warms the channels and stops bleeding. The two drugs mentioned above, as principal drugs, can also regulate menstruation to prevent miscarriage and cure metrorrhagia and stop metrostaxis. No. 3, No. 4, No. 5, and No. 6, as assistant drugs, enrich the blood, regulate menstruation, promote blood circulation to prevent forming blood stasis after bleeding has been stopped. No. 7, as a guiding drug, coordinates the actions of the other drugs. Moreover, combined with No. 1 it stops bleeding and combined with No. 4 it relieves

【组成】 阿胶6克，艾叶9克，当归9克，芍药12克，干地黄12克，川芎12克，甘草6克。

【用法】 水煎去滓，或加酒适量，入阿胶烊化，温服。

【功用】 补血止血，调经安胎。

【主治】 妇人冲任虚损所致的崩漏下血，月经过多，淋漓不止；或半产下血不绝；或妊娠胎漏下血，腹中疼痛。

先兆流产、习惯性流产、功能性子宫出血、产后子宫复旧不全出血不止等表现为冲任虚损者，可用本方加减治疗。

【方解】 方中阿胶补血、止血，艾叶温经止血，二药又可调经安胎，治崩止漏，共为主药。当归、芍药、干地黄、川芎补血调经，并能活血，以防血止留瘀，共为辅佐药。甘草调和诸药，并且配阿胶止血，配芍药缓急止痛，以治下血腹痛，为使药。

spasm and pain.

Modern researches have proved that the recipe has remarkable effects of stopping bleeding, improving the function of uterine and promoting the regeneration of red blood cells.

CAUTIONS: Patients with menorrhagia, metrorrhagia and metrostaxis marked by the syndrome of the blood-heat type are forbidden to use the recipe.

现代研究证实，本方止血作用显著，并有改善子宫机能、促进红细胞再生等作用。

【使用注意】 月经过多、崩漏等属血热妄行者禁用。

Chapter XI

Sedative Prescriptions

All those prescriptions, chiefly composed of sedative drugs or sedative tonics for nourishing the heart, having the effects of tranquilizing the mind and allaying excitement, and treating mental derangement, are generally known as sedative prescriptions.

In accordance with their effect, sedative prescriptions are divided into two types: the sedative recipes with heavy drugs and the sedative recipes with tonic drugs.

Section 1

Sedative Recipes with Heavy Drugs

This type of recipes is mainly composed of heavy materials used as sedatives, such as minerals or shells, having the effects of relieving palpitation and tranquilizing the mind. It is fit for treating the cases of fright, epilepsy, restlessness and others.

Sedative Bolus of Cinnabar

(Zhusha Anshen Wan)

SOURCE: *Inventions of Medicine*

INGREDIENTS:

No. 1 Cinnabar, *Cinnabaris* 15 g

No. 2 Goldthread root, *Rhizoma Coptidis* 18 g

第十一章

安　神　剂

凡主要由重镇安神或滋养心神的药物组成，具有镇静安神作用，以治疗神志不安诸证的方剂，统称安神剂。

安神剂根据功用分为重镇安神和滋养安神两类。

第一节　重镇安神剂

重镇安神剂是由重镇安神药为主组成，具有镇心安神作用，适用于惊恐、癫痫、躁扰不宁诸证。

朱砂安神丸

【来源】《医学发明》

【组成】 朱砂15克，黄连18克，当归8克，生地8克，炙甘

No. 3 Chinese angelica root, *Radix Angelicae Sinensis* 8 g
No. 4 Rehmannia root, *Radix Rehmanniae* 8 g
No. 5 Prepared licorice root, *Radix Glycyrrhizae Praeparata* 16 g

DIRECTIONS: Make the above-mentioned ingredients into boluses, take 6 or 9 grams a day before going to bed or decoct the drugs except No. 1 in water, with the dosage modified proportionally on the basis of the original recipe. No. 1 should be refined into powder with water, and taken with decoction.

FUNCTIONS: Relieving palpitation, tranquilizing the mind, removing pathogenic heat and nourishing the blood.

INDICATIONS: The flaming of heart-fire marked by mental irritability, insomnia, dreaminess, severe palpitation with fright, or nausea, heart-burn sensation in the chest, red tongue, rapid and thready pulse.

Insomnia, amnesia, palpitation due to neurosism or mental depression associated with the flaming of heart-fire can be treated by the modified recipe.

INTERPRETATION: No.1 in the recipe clears away heart-fire, relieves floating-*yang* and tranquilizes the mind; No. 2 clears away heart-fire and relieves restlessness. The combined use of the two drugs can clear away heart-fire to tranquilize the mind as principal drugs. No. 3 and No. 4, as assistant drugs, nourish *yin* and enrich blood while No. 4 can also replenish the kidney-*yin* to promote its flowing upward to clear away flaring heart-fire. No. 5 coordinates the actions of the other drugs, playing the part of a guiding drug.

Modern researches have proved that the recipe has the effects of tranquilizing the mind, inducing sleep, regulating the heart rate and nourishing the body.

CAUTIONS: No. 1 containing mercuric sulfide can not be taken in large dosage or for a long time to prevent mercurialism. It can not be decocted with other drugs in water.

草16克。

【用法】 上药为丸，每服6～9克，睡前服。亦可作汤剂，用量参考原方酌情增减，朱砂研末水飞，以药汤送服。

【功用】 镇心安神，清热养血。

【主治】 心火内扰证，表现为心烦神乱、失眠多梦、怔忡惊悸，甚则欲吐不吐，胸中懊憹，舌质红，脉细数。

神经衰弱之失眠、健忘、心悸或精神抑郁等证属心火内扰者可用本方加减治疗。

【方解】 方中朱砂清心火、镇浮阳、安心神，黄连清心火、除烦热，两药合用能清心安神，为主药。当归、生地滋养阴血，其中生地又可滋补肾阴，使肾水上济以制心火之亢，共为辅药。甘草调和诸药，为使药。

现代研究证实，本方具有镇静、催眠、调整心律及补养作用。

【使用注意】

朱砂含硫化汞，不宜多服、久服，以防汞中毒。亦不可入煎。

Pill of Magnetite and Cinnabar

(Cizhu Wan)

SOURCE: ***Prescriptions Worth a Thousand Gold for Emergencies***

INGREDIENTS:

No. 1 Magnetite, *Magnetium* 60g

No. 2 Cinnabar, *Cinnabaris* 30g

No. 3 Medicated leaven, *Massa Fermentata Medicinalis* 120 g

DIRECTIONS: Grind the above-mentioned ingredients into fine powder and then mix them with honey to make pills. Take 6 grams each time, twice a day with rice soup or boiled water.

FUNCTIONS: Relieving palpitation and tranquilizing the mind, suppressing sthenic *yang* and improving eyesight.

INDICATIONS: The syndrome of floating up of heart-*yang* marked by palpitation, insomnia, tinnitus, deafness, dizziness and so on. It can also be used to treat epilepsy.

Insomnia, vegetative nerve functional disturbance, neurosis, catarct, degeneration of optic nerve and others can be treated by the modified recipe.

INTERPRETATION: No. 1, acting on the kidney, can replenish *yin* to suppress sthenic *yang* and tranquilize the mind as a principal drug. No. 2, acting on the heart, can also tranquilize the mind. The combined use of the two drugs can cause the coordination between the heart-fire and the kidney-water. Therefore, the patient can fall asleep. If the patient gets sufficient kidney-essence, he can hear and see well. No. 3 promotes the activities of the spleen and the stomach. Mixed with honey to be made into bolus, it can not only regulate the stomach and supplement the middle-warmer but also prevent various metal and mineral drugs from interrupting the stomach.

Modern researches have proved that the recipe has very

磁 朱 丸

【来源】 《备急千金要方》

【组成】 磁石60克，朱砂30克，神曲120克。

【用法】 上药为末，炼蜜为丸，每次6克，1日2次，以米汤或开水送服。

【功用】 镇心安神，潜阳明目。

【主治】 心阳浮越证，表现为心悸失眠，耳鸣耳聋，视物昏花等。亦可治癫痫。

失眠、植物神经功能紊乱、神经官能症、白内障、视神经变性等，可用本方加减治疗。

【方解】 方中磁石入肾，能益阴潜阳，重镇安神，为主药。朱砂入心，能安神定志。两药合用，使水火既济，心肾交通，乃能入寐；肾精充足，则耳聪目明。神曲健脾胃、助运化，更以蜂蜜为丸，既可和胃补中，又防诸石药碍胃。

现代研究证实，本方具有很强的镇静作用。

strong sedative effect.

CAUTIONS:

1. The recipe is mainly used to treat ear or eye troubles due to floating up of *yang*. Patients with excessive internal fire due to *yin*-deficiency of the liver and kidney should not use this recipe.

2. Mineral and metal drugs offend the stomach, so patients with weakness of the spleen and stomach marked by dyspepsia should be prudent when using the recipe.

Section 2

Sedative Recipes with Tonic Drugs

This group of recipes is mainly composed of the drugs for nourishing *yin* and supplementing the blood and those for tranquilizing the mind. They are fit for the treatment of palpitation with fear or severe palpitation, restlessness of deficiency type, insomnia due to vexation.

Wild Jujube Seed Decoction

(Suanzaoren Tang)

SOURCE: ***Synopsis of Prescriptions of the Golden Chamber***

INGREDIENTS:

No. 1 Wild or spiny jujuba seed, *Semen Ziziphi Spinosae* 18 g
No. 2 Chuanxiong rhizome, *Rhizoma Ligustici Chuanxiong* 3 g
No. 3 Tuckahoe, *Poria* 6 g
No. 4 Rhizome of wind-weed, *Rhizoma Anemarrhenae* 6 g
No. 5 Licorice root, *Radix Glycyrrhizae* 3 g

DIRECTIONS: All the above drugs are to be decocted in water for oral administration

FUNCTIONS: Nourishing the blood and tranquilizing the

【使用注意】

1．本方以治浮阳外越之耳目病为主，若肝肾阴虚有火者不宜应用。

2．石药碍胃，故凡脾胃虚弱、消化不良者应慎用。

第二节 滋养安神剂

滋养安神剂主要由滋阴养血药与宁心安神药组成，具有滋养安神作用，适用于惊悸、怔忡、虚烦失眠等症。

酸枣仁汤

【来源】《金匮要略》

【组成】酸枣仁18克，川芎3克，茯苓6克，知母6克，甘草3克。

【用法】水煎服。

【功用】养血安神，清热除烦。

mind and clearing away pathogenic heat to relieve restlessness.

INDICATIONS: Symptoms due to asthenic diseases such as insomnia with vexation, palpitation, night sweat, dizziness, dry throat and mouth, thready and taut pulse.

Patients with neurosism, cardiac neurosis, paroxysmal tachycardia, climacteric syndrome and others marked by the above-mentioned symptoms can be treated by the modified recipe.

INTERPRETATION: No. 1, neutral in nature, sour in traste, related to the channels of heart and liver, can nourish the heart-blood and supplement the liver-blood to tranquilize the mind as a principal drug. No. 2, pungent and frangrant in flavor and warm in nature, strong in running and dispersing, can promote the flow of *qi* and blood circulation, regulate the liver-*qi*. The combined use of No. 1 and No. 2 can produce astringent and dispersing effects both being opposite and complementary to each other to nourish the blood, regulate the function of the liver and tranquilize the mind. No. 3 reinforces the spleen and tranquilizes the mind. No. 4 nourishes *yin* and reduces pathogenic fire to relieve restlessness. In addition, it can also moderate the pungent flavor and drastic nature of No. 2. No. 5 coordinates the actions of the other ingredients in the recipe. The joint use of the above drugs produces the effects of nourishing the blood to tranquilizing the mind and removing pathogenic heat to relieve restlessness.

Modern researches have proved that the recipe has the effects of tranquilizing the mind, inducing sleep and bringing down fever.

Cardiotonic Pill

(Tianwang Buxin Dan)

SOURCE: ***An Outline of Health Conservation***

【主治】 虚劳虚烦不眠，心悸盗汗，头晕目眩，咽干口燥，脉弦细。

神经衰弱、心神经官能症、阵发性心动过速、更年期综合征等有上述表现者，可用本方加减治疗。

【方解】 方中酸枣仁性平味酸，入心肝二经，能养血补肝，宁心安神，为主药。川芎辛温芳香，性善走散，行气活血，调达肝气，同酸枣仁配伍，一收一散，相反相成，以养血调肝安神。茯苓补脾宁心，知母滋阴降火除烦，又能缓和川芎之辛燥。甘草调和诸药。诸药合用，共奏养血安神、清热除烦之功。

现代研究证实，本方具有镇静、催眠、解热等作用。

天王补心丹

【来源】《摄生总要》

INGREDIENTS:

No. 1 Dried rehmannia root, *Radix Rehmanniae* 120 g
No. 2 Figwort root, *Radix Scrophulariae* 60g
No. 3 Red sage root, *Radix Salviae Miltiorrhizae* 60 g
No. 4 Chinese angelica root, *Radix Angelicae Sinensis* 60 g
No. 5 Ginseng, *Radix Ginseng* 60 g
No. 6 Tuckahoe, *Poria* 60 g
No. 7 Arborvitae seed, *Semen Biotae* 60 g
No. 8 Wild or spiny jujuba seed, *Semen Ziziphi Spinosae* 60 g
No. 9 Plolygala root, *Radix Polygalae* 60 g
No.10 Lucid asparagus root, *Radix Asparagi* 60 g
No.11 Lilyturf root, *Radix Ophiopogonis* 60 g
No.12 Magnolia vine fruit, *Fructus Schisandrae* 60 g
No.13 Root of balloonflower, *Radix Platycodi* 60 g

DIRECTIONS: Grind the above-mentioned ingredients into fine powder and mix the powder with honey to make pills coated with 15 to 20 grams of cinnabar. Take 9 grams three times a day. It can also be made into decoction, with the dosage modified proportionally according to the original recipe.

FUNCTIONS: Nourishing *yin* to remove heat and tonifying the blood to tranquilize the mind.

INDICATIONS: Deficiency-fire stirring up inside due to deficiency of *yin* and blood brought on by the hypofunction of heart and kindey marked by insomnia with vexation, palpitation, mental weariness, nocturnal emission, amnesia, dry stools, orolingual boil, reddened tongue with little fur, thready and rapid pulse.

Neurosism, paroxysmal tachycardia, hypertension, hyperthyroidism and others marked by the above-mentioned symptoms can be treated by the modified recipe.

INTERPRETATION: No. 1 is used in large dosage to nourish *yin* and blood, tonify the kidney and the heart; its combined use with No. 2 as principal drugs nourishes *yin* and clears pathogenic fire to get the deficiency-fire suppressed and

【组成】 生地120克，玄参、丹参、当归、人参、茯苓、柏子仁、酸枣仁、远志、天冬、麦冬、五味子、桔梗各60克。

【用法】 上药为末，炼蜜为丸，朱砂15～20克为衣。每服9克，1日3次。亦可作汤剂，用量参考原方比例酌定。

【功用】 滋养清热，养血安神。

【主治】 心肾不足，阴亏血少，虚火内扰，表现为虚烦少寐，心悸神疲，梦遗健忘，大便干燥，口舌生疮，舌红少苔，脉细而数。

神经衰弱、阵发性心动过速、高血压、甲亢等有上述证候者可用本方加减治疗。

【方解】 方中重用生地滋阴养血，补肾养心；配玄参滋阴清

the mind tranquilized. No. 3, No. 4, No. 5 and No. 6 invigorate *qi*, enrich the blood and tranquilize the mind. No. 7, No. 8 and No.9 reinforce the heart and the spleen to tranquilize the mind. No. 10 and No. 11, sweet in taste and cold in nature, produce an moistening effect to clear deficiency-fire. No.12 astringes *qi* and promotes the production of the body fluid to avoid the dissapation of the heart-*qi*. No. 13 carries all the ingredients in the recipe upward. cinnabar tranquilizes the mind. The joint use of all the drugs in the recipe can get *yin* and blood enriched, the fire of deficiency type reduced, thus, with the mind tranquilized spontaneously.

Modern researches have proved that the recipe has a better effect of regulating the cerbral cortex. It can tranquilize the mind to induce sleep without causing listlessness and achieve the effects of enriching the blood and relieving the symptoms of coronary heart disease.

CAUTIONS: The recipe is composed of nourishing, greasy drugs which affect the stomach, so it is not fit to take for a long time.

火，使虚火伏而心神安，共为主药。丹参、当归、人参、茯苓益气、补血、安神。柏子仁、酸枣仁、远志补益心脾，安神益志。天冬、麦冬甘寒滋润以清虚火。五味子敛气生津，以防心气耗散。桔梗载药上浮。朱砂镇心安神。诸药合用，使阴血得补，虚火得降而心神自安。

现代研究证实，本方具有较好的调节大脑皮层作用。既能镇静催眠，又不致使人精神萎靡不振。并具有补血及改善冠心病症状的作用。

【使用注意】 本方药物多滋腻碍胃，不宜长期服用。

Chapter XII

Prescriptions for Resuscitation

This type of prescriptions is composed of aromaric stimulants has the effect of inducing resuscitation to treat loss of consciousness. The prescription is divided into two kinds: the cold-natured recipe for inducing resuscitation and the warm-natured recipe for inducing resuscitation.]

Section 1

Cold-natured Recipes for Inducing Resuscitation

This group of recipes is usually composed of aromatic stimulants combined with the heart-clearing and blood-cooling drugs or the heat-clearing and fire-purging drugs. They are indicated for heat syndrome of coma due the to attack of pericardium by pathogenic warm or heat.

Bezoar Bolus for Resurrection

(Angong Niuhuang Wan)

SOURCE: ***Treatise on Differentiation and Treatment of Epidemic Febrile Diseases***

INGREDIENTS:

No. 1 Cow-bezoare, *Calculus Bovis* 30 g

No. 2 Musk, *Moschus* 7.5 g

No. 3 Rhinoceros horn, *Cornu Rhinocerotis* 30 g

第十二章

开　窍　剂

凡以芳香开窍药为主组成，具有开窍醒神作用，治疗神昏闭证的方剂，统称开窍剂。开窃剂分为凉开剂和温开剂两类。

第一节　凉　开　剂

凉开剂一般由芳香开窍药配伍清心凉血药、清热泻火药组成，适用于温邪热毒内陷心包的热闭证。

安宫牛黄丸

【来源】《温病条辨》

【组成】 牛黄30克，麝香7.5克，犀角、黄连、黄芩、山栀各

No. 4 Goldthread root, *Rhizoma Coptidis* 30 g
No. 5 Scutellaria root, *Radix Scutellariae* 30 g
No. 6 Capejasmine fruit, *Fructus Cardeniae* 30 g
No. 7 Borneol, *Borneolum* 7.5 g
No. 8 Curcuma root, *Radix Curcumae* 30 g
No. 9 Cinnabar, *Cinnabaris* 30 g
No.10 Pearl, *Margarita* 15 g
No.11 Realgar, *Realgar* 30g
No.12 Gold foil (appropriate amount)

DIRECTIONS: Grind the above-mentioned ingredients into fine powder, mix them with honey to make boluses, with each weighing 3 grams, coated with gold foil, enveloped with wax shell. Take one bolus each time with warm boiled water.

FUNCTIONS: Clearing away heat and toxins and eliminating phlegm to induce resuscitation.

INDICATIONS: Attack of pericardium by pathogenic heat occurring in the course of epidemic febrile diseases or accumulation of phlegm-heat in the heart manifested as high fever, dysphoria, coma and delirium or coma due to apoplexy, infantile convulsion and so on.

Patients with encephalitis B, epidemic encephalitis, toxic pneumonia, toxic dysentery, uremia, cerebrovascular accident, toxic hepatitis, hepatic coma and others marked by stagnation of phlegm and heat in the interior can be treated by the recipe.

INTERPRETATION: No. 1 in the recipe, functions in clearing away pathogenic heart-fire and toxins and eliminating phlegm to induce resuscitation. No. 2 has the functions of inducing resuscitation and restoring consciousness. The two drugs are used as principal drugs. No. 3 clears away heart-fire, blood-heat and toxins. No. 4, No. 5 and No. 6 clear away pathogenic fire and toxins to assist No. 1 in clearing away pathogenic fire accumulating in the pericardium. No. 7 and No. 8 dispel turbid pathogens and induce resuscitation by means of

30克，冰片7.5克，郁金30克，朱砂30克，珍珠15克，雄黄30克，金箔衣适量。

【用法】 共为极细末，炼蜜为丸，每丸重3克，金箔为衣，蜡护。温开水送服。每次1丸。

【功用】 清热解毒，豁痰开窍。

【主治】 温热病，热邪内陷心包，或痰热壅闭心窍所致的高热烦躁、神昏谵语以及中风昏迷，小儿惊厥等。

“乙脑”、“流脑”、中毒性肺炎、中毒性痢疾、尿毒症、脑血管意外、中毒性肝炎、肝昏迷等证属痰热内闭者可用本丸剂治疗。

【方解】 方中牛黄清心解毒，豁痰开窍；麝香开窍醒神，共为主药。犀角清心凉血解毒，黄连、黄芩、山栀清热泻火解毒，助牛黄清心包之火。冰片、郁金芳香辟秽，通窍开闭，以加强麝香

aroma to reinforce the effect of No. 2 in inducing resuscitation. No. 9 and No. 10 relieve palpitation and tranquilize the mind to remove dysphoria. No. 11 assists No. 1 in eliminating phlegm and clearing away toxins. No. 12, as coating, has the effect of tranquilization.

Modern researches have proved that the recipe has the functions of bringing down fever, resisting inflammation, virus, shock, and bacteria, tranquilizing the mind, relieving spasm and inducing resuscitation.

CAUTIONS: The recipe is rarely used alone. The joint use of the recipe and others consisting of the cold-natured or cool-natured drugs can produce much more curative effect.

Purple Snowy Powder

(Zixue Dan)

SOURCE: ***The Medical Secrets of an Official***

INGREDIENTS:

No. 1 Gypsum, *Gypsum Fibrosum* 1500 g
No. 2 Calcite, *Calcitum* 1500 g
No. 3 Talc, *Talcum* 1500 g
No. 4 Scrophularia root, *Radix Scrophulariae* 500 g
No. 5 Bugbane rhizome, *Rhizoma Cimicifugae* 500 g
No. 6 Licorice root, *Radix Glycyrrhizae* 240 g
No. 7 Rhinoceros horn, *Cornu Rhinocerotis* 150 g
No. 8 Musk, *Moschus* 1.5 g
No. 9 Dutchmanspipe root, *Radix Aristolochiae* 150 g
No.10 Eagle wood, *Lignum Aquilariae Resinatum* 150 g
No.11 Cloves, *Flos Caryophylli* 30 g
No.12 Antelope's horn, *Cornu Saigae Tataricae* 150 g
No.13 Cinnabar, *Cinnabaris* 90 g
No.14 Magnetite, *Magnetitum* 1500 g
No.15 Glauber's salt, *Natrii Sulphas* 5000 g

开窍醒神之效。朱砂、珍珠镇心安神，以除烦躁不安。雄黄助牛黄豁痰解毒。金箔为衣，有重镇安神之功。

现代研究证实，本方具有解热、抗炎、抗病毒、抗休克、抗菌、镇静、镇痉、醒脑等作用。

【使用注意】 本方很少单独使用，若与其他寒凉剂配用则疗效更佳。

紫雪丹

【来源】《外台秘要》

【组成】 石膏、寒水石、滑石各1500克，玄参、升麻各500克，甘草240克，犀角150克，麝香1.5克，青木香、沉香各150克，丁香30克，羚羊角150克，朱砂90克，磁石1500克，朴硝5000克，硝

No. 16 Niter, *Nitrum* 96 g

No. 17 Gold 3000 g

DIRECTIONS: Grind the above drugs into fine powder, take 1.5 to 3 grams each time, one or twice a day.

FUNCTIONS: Waking up the patient from unconsciousness by clearing away pathogenic heat, tranquilizing the mind and allaying excitement.

INDICATIONS: Heat-syndrome of coma due to excessive heat marked by high fever, convulsion, unconsciousness, delirium, restlessness, thirst with parched lips, dark brown urine, constipation, infantile convulsion.

All kinds of febrile diseases, such as crisis of encephalitis B, or epidemic cerebrospinal meningitis, severe pneumonia, and septicemic stage of pyogenic infection, typhus, scarlet fever and others marked by the above symptoms may be treated with the recipe.

INTERPRETATION: No. 1 ,No. 2 and No. 3, sweet in taste and cold in nature, function in clearing pathogenic heat. No. 4, No. 5 and No. 6 are the heat-clearing and detoxicating drugs, while No. 4 replenishes *yin* to promote the production of body fluid and No. 6 regulates the stomach. No. 7 clears away heart-heat and toxins. No. 8, No. 9, No. 10 and No. 11 promote the circulation of *qi* and induce resuscitation. The above-mentioned drugs are the main ingredients in the recipe. No. 12 removes liver-heat and calms endopathic wind to treat spasm and syncope. No. 13 and No. 14 are heavy materials for tranquilization to reinforce the actions of the other drugs in relieving restlessness and tranquilizing the mind. No. 15 and No. 16 purge the accumulation of excessive heat just like removing the burning wood from under the boiler. No.17 tranquilizes the mind and clears away toxins. The drugs from No. 12 to No. 17 are assistant drugs.

Modern researches have proved that the recipe has a strong effect of relieving spasm and the effects of tranquilizing

石96克，黄金3000克。

【用法】 制成散剂，日服1～2次，每次1.5～3克。

【功用】 清热开窍，镇静安神。

【主治】 热盛内闭证，表现为高热抽搐，神昏谵语，狂躁，口渴唇焦，尿赤便闭以及小儿热盛惊厥。

各种发热性传染病及感染性热病，如“乙脑”、“流脑”等的极期，重症肺炎及化脓性感染的败血症期，斑疹伤寒，猩红热等证属邪热内陷心包者，可配用本药治疗。

【方解】 方中石膏、寒水石、滑石甘寒清热。玄参、升麻、甘草清热解毒，其中玄参尤能养阴生津，甘草兼能和胃安中。犀角清心解毒。麝香、青木香、沉香、丁香行气开窍。以上是方中的主要组成部分。羚羊角清肝熄风以治痉厥。朱砂、磁石重镇安神，加强除烦安神之效。朴硝、硝石泻热散结，釜底抽薪。黄金镇心安神解毒。以上为方中辅助部分。

现代研究证实，本方镇痉作用较强，并具有镇静、消炎、抗

the mind, relieving inflammation, resisting bacteria and virus, bringing down fever and inducing resuscitation.

CAUTIONS: Never take an overdose of this medicine. Stop taking it as soon as the disease is cured.

Treasured Bolus

(Zhibao Dan)

SOURCE: ***Prescription of Peaceful Benevolent Dispensary***

INGREDIENTS:

No. 1 Musk, *Moschus* 7.5 g
No. 2 Borneol, *Borneolum* 7.5 g
No. 3 Benzoin, *Benzoinum* 4.5
No. 4 Rhinoceros horn, *Cornu Rhinocerotis* 30 g
No. 5 Cow-bezoare, *Calculus Bovis* 15 g
No. 6 Tortoise shell, *Carapax Eretmochelydis* 30 g
No. 7 Cinnabar, *Cinnabaris* 20 g
No. 8 Amber, *Succinum* 30 g
No. 9 Realgar, *Realgar* 30g
No.10 Gold foil 50 pieces
No.11 Silver foil 50 pieces

DIRECTIONS: Grind the above-mentioned drugs into fine powder to make boluses, each weighing 3 grams. Take one bolus each time with boiled water.

FUNCTIONS: Eliminating turbid pathogenic factor to induce resuscitation and clearing away heat and toxins.

INDICATIONS: Stagnation of phlegm-heat in the interior marked by coma and delirium, feverish body and irritability, abundant expectoration, harsh respiration, red tongue with yellow, thick and greasy fur, slippery and rapid pulse, and infantile convulsion associated with the above syndrome.

Encephalitis B, epidemic cerebrospinal meningitis, cerebrovascular accident, hepatic coma and other diseases belonging to stagnation of phlegm-heat in the interior or other diseases

菌、抗病毒、解热、醒脑等作用。

【使用注意】 本药不可过量服用，中病即止。

至宝丹

【来源】《太平惠民和剂局方》

【组成】 麝香、冰片各7.5克，安息香4.5克，犀角30克，牛黄15克，玳瑁30克，朱砂20克，琥珀、雄黄各30克，金箔、银箔各50克。

【用法】 研末为丸，每丸重3克。每次1丸，温开水送服。

【功用】 化浊开窍，清热解毒。

【主治】 痰热内闭证，表现为神昏谵语，身热烦躁，痰盛气粗，舌红，苔黄厚腻，脉滑数，以及小儿惊厥属痰热内闭者。

“乙脑”、“流脑”、脑血管意外、肝昏迷等证属痰热内闭或昏

marked by severe coma can be treated with the recipe.

INTERPRETATION: No. 1, No. 2 and No. 3 induce resuscitation and remove turbid pathogenic factor by means of aroma. No. 4, No. 5 and No. 6 clear away pathogenic heat and toxins while No. 5 can also resolve phlegm and relieve convulsion. The above drugs are all the principal ingredients in the recipe. No. 7 and No. 8 tranquilizes the mind and No. 9 eliminates phlegm for resuscitation and clears away toxins as assistant drugs. No. 10 and No. 11 can strengthen the action of No. 7 and No. 8 in tranquilizing the mind.

Modern researches have proved that the recipe has remarkable effect of relieving spasm and better effects of tranquilizing the mind, allaying fever, relieving inflammation, and resisting bacteria.

Section 2

Warm-natured Recipes for Inducing Resuscitation

This group of recipes is mainly composed of the resuscitation-inducing drugs with aroma and the *qi*-regulating drugs with a pungent flavor and warm nature. They are indicated for apoplexy, cold stroke, phlegm syncope and others belonging to the cold syndrome of coma.

Storax Pill

(Suhexiang Wan)

SOURCE: ***Prescription of Peaceful Benevolent Dispensary***

INGREDIENTS:

No. 1 Oriental sweetgum resin, *Resina Liquidambaris Orien-*

迷较重者可用本方治疗。

【方解】 方中麝香、冰片、安息香芳香开窍，辟秽化浊。犀角、牛黄、玳瑁清热解毒，其中牛黄又能化痰镇惊。以上是方中的主要组成部分。朱砂、琥珀镇心安神，雄黄豁痰解毒，均为辅助药。金箔、银箔加强朱砂、琥珀镇心安神之效。

现代研究证实，本方镇痉作用突出，镇静、解热、消炎、抗菌作用也较明显。

第二节 温开剂

温开剂主要由芳香开窍药配合辛温行气药组成，适用于中风、中寒、痰厥等证属寒闭者。

苏合香丸

【来源】 《太平惠民和剂局方》

talis (mixed with the extract of Benzoinum) 30 g

No. 2 Musk, *Moschus* (ground) 60 g

No. 3 Borneol, *Borneolum* (ground) 30 g

No. 4 Benzoin, *Benzoinum* (ground into powder, decocted in a Chinese *Sheng* of limeless liquor into extract) 60 g

No. 5 Dutchmanspipe root, *Radix Aristolochiae* 60 g

No. 6 White sandal wood, *Lignum Santali* 60 g

No. 7 Eagle Wood, *Lignum Aquilariae Resinatum* 60 g

No. 8 Cloves, *Flos Caryophylli* 60 g

No. 9 Nutgrass flatsedge rhizome, *Rhizoma Cyperi* (stir-fried, remove the hair) 60 g

No.10 Olibanum, *Resina Olibani* (ground alone) 30 g

No.11 Long pepper, *Fructus Piperis Longi* 60 g

No.12 Rhinoceros horn, *Cornu Rhinocerotis* 60 g

No.13 Cinnabar, *Cinnabaris* (ground, refined with water) 60 g

No.14 Bighead atractylodes rhizome, *Rhizoma Atractylodis Macrocephalae* 60 g

No.15 Myrobalan fruit, *Fructus Chebulae* (roasted in ashes) 60 g

DIRECTIONS: Make pills with honey, each weighing 3 grams. Take one pill each time with warm boiled water.

FUNCTIONS: Inducing resuscitation with aromatics, promoting the circulation of *qi* to relieve pain.

INDICATION: Cold syndrome of coma marked by sudden fainting, trismus, unconsciousness, or fullness with cold sensation in the chest and abdomen, nausea and so on.

Cerebrovascular accident, hysterical syncope, psychognic syncope, epilepsy, and concussion of brain during the stage of syncope marked by cold syndrome of coma can be treated with the recipe.

INTERPRETATION: No. 1, No. 2, No. 3 and No. 4 are aromatics to induce resuscitation as principal ingredients. No. 5, No. 6, No. 7, No. 8, No. 9 and No. 10 promote the cir-

【组成】 苏合香油（入安息香膏内）30克，麝香（研）30克，冰片（研）30克，安息香（研为末，用无灰酒一升熬膏）30克，青木香、白檀香、沉香、丁香、香附（炒，去毛）各60克，乳香（另研）30克，荜茇、犀角、朱砂（研，水飞）、白术、诃子（煨，去皮）各60克。

【用法】 炼蜜为丸，每丸3克，每次1丸，温开水送服。

【功用】 芳香开窍，行气止痛。

【主治】 寒邪内闭证，表现为突然昏倒，牙关紧闭，不省人事，或心腹满闷而冷，欲吐而不得。

脑血管意外、癔病性昏迷、突受精神刺激而昏厥、癫痫、脑震荡（昏厥期）等表现为寒邪内闭者可用本方治疗。

【方解】 方中苏合香、麝香、冰片、安息香芳香开窍，为主要

culation of *qi* and alleviate mental depression, expel cold and dissolve the turbid pathogenic factor. Combined use of the above ingredients with No. 11 can strengthen the effects of dispelling cold, relieving pain and alleviating mental depression. No. 12 clears away heart-heat and toxins. No.13 tranquilizes the mind. No. 14 eliminates dampness, invigorates the spleen and dissolves turbid pathogenic factor. No.15 can produce the effect of astringing *qi* and combined with various aromatics, it can prevent excessive effect of pungent and aromatic drugs from causing dissipation of the vital *qi*.

Modern researches have proved that the recipe has the effects of relieving convultion and pain and tranquilizing the mind.

Supplementary Recipe:

Storax Pill for Coronary Heart Disease (from the book, ***Chinese Pharmacopoeia*** published in 1977)

INGREDIENTS:

No. 1 Storax, *Styrax Liquidus* 50 g

No. 2 Borneol, *Borneolum* 105 g

No. 3 Prepared olibanum, *Resina Olibani Praeparata* 105 g

No. 4 Sandal wood, *Lignum Santali* 210 g

No. 5 Dutchmanspipe root, *Radix Aristolochiae* 210 g

DIRECTIONS: Grind No. 3, No. 4 and No. 5 into fine powder; then grind the powder together with the fine powder of the ground No. 2, screen the powder and then mix well; take some honey and heat it slightly. Add it to No. 1, stir up and then mix it well with the above powder to make 1000 pills. Suck or swallow a pill after chewing it well. Take it before going to bed or during an attack, or one pill each time, one to three times a day.

FUNCTIONS: Inducing the resuscitation with aromatics and promoting the flow of *qi* to relieve pain.

INDICATIONS: Angina pectoris marked by oppressed feeling in the chest belonging to the syndrome of turbid phlegm and accumulation of *qi* in the chest.

组成部分。配以青木香、白檀香、沉香、丁香、香附、乳香行气解郁，散寒化浊。荜茇与上述诸药合用，可增强其散寒、止痛、开郁作用。犀角清心解毒。朱砂镇心安神。白术燥湿、健脾、化浊。诃子收涩敛气，与诸香药配伍，防其辛香太过，耗散正气。

现代研究证实，本方具有解痉、镇静、镇痛作用。

【附方】

冠心苏合丸 （《中国药典》1977年版）

【组成】 苏合香50克，冰片105克，乳香（制）105克，檀香210克，青木香210克。

【用法】 乳香、檀香、青木香三味粉碎成细末；将冰片研细与上述粉末配研，过筛，混匀；另取炼蜜适量微温后，加入苏合香搅匀。再与上述粉末混匀，制成1000丸。含服或嚼碎后咽服，1次1丸，每日1～3次。亦可在睡前或发病时服用。

【功用】 芳香开窍，行气止痛。

【主治】 心绞痛症见胸闷、憋气，属于痰浊气阻者。

Chapter XIII

Prescriptions for Calming wind

This type of prescriptions, mainly composed of the wind-dispelling drugs with a pungent flavor, or the *yin*-nourishing and hyperactive-*yang*-suppressing and wind-calming drugs, has the effect of dispelling exopathic wind or calming interior wind.

Section 1

Recipes for Dispelling Exopathic Wind

This group of recipes is mainly composed of the wind-dispelling drugs with a pungent flavor and is indicated for diseases due to exopathic wind.

Chuanxiong Mixture

(Chuanxiong Chatiao San)

SOURCE: ***Prescription of Peaceful Benevolent Dispensary***

INGREDIENTS:

No. 1 Chuanxiong rhizome, *Rhizoma Ligustici Chuanxiong* 120 g
No. 2 Schizonepeta, *Herba Schizonepetae* (remove stem) 120 g
No. 3 Dahurian angelica root, *Radix Angelicae Dahuricae* 60 g
No. 4 Notopterygium root, *Rhizoma seu Radix Notopterygii* 60 g
No. 5 Licorice root, *Radix Glycyrrhizae* 60 g
No. 6 Wild ginger, *Herba Asari* 30 g
No. 7 Ledebouriella root, *Radix Ledebouriellae* 45 g

第十三章

治　风　剂

凡主要由辛散疏风或滋阴潜阳熄风药物所组成，具有疏散外风或平熄内风作用的方剂，统称为治风剂。

第一节　疏散外风剂

疏散外风剂主要由辛散祛风的药物组成，适用于外风所致诸病。

川芎茶调散

【来源】《太平惠民和剂局方》

【组成】川芎、荆芥(去梗)各120克，白芷、羌活、甘草各60

No. 8 Peppermint, (herb) *Herba Menthae* (un-baked) 240 g

DIRECTIONS: Grind the drugs into fine powder, take 6 grams each time, twice a day, after mixing well with tea. It can also be decocted in water for oral administration but the dosage should be reduced proportionally on the basis of the original recipe.

FUNCTIONS: Dispelling exopathic wind to relieve pain.

INDICATIONS: Attacks of exopathic wind marked by headache, migraine, or pain on the top of head, aversion to cold with fever, obstruction of nose, dizziness, thin and white fur of the tongue, floating and slippery pulse.

The common cold, migraine, nervous headache, headache due to chronic rhinitis, marked by the symptoms of the attack of exopathic wind can be treated by the modified recipe.

INTERPRETATION: As principal drugs, No.1 is effective for *shaoyang* headache and *jueyin* headache (pain in the temples or pain on the top of the head), No. 4, for *taiyang* headache (posterior pain of the head), No. 3 for *yangming* headache (pain in the frontal bone and superciliary ridge), No. 6 for *shaoyin* headache (dizziness and pain radiating to the cheeks). As assistant drugs, No.8, No. 2 and No.7 with an elevating and dispelling effect, can be used to refresh the mind, dispel exopathic wind in assisting the principal drugs to strengthen the effect of dispelling the wind to relieve pain and induce mild diaphoresis. No. 5 regulates the stomach and supplements *qi*, coordinates the actions of all the other drugs to prevent their excessive disitpation of *qi*. Taking the medicine with tea is aimed at making use of its bitter taste and cold nature to prevent the excessive warm-dryness and the excessive elevating and dispelling actions of the wind-dispelling drugs and moderate the elevating and lowering effects. They are all used as adjuvant drugs.

Modern researches have proved that the recipe has the effects of relieving pain, inducing diaphoresis, bringing down

克，细辛30克，防风45克，薄荷叶（不见火）240克。

【用法】 共为细末，每服6克，每日2次，清茶调下。亦可水煎服，用量按原方比例酌减。

【功用】 疏风止痛。

【主治】 外感风邪，偏正头痛或巅顶作痛，恶寒发热，鼻塞目眩，舌苔薄白，脉浮滑。

感冒、偏头痛、神经性头痛、慢性鼻炎引起的头痛，表现为外感风邪头痛证者，可用本方加减治疗。

【方解】 方中川芎善治少阳经、厥阴经头痛（两侧痛或头顶痛），羌活善治太阳经头痛（后头痛），白芷善治阳明经头痛（眉棱、额骨痛），细辛善治少阴经头痛（晕痛连两颐），均为主药；薄荷、荆芥、防风升散上行，以清利头目，疏散风邪，协助主药以增强疏风止痛之效，并能解表，均为辅药。甘草和中益气，调和诸药，使升散不致耗气。用茶水调服，是取其苦寒之性味，既可上清风热，又能防止风药过于温燥、升散，使升中有降，均为佐使药。

现代研究证实，本方具有镇痛、发汗、解热、镇静等作用。

fever and tranquilizing the mind.

CAUTIONS: Since it consists of more drugs with a pungent flavor which induce perspiration, the recipe is not indicated for insufficiency of *qi* and blood due to persistent illness or headache caused by up-stirring of liver-wind or hyperactivity of liver-*yang*.

Major Gentian Decoction

(Da Qinjiao Tang)

SOURCE: ***Etiology and Health Preserving in Plain Questions***

INGREDIENTS:

No. 1 Root of large-leaf gentian, *Radix Gentianae Macrophyllae* 90 g

No. 2 Licorice root, *Radix Glycyrrhizae* 60 g

No. 3 Chuanxiong rhizome, *Rhizoma Ligustici Chuanxiong* 60 g

No. 4 Chinese angelica root, *Radix Angelicae Sinensis* 60 g

No. 5 White peony root, *Radix Paeoniae Alba* 60 g

No. 6 Wild ginger, *Herba Asari* 15 g

No. 7 Notopterygium root, *Rhizoma seu Radix Notopterygii* 30 g

No. 8 Ledebouriella root, *Radix Ledebouriellae* 30 g

No. 9 Skullcap root, *Radix Scutellariae* 30 g

No.10 Gypsum, *Gypsum Fibrosum* 60 g

No.11 Dahurian angelica root, *Radix Angelicae Dahuricae* 30 g

No.12 Large-headed atractylodes rhizome, *Rhizoma Atractylodis Macrocephalae* 30 g

No.13 Dried root of rehmannia, *Radix Rehmanniae* 30 g

No.14 Prepared rehmannia root, *Radix Rehmanniae Praeparata* 30 g

No.15 Tuchahoe, *Poria* 30 g

No.16 Pubescent angelica root, *Radix Angelicae Pubescentis* 60 g

DIRECTIONS: Grind the above drugs into powder, take

【使用注意】 本方的辛散药物较多，凡久病气虚、血虚，或因肝风、肝阳而引起的头痛，均非本方所宜。

大秦艽汤

【来源】《素问病机气宜保命集》

【组成】 秦艽90克，甘草60克，川芎60克，当归60克，白芍60克，细辛15克，羌活、防风、黄芩各30克，石膏60克，白芷30克，白术30克，生地30克，熟地30克，白茯苓30克，独活60克。

【用法】 上药为散，每次30克，水煎去滓服。或作汤剂，水煎

30 grams each time after being decocted in water and discarding the residue, or make decoction in water for oral administration. Its dosage is modified proportionally on the basis of the original recipe.

FUNCTIONS: Dispersing exopathic wind and clearing away pathogenic heat.

INDICATIONS: Attacks of exopathic wind on the channels marked by numbness of muscles, skin, hands and feet, sudden deviation of the eye and mouth, rigidity of the extremities, failure to move the hands and feet, or accompanied by exterior syndrome of cold type or exterior syndrome of heat type marked by white tongue fur and floating pulse.

INTERPRETATION: No. 1 dispels exopathic wind to remove obstruction in the channels as a principal drug. No. 7, No.16, No.8, No.11, No.6, pungent in flavor and warm in nature, are used as assistant drugs to expel exopathic wind and other pathogens. No. 4, No. 5 and No. 14 nourish the blood and strengthen the muscles and tendon, expel pathogenic wind without impairing the body fluid; No. 3 reinforces the effects of No. 4 and No. 5 in promoting blood flow and activating the channels; No. 12 and No. 15 replenish *qi* and invigorate the spleen to support the source of growth and the development of *qi* and blood. No. 9, No. 10 and No. 13 clear away pathogenic heat from the blood. All the drugs mentioned above are used as adjuvant drugs. Besides, No. 2 coordinates the effects of all the other drugs as a guiding drug.

Modern researches have proved that the recipe has the effects of relieving inflammation, allaying fever, tranquilizing the mind, arresting pain and promoting blood circulation.

CAUTIONS: The recipe is mainly composed of drugs with warm and dry nature, so it is contraindicated in patients with convulsion due to endogenous wind.

服，用量按原方比例酌情增减。

【功用】 祛风清热，养血活血。

【主治】 风中经络证，表现为肌肤不仁，手足麻木，突然口眼歪斜，肢体拘急，手足不能运动，或兼寒热表证，苔白脉浮。

【方解】 方中秦艽祛风而通行经络，为主药。羌活、独活、防风、白芷、细辛，均为辛温之品，祛风散邪，俱为辅药。当归、白芍、熟地养血柔筋，使祛风而不伤津；川芎协助当归、白芍、活血通络；白术、茯苓益气健脾，以助生化之源；黄芩、石膏、生地凉血清热，以上俱为佐药。另以甘草调和诸药为使。

现代研究证实，本方具有抗炎、解热、镇静、镇痛、促进血液循环等作用。

【使用注意】 本方药多温燥，内风证忌用。

Powder for Dispersing Pathogenic Wind

(Xiaofeng San)

SOURCE: ***Orthodox Manual of External Diseases***

INGREDIENTS:

No. 1 Chinese angelica root, *Radix Angelicae Sinensis* 3 g
No. 2 Dried root of rehmannia, *Radix Rehmanniae* 3 g
No. 3 Ledebouriella root, *Radix Ledebouriellae* 3 g
No. 4 Cicada slough, *Periostracum Cicadae* 3 g
No. 5 Rhizome of wind-weed, *Rhizoma Anemarrhenae* 3 g
No. 6 Flavescent sophora root, *Radix Sophorae Flavescentis* 3 g
No. 7 Sesame seed, *Semen Sesami* 3 g
No. 8 Schizonepeta, *Herba Schizonepetae* 3 g
No. 9 Atractylodes rhizome, *Rhizoma Atractylodis* 3 g
No.10 Arctium fruit, *Fructus Arctii* (parched and ground) 3 g
No.11 Gypsum, *Gypsum Fibrosum* (calcined) 3g
No.12 Licorice root, *Radix Glycyrrhizae* 1.5 g
No.13 Fiveleaf akebia (stem), *Caulis Akebiae* 1.5 g

DIRECTIONS: The above-mentioned drugs should be decocted in water. The decoction should be taken with an empty stomach.

FUNCTIONS: Dispelling pathogenic wind, nourishing the blood, clearing away heat and removing dampness.

INDICATIONS: Endogenous stagnation of pathogenic wind marked by eczema, rubella, red skin rash with pruritus, exudation of the body fluid after being injured by scratching, white or yellow tongue fur, floating, rapid and forceful pulse.

Patients with eczema, rubella, urticaria, allergic dermatitis and neurodermatitis marked by endogenous stagnation of pathogenic wind can be treated by the modified recipe.

INTERPRETATION: No.8, No.3, No.10, and No.4 dispel pathofenic wind and other pathogens from the exterior as principal drugs. No. 9 also expels the wind and removes damp-

消 风 散

【来源】《外科正宗》

【组成】当归、生地、防风、蝉蜕、知母、苦参、胡麻、荆芥、苍术、牛蒡子(炒研)、石膏(煅)各3克，甘草、木通各1.5克。

【用法】水煎，空腹服。

【功用】疏风养血，清热除湿。

【主治】风毒内郁证，表现为湿疹、风疹，皮肤疹出色红，瘙痒，抓破后渗出津水，舌苔白或黄，脉浮数有力。

湿疹、风疹、荨麻疹、过敏性皮炎、神经性皮炎，表现为风毒内郁者，可用本方加减治疗。

【方解】方中荆芥、防风、牛蒡子、蝉蜕疏风透表，以除在表

ness. No. 6 clears way pathogenic heat and dampness. No. 13 excretes dampness and heat. No.11 and No. 5 clear away pathogenic heat and fire. All of these are used as assistant drugs. No. 2 ,No. 1 an No. 7 nourish the blood and promote blood circulation, replenish *yin* essence and moisturize the viscera as adjuvant drugs. No. 12 clears away pathogenic heat and toxins and coordinates the effects of all the drugs as a guiding drug. Joint use of all the drugs can dispel pathogenic wind and nourish the blood, clear away pathogenic heat and eliminate dampness.

Modern researches have proved that the recipe has the effects of relieving inflammation, allaying fever, relieving itching, resisting bacteria and reducing the exudation of body fluid.

CAUTIONS:

1. The recipe is contraindicated in patients with deficiency of both *qi* and blood.

2. When taking the recipe, the patient should refrain from pungent food, fish, smoking, wine and strong tea.

3. The combined use of the recipe with drugs for external application is preferable.

Bolus for Activating Energy Flow in the Channels and Collaterals

(Xiao Huo Luo Dan)

SOURCE: ***Prescription of Peaceful Benevolent Dispensary***

INGREDIENTS:

No 1 Prepared sichuan aconite root. *Radix Aconiti Praeparata* 180 g

No. 2 Prepared wild aconite root, *Radix Aconiti Kusnezoffii Praeparata* 180 g

No. 3 Earth worm, *Lumbricus* 180 g

No. 4 Prepared arisaema root, *Rhizoma Arisaematis* 180 g

之风邪，为主药。苍术散风除湿，苦参清热燥湿，木通渗利湿热，石膏、知母清热泻火，俱为辅药。生地、当归、胡麻养血活血，滋阴润燥，为佐药。生甘草清热解毒，调和诸药，为使药。诸药合用，疏风养血，清热除湿。

现代研究证实，本方具有消炎、解热、止痒、抗菌、减少渗出等作用。

【使用注意】

1．气血虚弱者不宜用。

2．服用本方时，不宜食辛辣、鱼腥、烟酒、浓茶等。

3．使用本方宜配合外用药。

小活络丹

【来源】《太平惠民和剂局方》

【组成】 制川乌、制草乌、地龙、制天南星各180克，乳香、没

No. 5 Olibanum, *Resina Olibani* 66 g
No. 6 Myrrh, *Myrrha* 66 g

DIRECTIONS: Make the above drugs into boluses, each weighing 3 grams. Take one bolus each time, one or two times a day. Take it on an empty stomach and with old wine or warm boiled water.

FUNCTIONS: Warming the channels and activating the collaterals, dispelling pathogenic wind-dampness and removing phlegm and blood stasis.

INDICATIONS: Stagnation of wind-dampness in the channels and collaterals marked by prolonged numbness of hands and feet without recovery, or pain of limbs, muscles and bones without fixed spots, or pain of arms or legs.

Arthritis, lumbago, neck-shoulder-wrist syndrome, periarthritis of shoulder, arthrosis deformans, chronic rheumatic arthritis and others marked by stagnation of wind-dampness in the channels and collaterals, or cerebral thrombosis and disturbance of cerebral circulation marked by apoplexy due to phlegm-dampness in the channels and collaterals.

INTERPRETATION: No. 1 and No. 2 with a pungent and hot nature dispel wind-dampness, warm the channels and collaterals to relieve pain as principal drugs. No. 4, as an assistant drug, dries dampness and resolves phlegm to alleviate pain. No, 5 and No. 6 promote the flow of *qi* and blood circulation to remove blood stasis from the channels and collaterals. No. 3 is especially predominant in clearing and activating the channels and collaterals. The three drugs act as adjuvant drugs. Old liquor can reinforce the effects of the drugs and guides other drugs in the recipe to the affected region as a guiding drug.

Modern researches have proved that the recipe has the effects of relieving pain and spasm, tranquilizing the mind, relieving inflammation, removing phlegm, inducing diuresis, promoting blood circulation, etc.

药各66克。

【用法】 为丸，每丸重3克，每服1丸，每日1～2次，空腹用陈酒或温开水送服。

【功用】 温经活络，搜风除湿，祛痰逐瘀。

【主治】 风湿阻络证，表现为手足麻木不仁，日久不愈，或四肢筋骨疼痛，游走不定，或腿臂作痛。

关节炎、腰痛、颈-肩-腕综合征、肩关节周围炎、变形性关节病、慢性风湿性关节炎等，表现为风湿阻络者，或脑血栓表现为痰湿阻络者，可用本方治疗。

【方解】 方中川乌、草乌为辛热之品，祛风除湿，温经止痛，为主药。天南星燥湿化痰而止痛，为辅药。乳香、没药行气活血，以化络中瘀血，使气血流畅；地龙尤善通经活络，共为佐药。酒助药势，可引诸药直达病所，为使药。

现代研究证实，本方具有镇痛、解痉、镇静、消炎、祛痰、利尿、改善血液循环等作用。

CAUTIONS: The recipe, consisting of drastic drugs, is indicated for persistent cases without deficiency symptoms. It is contraindicated in patients with fever due to deficiency of *yin* and in pregnancy.

Section 2

Recipes for Calming Endogenous Wind

Thie group of recipes is mainly composed of drugs for calming the liver to stop convulsion and some heat-clearing, phlegm-resolving, and blood-nourishing drugs. It has the effect of calming endogenous wind and is indicated for endogenous-wind syndrome.

Decoction of Antelope's Horn and Uncaria Stem

(Lingjiao Gouteng Tang)

SOURCE: ***Popular Treatise on Febrile Diseases***

INGREDIENTS:

No. 1 Antelope's horn, *Cornu Saigae Tataricae* (decocted first) 4.5 g

No. 2 Uncaria stem with hooks, *Ramulus Uncariae Cum Uncis* (decocted later) 9 g

No. 3 Mulberry leaf, *Folium Mori* 6 g

No. 4 Sichuan fritillary bulb, *Bulbus Fritillariae Cirrhosae* 12 g

No. 5 Fresh root of rehmannia, *Radix Rehmanniae* 15 g

No. 6 Bamboo shavings, *Caulis Bambusae in Taenis* (fresh and prepared, decocted first with No.1 in water) 9 g

No. 7 Chrysanthemum flower, *Flos Chrysanthemi* 9 g

No. 8 White peony root, *Radix Paeoniae Alba* 9 g

【使用注意】 本方药力颇峻，以日久不愈而体质壮实者为宜。若阴虚有热及孕妇忌用。

第二节 平熄内风剂

平熄内风剂以平肝熄风药为主，配伍清热、化痰、养血之品组成，有平熄内风的作用，适用于内风病证。

羚角钩藤汤

【来源】《通俗伤寒论》

【组成】 羚羊角4.5克（先煎），双钩藤（后入）9克，桑叶 6 克，川贝母12克，鲜生地15克，竹茹（鲜刮，与羚羊角先煎代水）、菊

No. 9 Poria with hostwood, *Poria cum Ligno Hospite* 9 g
No.10 Licorice root, *Radix Glycyrrhizae Recens* 3 g

DIRECTIONS: All the above drugs are to be decocted in water for oral administration.

FUNCTIONS: Removing pathogenic heat from the liver and calming endogenous wind and increasing body fluid to relax muscles and tendons.

INDICATIONS: Occurrence of wind syndrome in case of extreme heat marked by persistent high fever, restlessness and convulsion, or coma in serious case, dry and deep-red tongue, or prickled and parched tongue, taut and rapid pulse.

Hypertension, functional disturbance of vegetative nerve, cerebrovascular accident, hyperthyroidism, epilepsy and vertigo marked by occurrence of wind syndrome in case of extreme heat can be treated by the modified recipe.

INTERPRETATION: No. 1 and No.2, as principal drugs, cool the liver to calm endogenous wind, remove pathogenic heat to relieve convulsion. No.3 and No.7 strengthen the wind-calming effect as assistant drugs. No.8 and No.5 replenish *yin* and body fluid to nourish the liver and relax the muscles and tendons; No.4 and No.6 remove heat to resolve phlegm; No.9 calms the liver and tranquilizes the mind. The above ingredients act as adjuvant drugs. No.10 coordinates the effects of all the other drugs in the recipe as a guiding drug. When combined with No.8 it can promote the production of *yin*, relax the muscles and tendons and relieve spasm.

Modern researches have proved that all the drugs in the recipe have the effects of lowering high blood pressure and tranquilizing the mind.

CAUTIONS: The recipe is not indicated for stirring up of endopathic wind of deficiency type caused by the retention cf pathogenic heat and impairment of genuine *yin* due to

花、白芍、茯神木各9克，生甘草3克。

【用法】 水煎服。

【功用】 凉肝熄风，增液舒筋。

【主治】 热盛风动证，表现为高热不退，烦闷躁扰，痉厥抽搐，甚则神昏，舌质绛而干，或舌焦起刺，脉弦而数。

高血压病、植物神经失调、脑血管意外、甲状腺机能亢进、癫痫、眩晕等，表现为热盛风动证者，可用本方加减治疗。

【方解】 方中羚羊角、钩藤凉肝熄风，清热解痉，为主药。桑叶、菊花有加强熄风之效，为辅药。白芍、生地养阴增液以柔肝舒筋；贝母、竹茹清热化痰；茯神木平肝、宁心安神，俱为佐药。生甘草调和诸药为使药，与白芍相配，又能酸甘化阴，舒筋缓急。

现代研究证实，本方几乎所有药物都有降压作用，还有镇静效果。

【使用注意】 若温热病邪热羁留，灼伤真阴，以致虚风内动，

epidemic febrile disease marked by spasm of the muscles and involuntary movement of limbs.

Tranquilizing Liver-wind Decoction

(Zhengan Xifeng Tang)

SOURCE: ***Records of Traditional Chinese and Western Medicine in Combination***

INGREDIENTS:

No. 1 Achyranthes root, *Radix Achyranthis Bidentatae* 30 g

No. 2 Red ochre, *Ochra Haematitum* (ground into fine powder) 30 g

No. 3 Dragon's bone, *Os Draconis Fossilia Ossis Mastodi* (smashed) 15 g

No. 4 Oyster shell, *Concha Ostreae* (smashed) 15 g

No. 5 Tortoise plastron, *Plastrum Testudinis* (smashed) 15g

No. 6 White peony root, R*adix Paeoniae Alba* 15 g

No. 7 Scrophularia root, *Radix Scrophulariae* 15 g

No. 8 Lucid asparagus root, *Radix Asparagi* 15 g

No. 9 Sichuan chinaberry, *Fructus Meliae Toosendan* (smashed) 6 g

No.10 Germinated barley, *Fructus Hordei Germinatus* 6 g

No.11 Oriental wormwood, *Herba Artemisiae Capillaris* 6 g

No.12 Licorice root, *Radix Glycyrrhizae* 4 g

DIRECTIONS: The drugs described above should be decocted in water for oral administration.

FUNCTIONS: Tranquilizing the liver to calm endogenous wind.

INDICATIONS: Syndrome of wind stirring inside due to excess of *yang* marked by vertigo, swollen eyes and tinnitus, pain and heat sensation in the head, flushed face, restlessness, or eructation, or the limited sensation in the movement of limbs or wry mouth by degrees, or even falling down due to faint, coma, coming round when moved but failing to recover, taut and forceful

筋脉拘急，手足蠕动者，则非本方所宜。

镇肝熄风汤

【来源】《医学衷中参西录》

【组成】怀牛膝30克，生赭石(轧细)30克，生龙骨(捣细)15克，生牡蛎、生龟板(捣细)、生杭芍、玄参、天冬各15克，川楝子(捣细)6克，生麦芽6克，茵陈6克，甘草4克。

【用法】水煎服。

【功用】镇肝熄风。

【主治】阳亢风动证，表现为头目眩晕，目胀耳鸣，脑中热痛，面色如醉，心中烦热，或时常噫气，或肢体渐觉不利，口角渐形歪斜；甚或眩晕颠仆，昏不知人，移时始醒，或醒后不能复原，脉弦有力。

pulse.

Hypertension, cerebrovascular accident, hypertensive encephalopathy and so on marked by endogenous wind due to excess of *yang* can be treated by the modified recipe.

INTERPRETATION: No.1 in the recipe ensures proper downward flow of the blood from the head and invigorates the liver and kidney as a principal drug. No.2, No.3 and No. 4 as assistant drugs lower the adverse flow of *qi*, check exuberance of *yang* and tranquilize the liver-wind. No.5, No.6, No.7 and No.8 nourish *yin*-fluid to check exuberance of *yang*. No.11, No.9 and No.10 clear away liver-*yang* to regulate the liver-*qi*. No.12 coordinates the effects of all the other drugs in the recipe. Its combined use with No.10 can regulate the stomach to prevent metal and mineral drugs from affecting the stomach. They are all used as adjuvant and guiding drugs.

Modern researches have proved that the recipe has the effects of inhibiting the excitation process of the brain and reducing its congestion.

Decoction of Gastrodia and Uncaria

(Tianma Gouteng Yin)

SOURCE: ***New Standards for Diagnosis and Treatment of Miscellaneous Diseases***

INGREDIENTS:

No. 1 Gastrodia tuber, *Rhizoma Gastrodiae* 9 g

No. 2 Uncaria stem with hooks, *Ramulus Uncariae Cum Uncis* (decocted later) 12 g

No. 3 Abalone shell or sea-ear shell, *Concha Haliotidis* (decocted first) 18 g

No. 4 Capejasmine fruit, *Fructus Gardeniae* 9 g

No. 5 Scutellaria root, *Radix Scutellariae* 9 g

No. 6 Achyranthes root, *Radix Achyranthis Bidentatae* 12 g

高血压病、脑血管意外、高血压性脑病等，表现为阳亢风动证者，可用本方加减治疗。

【方解】 方中怀牛膝引血下行，并有补益肝肾之效，为主药。代赭石、龙骨、牡蛎降逆潜阳，镇肝熄风，为辅药。龟板、玄参、天冬、白芍滋养阴液，以制阳亢；茵陈、川楝子、生麦芽等清泄肝阳，条达肝气；甘草调和诸药，与麦芽相配，并能和胃调中，防止金石类药物碍胃之弊，均为佐使药。

现代研究证实，本方具有抑制脑的兴奋过程、改善充血状态的作用。

天麻钩藤饮

【来源】 《杂病证治新义》

【组成】 天麻 9 克，钩藤(后下)12克，石决明(先煎)18克，山

No. 7 Bark of eucommia, *Cortex Eucommiae* 9 g
No. 8 Motherwort (whole plant), *Herba Leonuri* 9 g
No. 9 Loranthus mulberry mistletoe, *Ramulus Loranthi* 9 g
No.10 Fleece-flower stem, *Caulis Polygoni Multiflori* 9 g
No.11 Poria with hostwood, *Poria cum Ligno Hospite* 9 g

DIRECTIONS: The drugs described above should be decocted in water for oral administration.

FUNCTIONS: Calming the liver to stop endogenous wind, clearing away pathogenic heat, promoting blood circulation and nourishing the liver and kidney.

INDICATIONS: Wind-syndromes caused by hyperactivity of the liver-*yang* marked by headache, vertigo, tinnitus and dim eyesight, involuntary movement of limbs, insomnia, or even hemiplegia, red tongue, taut and rapid pulse.

Hypertension, functional disturbance of vegetative nerve, cerebrovascular accident, hyperthyroidism, epilepsy and vertigo marked by wind-syndrome caused by hyperactivity of the liver-*yang* can be treated by the modified recipe.

INTERPRETATION: No.1, No.2 and No.3 calm the liver to stop the wind as principal drugs. No.4 and No.5 clear away heat and purge fire from the liver channel as assistant drugs. No.8 promotes blood circulation and induces diuresis. No.6 ensures proper downward flow of the blood from the head. No.7 and No.9 nourish the liver and kidney. No.10 and No.11 tranquilize the mind. The drugs mentioned above are used as adjuvant and guiding drugs.

Modern researches have proved that the recipe has the effects of tranquilizing the mind, relieving spasm, resisting epilepsy, dilating blood vessels and lowering high blood pressure. It also has the fever-allaying, antibacterial and anti-inflammatory effects.

栀、黄芩各9克，川牛膝12克，杜仲、益母草、桑寄生、夜交藤、茯神各9克。

【用法】 水煎服。

【功用】 平肝熄风，清热活血，补益肝肾。

【主治】 肝阳化风证，表现为头痛，眩晕，耳鸣眼花，手足震颤，失眠，甚或半身不遂，舌红脉弦数。

高血压、植物神经功能失调、脑血管意外、甲状腺机能亢进、癫痫、眩晕等，表现为肝阳化风症状者，可用本方加减治疗。

【方解】 方中天麻、钩藤、石决明平肝熄风，为主药。山栀、黄芩清热泻火，以清肝经之热，为辅药。益母草活血利水，牛膝引血下行，杜仲、桑寄生补益肝肾，夜交藤、茯神安神定志，俱为佐使药。

现代研究证实，本方具有镇静、镇痉、抗癫痫、扩张血管和降压等作用，同时还有一定的解热、抗菌及消炎效果。

Chapter XIV

Prescriptions for Treating Dryness Syndrome

Those mainly composed of drugs with moistening effect, functioning in promoting the production of body fluids to moisturize the viscera and treating dryness syndromes are generally known as prescriptions for treating dryness syndrome.

Dryness syndrome is divided into exopathic dryness and endogenous dryness syndromes. The former is mainly caused by attack of pathogenic dryness in autumn while the latter by deficiency of body fluids of the viscera. Exopathic dryness syndrome should be treated by facilitating the flow of the lung-*qi* with drugs of mild effect while endogenous dryness syndrome should be treated with drugs moisturizing the viscera. The prescription for treating dryness syndrome is divided into two types: recipes for slightly facilitating the flow of lung-*qi* and moistening exopathic dryness; and those for moistening endogenous dryness.

Section 1

Recipes for Slightly Facilitating the Flow of Lung-*qi* and Moistening Exopathic Dryness

Exopathic dryness syndrome is subdivided into cool-dryness syndrome and warm-dryness syndrome. Cool-dryness

第十四章

治 燥 剂

凡主要由润燥药物组成，具有滋生津液、润泽脏腑的作用，治疗燥证的方剂，称为治燥剂。

燥证有外燥、内燥之分。外燥多系感受秋令燥邪所致。内燥多由脏腑津液亏损而成。治疗方法，外燥宜轻宣，内燥宜滋润，治燥剂分为轻宣外燥剂和滋润内燥剂两类。

第一节 轻宣外燥剂

外燥又有凉燥、温燥之分。凉燥是感受秋天风寒燥邪，肺气

syndrome is caused by the obstruction of lung-*qi* due to the attack of coolness and dryness in autumn. It is usually treated with drugs of warm nature and mild effect. Its representative recipe is Apricot Kernel and Perilla Powder. Warm-dryness syndrome is caused by the impairment of lung-fluid due to the attack of exopathic dryness and heat in autumn. It is usually treated by using drugs of cool nature and mild effect. Its representative recipes are Decoction of Mulberry Leaf and Apricot Kernel and Decoction for Relieving Dryness of the Lung.

Apricot Kernel and Perilla Powder

(Xing Su San)

SOURCE: ***Treatise on Differentiation and Treatment of Epidemic Febrile Diseases***

INGREDIENTS:

No. 1 Perilla leaf, *Folium Perillae* 6 g
No. 2 Pinellia tuber, *Rhizoma Pinelliae* 6 g
No. 3 Poria, *Poria* 6 g
No. 4 Root of purple-flowered peucedanum, *Radix Peucedani* 6 g
No. 5 Balloonflower root, *Radix Platycodi* 6 g
No. 6 Fruit of citron or trifoliate orange, *Frucutus Aurantii* 6 g
No. 7 Licorice root, *Radix Glycyrrhizae* 6 g
No. 8 Fresh ginger, *Rhizoma Zingiberis Recens* 6 g
No. 9 Tangerine peel, *Pericarpium Citri Reticulatae* 6 g
No.10 Apricot kernel, *Semen Armeniacae* 6 g
No.11 Chinese dates, *Fructus Ziziphi Jujubae* 2 pcs.

DIRECTIONS: The drugs described above should be decocted in water for oral administration.

不宣所致，多用轻灵性温的药物治疗，代表方为杏苏散。温燥是感受秋令燥热，损伤肺津所致，多用轻清性凉的药物治疗，代表方为桑杏汤、清燥救肺汤。

杏 苏 散

【来源】《温病条辨》

【组成】 苏叶、半夏、茯苓、前胡、苦桔梗、枳壳、甘草、生姜、橘皮、杏仁各6克，大枣2枚。

【用法】 水煎服。

FUNCTIONS: Dispelling pathogenic cool-dryness removing pathogenic heat from the lung and dissolving phlegm.

INDICATIONS: Cool-dryness syndrome caused by exopathic factors marked by slight headache, chills, absence of sweating, cough with thin sputum, stuffy nose, dry sensation in pharynx, white tongue fur and taut pulse.

The common cold, bronchitis and other diseases marked by the symptoms of cool-dryness syndrome can be treated by the modified recipe.

INTERPRETATION: No.1 and No.4 relieve exterior syndrome and eliminate pathogenic factors by inducing slight diaphoresis. No.10 and No.5 promote the function of the lung to disperse pathogens and the circulation of *qi* to relieve cough. No.2 and No.3 eliminate dampness and dissolve phlegm. No.6 and No.9 regulate the flow of *qi* and relieve the depression in the chest. No.8, No.11 and No.7 regulate *ying* and *wei*, and coordinate the effects of all the other ingredients in the recipe.

Modern researches have proved that the recipe has remarkable effects of relieving cough and eliminating phlegm as well as the effects of slightly inducing diaphoresis and clearing heat.

CAUTIONS: Since it is composed of pungent and warm-natured drugs, the recipe is only indicated for cool-dryness syndrome due to pathogenic wind-cold, not for wind-warm syndrome. Therefore, it can not be used as an ordinary recipe for the treatment of cough due to the common cold.

Decoction of Mulberry Leaf and Apricot Kernel

(Sang Xing Tang)

SOURCE: ***Treatise on Differentiation and Treatment of Epidemic Febrile Diseases***

【功用】 轻宣凉燥，清肺化痰。

【主治】 外感凉燥证，表现为头微痛，恶寒无汗，咳嗽痰稀，鼻塞嗌干，苔白，脉弦。

感冒、支气管炎等表现为外感凉燥证者，可用本方加减治疗。

【方解】 方中苏叶、前胡解表散邪，微发其汗。杏仁、桔梗宣肺达邪，利气止咳。半夏、茯苓祛湿化痰。枳壳、橘皮理气宽胸。生姜、大枣、甘草调营卫，和诸药。

现代研究证实，本方在轻度发汗、解热的同时，还有很强的镇咳、祛痰作用。

【使用注意】 本方辛温，只宜于风寒凉燥之证，不宜于风温，故不能作为伤风咳嗽通用之方。

桑杏汤

【来源】《温病条辨》

INGREDIENTS:

No. 1 Mulberry leaf, *Folium Mori* 6 g
No. 2 Apricot kernel, *Semen Pruni Armeniacae* 9 g
No. 3 Ladybell root, *Radix Adenophorae* 12g
No. 4 Fritillary bulb, *Bulbus Fritillariae Thunbergii* 6 g
No. 5 Prepared soybean, *Semen Sojae Praeparatum* 6 g
No. 6 Capejasmine fruit, *Fructus Gardeniae* 6 g
No. 7 Pear peel 6 g

DIRECTIONS: The drugs described above should be decocted in water for oral administration.

FUNCTIONS: Expelling pathogenic dryness-heat and moistening the lung to arrest cough.

INDICATIONS: Warm-dryness syndrome caused by exopathogen marked by headache, fever, thirst, dry cough or with a small amount of mucilaginous sputum, red tongue with thin, white and dry fur, and floating and rapid pulse.

The common cold, pharyngitis, bronchitis, bronchiectasis and other diseases marked by symptoms of warm-dryness syndrome caused by exopathogen can be treated by the modified recipe.

INTERPRETATION: No.1 and No.5 in the recipe ventilate the lung to dispel pathogenic factors. No.2 ventilates the lung and promotes the flow of *qi*. No.3, No.4 and No.7 moisten the lung to arrest cough. No.6 clears away pathogenic heat in the chest.

Modern researches have proved that the recipe has the effects of allaying fever, eliminating phlegm, arresting cough, subduing inflammation and bacteria.

Decoction for Relieving Dryness of the Lung

(Qingzao Jiufei Tang)

SOURCE: ***Principle and Prohibition for Medical Profession***

【组成】 桑叶6克，杏仁9克，沙参12克，浙贝母6克，淡豆豉6克，山栀子6克，梨皮6克。

【用法】 水煎服。

【功用】 轻宣燥热，润肺止咳。

【主治】 外感温燥证，表现为头痛身热，口渴，干咳无痰，或痰少而粘，舌红，苔薄白而燥，脉浮数。

感冒、咽炎、支气管炎、支气管扩张等表现为外感温燥证者，可用本方加减治疗。

【方解】 方中桑叶、豆豉宣肺散邪；杏仁宣肺利气；沙参、贝母、梨皮润肺止咳；栀子清泄胸膈之热。

现代研究证实，本方具有解热、祛痰、镇咳、消炎、抗菌等作用。

清燥救肺汤

【来源】 《医门法律》

INGREDIENTS:

No. 1 Mulberry leaf, *Folium Mori* 9 g

No. 2 Gypsum, *Gypsum Fibrosum* 7.5 g

No. 3 Ginseng, *Radix Ginseng* 2 g

No. 4 Licorice root, *Radix Glycyrrhizae* 3 g

No. 5 Sesame seed, *Semen Sesami* (fried and ground) 3 g

No. 6 Donkey-hide gelatin, *Colla Corii Asini* 2.4 g

No. 7 Lilyturf root, *Radix Ophiopogonis* (core removed) 3.6 g

No. 8 Apricot kernel, *Semen Pruni Armeniacae* (skin removed, fried) 2 g

No. 9 Loquat leaf, *Folium Eriobotryae* (hair removed, honey-fried to yellow) 3 g

DIRECTIONS: The drugs should be decocted in water for oral administration.

FUNCTIONS: Dispelling pathogenic dryness and moistening the lung.

INDICATIONS: Impairment of the lung caused by pathogenic warm-dryness which has invaded the *qi* system marked by headache, fever, dry cough, asthma, dryness of the pharynx and nasal cavity, fullness sensation in the chest and pain in the hypochondrium, vexation, thirst, dry and uncoated tongue, feeble, large and rapid pulse.

Pharyngitis, bronchitis, Bronchiectasis, pulmonary tuberculosis and other diseases marked by the syndrome of impairment of the lung caused by warm-dryness which has invaded the *qi* system can be treated by the modified recipe.

INTERPRETATIONS: No.1 clears away lung dryness as a principal drug. No.2 and No. 7 as assistant drugs clear away pathogenic heat from the lung and moisten the dryness. No.8 and No.9 promote the circulation of the lung *qi*; No.6 and No.5 moisten the lung and replenish *yin*; No. 3 and No. 4 supplement *qi* and regulate the stomach. These ingredients act as adjuvant drugs.

Modern researches have proved that the recipe has the

【组成】 冬桑叶9克，石膏7.5克，人参2克，甘草3克，胡麻仁（炒，研）3克，真阿胶2.4克，麦门冬（去心）3.6克，杏仁（去皮尖，炒）2克，枇杷叶（刷去毛，蜜涂炙黄）3克。

【用法】 水煎服。

【功用】 清燥润肺。

【主治】 温燥伤肺，邪入气分证，表现为头痛身热，干咳无痰，气逆而喘，咽喉干燥，鼻燥，胸满胁痛，心烦口渴，舌干无苔，脉虚大而数。

咽炎、支气管炎、支气管扩张、肺结核等表现为温燥伤肺，邪入气分证者，可用本方加减治疗。

【方解】 方中桑叶清宣肺燥，为主药。石膏、麦冬清润肺之热燥，为辅药。杏仁、枇杷叶利肺气；阿胶、胡麻仁润肺养阴；人参、甘草益气和中，均为佐药。

现代研究证实，本方具有消炎、解热、滋养强壮、促进机能

effects of relieving inflammation, bringing down fever, tonifying the body, promoting functional activities, eliminating phlegm and relieving cough.

Section 2

Recipes for Moistening Endogenous Dryness

This group of recipes is mainly composed of drugs for replenishing *yin* and moistening the viscera. **It** has the effects of replenishing *yin* and moistening dryness and is indicated for endogenous dryness syndrome due to insufficiency of viscera fluids.

Lily Decoction for Strengthening the Lung

(Eaihe Gujin Tang)

SOURCE: Created by Dr. Zhao Jian but recorded in ***Collection of Prescription with Notes***

INGREDIENTS:

No. 1 Dried rehmannia root, *Radix Rehmanniae* 6 g

No. 2 Prepared rehmannia root, *Radix Rehmanniae Praeparata* 9 g

No. 3 Lilyturf root, *Radix Ophiopogonis* 5 g

No. 4 Lily bulb, *Bulbus Lilii* 3 g

No. 5 White peony root, *Radix Paeoniae Alba* (parched) 3 g

No. 6 Chinese angelica root, *Radix Angelicae Sinensis* 3 g

No. 7 Bulb of fritillary, *Bulbus Fritillariae* 3 g

No. 8 Licorice root, *Radix Glycyrrhizae* 3 g

No. 9 Figwort root, *Radix Scrophulariae* 3 g

No.10 Root of Balloon flower, *Radix Platycodi* 3 g

DIRECTONS: All the above drugs are to be decocted in water for oral administration.

FUNCTIONS: Nourishing *yin* to moisten the lung and resolving phlegm to arrest cough.

以及祛痰、镇咳作用。

第二节 滋润内燥剂

滋润内燥剂主要由滋阴润燥药组成，有滋阴润燥作用，适用于脏腑津液不足之内燥证。

百合固金汤

【来源】 《医方集解》引赵蕺庵方。

【组成】 生地黄6克，熟地黄9克，麦冬5克，百合、白芍(炒)、当归、贝母、生甘草各3克，玄参、桔梗各3克。

【用法】 水煎服。

【功用】 养阴润肺，化痰止咳。

INDICATIONS: Syndrome of cough due to dryness of the lung marked by sore throat, dryness of the pharynx, cough, dyspnea, bloody sputum, dysphoria with feverish sensation in the palms and soles, reddish tongue with little fur and thready and rapid pulse.

Pulmonary tuberculosis, chronic bronchitis, brochiectasis, chronic pharyngitis and other diseases marked by the syndrome of cough due to dryness of the lung can be treated by the modified recipe.

INTERPRETATION: No.1 and No.2, as principal drugs in the recipe, nourish *yin* to supplement the kidney and remove heat from the blood to arrest bleeding. No.3, No.4 and No.7 moisten the lung and replenish *yin*, resolve phlegm and arrest cough, acting as assistant drugs. As adjuvant drugs, No.9 nourishes *yin* and clears away heat from the blood to dispel fire of deficiency type; No.6 enriches the blood and moistens dryness, No.5 enriches the blood to strengthen *yin*; and No.10 promotes the circulation of the lung-*qi* to arrest cough and resolve phlegm. No.8, as a guiding drug, coordinates the effects of all the other ingredients in the recipe and the combined use of it with No.10 can relieve sore throat.

Modern researches have proved that the recipe has the effects of strengthening the constitution, inhibiting dissimilation, subduing inflammation, relieving cough and eliminating phlegm.

CAUTIONS: Most of the drugs in the recipe are of sweet taste and cold and greasy nature with moistening effect, so it should be applied with great care or should not be applied at all to patients with loose stools, abdominal distention and pain poor appetite due to hypofunction of the spleen.

【主治】 肺燥咳嗽证，表现为咽喉燥痛，咳嗽气喘，痰中带血，手足烦热，舌红少苔，脉细数。

肺结核、慢性支气管炎、支气管扩张、慢性咽炎等表现为肺燥咳嗽证者，可用本方加减治疗。

【方解】 方中生地黄、熟地黄滋阴补肾，凉血止血，为主药。麦冬、百合、贝母润肺养阴，且能化痰止咳，为辅药。玄参滋阴凉血清虚火；当归养血润燥；白芍养血益阴；桔梗宣利肺气而止咳化痰，为佐药。甘草调和诸药，与桔梗合用，更利咽喉，为使药。

现代研究证实，本方具有滋养强壮、抑制异化作用及消炎、镇咳、祛痰作用。

【使用注意】 本方药物多属甘寒滋润滞腻之品，若脾虚便稀、腹满胀痛、食欲不振者，慎用或忌用。

Decoction for Nourishing *Yin* and Clearing Lung-heat

(Yangyin Qingfei Tang)

SOURCE: *Jade Key to the Secluded Chamber*

INGREDIENTS:

No. 1 Dried rehmannia root, *Radix Rehmanniae* 6 g
No. 2 Lilyturf root, *Radix Ophiopogonis* 5 g
No. 3 Licorice root, *Radix Glycyrrhizae* 2 g
No. 4 Scrophularia root, *Radix Scrophulariae* 5 g
No. 5 Bulb of fritillary, *Bulbus Fritillariae* (core removed) 3 g
No. 6 Moutan bark, *Cortex Moutan Radicis* 3 g
No. 7 Peppermint, *Herba Menthae* 2 g
No. 8 White peony root, *Radix Paeoniae Alba* (parched) 3 g

DIRECTIONS: All the drugs are to be decocted in water for oral use.

FUNCTIONS: Nourishing *yin* and clearing away lung-heat.

INDICATIONS: Diphtheria due to deficiency *yin* marked by fever, dryness of the nasal cavity and lips, cough or absence of cough, difficult breath, and false membrane in the throat which is not easy to remove.

Diphtheria, acute pharyngitis, acute tonsillitis, chronic bronchitis, chronic pharyngitis and others marked by the syndrome of *yin* deficiency can be treated by the modified recipe.

INTERPRETATION: The recipe is specially indicated for the treatment of diphtheria. No.1 in the recipe nourishes the kidney-*yin*. No.2 nourishes the lung-*yin*. No.4 clears away fire of deficiency type and removes toxins. No.6 clears away heat from the blood to subdue swelling. No.5 nourishes the lung to resolve phlegm. No.8 astringes *yin* fluid and purges away heat and No.7, small in dosage, disperses pathogenic factors to relieve sore-throat. No.3 coordinates the effects of other drugs in the recipe and removes toxins.

养阴清肺汤

【来源】《重楼玉钥》

【组成】大生地6克，麦冬5克，生甘草2克，玄参5克，贝母(去心)3克，丹皮3克，薄荷2克，炒白芍3克。

【用法】水煎服。

【功用】养阴清肺。

【主治】白喉阴虚证，表现为发热，鼻干，唇燥，或咳或不咳，呼吸不利，似喘非喘，喉间起白膜如腐，不易拨去。

白喉、急性咽炎、急性扁桃体炎、或慢性支气管炎、慢性咽炎等表现为白喉阴虚证者，可用本方加减治疗。

【方解】本方为治疗白喉的专用方。方中生地养肾阴，麦冬养肺阴，玄参清虚火而解毒，丹皮凉血而消肿，贝母润肺化痰，白芍敛阴泄热，少佐薄荷散邪利咽，甘草和药解毒。

modern researches have proved that the recipe has the effects of strengthening the constitution by means of tonics, relieving inflammation and cough, eliminating phlegm and risisting bacillus diphtheriae.

Ophiopogon Decoction

(Maimendong Tang)

SOURCE: ***Synopsis of Prescriptions of the Golden Chamber***

INGREDIENTS:

No. 1 Lilyturf root, *Radix Ophiopogonis* 60 g
No. 2 Pinellia tuber, *Rhizoma Pinelliae* 9 g
No. 3 Ginseng, *Radix Ginseng* 6g
No. 4 Licorice root, *Radix Glycyrrhizae* 4 g
No. 5 Glutinous rice, *Oryza Glutinosae* 6 g
No. 6 Chinese-dates, *Fructus Ziziphi Jujubae* 3 pcs.

DIRECTIONS: All the drugs are to be decocted in water for oral administration.

FUNCTIONS: Nourishing the lung and the stomach, lowering the adverse flow of *qi* and regulating the stomach.

INDICATIONS: Consumptive lung disease marked by cough, whitish frothy sputum, shortness of breath, dryness of the mouth and pharynx, thirst, dryness of the tongue red in colour with little fur and weak and rapid pulse.

Chronic bronchitis, chronic pharyngitis, pulmonary tuberculosis, bronchiectasis, chronic gastritis, atrophic gastritis, and epidemic febrile diseases in the recover stage marked by deficiency of both the stomach-*qi* and stomach-*yin* can be treated by the modified recipe.

INTERPRETATION: No.1 in the recipe, used in large dosage as a principal drug, sweet in taste and cold in nature, nourishes the lung-*yin* and stomach-*yin* and clears away the fire of deficiency type. No.2 is aimed at lowering the adverse

现代研究证实，本方具有滋养强壮、消炎、镇咳、祛痰、抗白喉杆菌等作用。

麦门冬汤

【来源】 《金匮要略》

【组成】 麦门冬60克，半夏9克，人参6克，甘草4克，粳米6克，大枣3枚。

【用法】 水煎服。

【功用】 滋养肺胃，降逆和中。

【主治】 肺痿证，表现为咳唾涎沫，气喘短气，咽干口燥而渴，舌干苔少质红，脉虚数。

慢性支气管炎、慢性咽喉炎、肺结核、支气管扩张、慢性胃炎、萎缩性胃炎、热病恢复期等表现为肺胃气阴两虚者，可用本方加减治疗。

【方解】 方中重用麦门冬为主药，味甘性寒，滋养肺胃之阴，

flow of *qi* to resolve phlegm, as an assistant drug. In spite of its dry nature, when it is used in combination with a large dosage of No.1, its dry nature is reduced but its effect of lowering the adverse flow of *qi* remained. It also enables No.1 to keep its tonic effect and lose its greasy nature. No.3 replenishes and restores the middle-warmer *qi*. When it is used in combination with No.1, its effects of invigorating *qi* and producing body fluids can be strengthened. No.5, No.6 and No.4, as adjuvant and guiding drugs, tonify the spleen and benefit the stomach.

Modern researches have proved that the recipe has the effects of nourishing and moistening the human body, relieving cough and eliminating phlegm.

CAUTIONS: The recipe is contraindicated in patients with consumptive lung disease belonging to the cold of insufficiency type.

且清虚火。半夏为辅药意在降逆化痰，其性虽燥，但与大量麦冬配伍，则燥性减而降逆之性存，取其善降肺胃虚逆之气，又使麦门冬滋而不腻。人参补益中气，与麦门冬配伍，补气生津之力增强，复加粳米、大枣、甘草补脾益胃，共为佐使之药。

现代研究证实，本方具有滋润营养、镇咳、祛痰等作用。

【使用注意】 肺痿属于虚寒者，忌用。

Chapter XV

Phlegm-eliminating Prescriptions

Those composed of phlegm-eliminating drugs, with the effect of removing the retention of phlegm and fluids and for the treatment of various phlegm diseases, are generally known as phlegm-eliminating prescriptions.

Phlegm, being of many kinds, can be divided in accordance with its nature into damp phlegm, heat phlegm, sticky phlegm, cold phlegm and wind phlegm. Phlegm-eliminating prescriptions can be divided into five kinds: the recipes for removing dampness to reduce phlegm, the recipes for removing heat-phlegm, the recipes for moistening the lung to resolve phlegm, the recipes for warming the lung to resolve cold phlegm and the recipes for expelling wind and resolving phlegm.

Section 1

Recipes for Removing Dampness to Reduce Phlegm

This group of recipes is composed of the drugs for removing dampness to reduce phlegm and those for removing dampness by means of their bitter taste, warm and dry natures or those for promoting diuresis by means of their sweet or insipid taste. It is indicated for damp-phlegm syndrome.

第十五章

祛 痰 剂

凡以痰祛药为主组成，具有消除痰饮作用，治疗各种痰病的方剂，统称为祛痰剂。

痰的种类很多，根据痰的性质可分为湿痰、热痰、燥痰、寒痰、风痰等。祛痰剂可分为燥湿化痰、清热化痰、润燥化痰、温化寒痰、祛风化痰等五类。

第一节 燥湿化痰剂

燥湿化痰剂由苦温燥湿或甘淡利湿与燥湿化痰药组成，适用于湿痰证。

Two Old Drugs Decoction

(Erchen Tang)

SOURCE: ***Prescription of Peaceful Benevolent Dispensary***

INGREDIENTS:

No. 1 Pinellia tuber, *Rhizoma Pinelliae* 15 g

No. 2 Tangerine peel, *Pericarpium Citri Reticulatae* 15 g

No. 3 Tuckahoe, *Poria* 9 g

No. 4 Prepared licorice root, *Radix Glycyrrhizae Praeparata* 3 g

DIRECTIONS: Add 3 grams of fresh ginger and a piece of black plum into the above recipe, and then decoct them in water for oral use.

FUNCTIONS: Removing dampness to resolve phlegm, and regulating the stomach.

INDICATIONS: Damp-phlegm syndrome marked by cough with profuse whitish sputum, fullness sensation in the chest, nausea, vomiting, dizziness, palpitation, whitish and moist fur of the tongue and slippery pulse.

Bronchitis, gastritis, catarrhal gastritis and other diseases marked by damp-phlegm syndrome can be treated by the modified recipe.

INTERPRETATION: No.1, with a pungent flavor and warm and dry nature, is effective in removing dampness to resolve phlegm and lowering the adverse flow of *qi* and regulating the stomach to arrest vomiting, as a principal drug. No.2 as an assistant drug, with the effect of regulating *qi* to remove dampness, enables the *qi* to flow normally and gets the phlegm cleared away. No.3 strengthens the spleen and eliminates dampness; fresh ginger, being able to lower the adverse flow of *qi* and resolve phlegm, can not only reduce the toxic effect of No.1 but also strengthen the effects of promoting *qi*-flow and resolving phlegm of No.1 and No.2. A small amount of black plum astringes the lung-*qi*. The three drugs above are used

二陈汤

【来源】《太平惠民和剂局方》

【组成】半夏、橘红各15克，白茯苓 9 克，甘草(炙) 3 克。

【用法】加生姜 3 克，乌梅一个，水煎服。

【功用】燥湿化痰，理气和中。

【主治】湿痰证，表现为咳嗽痰多色白，胸膈胀满，恶心呕吐，头眩心悸，舌苔白润，脉滑。

支气管炎、胃炎、胃卡他性炎等表现为湿痰证者，可用本方加减治疗。

【方解】方中半夏辛温性燥，善燥湿化痰，且可降逆和胃而止呕，为主药。橘红理气燥湿，使气顺而痰消，为辅药。茯苓健脾渗湿；生姜降逆化饮，既可制半夏之毒，又能助半夏、橘红行

as adjuvant drugs. No.4, as a guiding drug, coordinates the effects of the other drugs, moistens the lung and regulates the stomach.

Modern researches have proved that the recipe has the effects of strengthening the stomach to arrest vomiting, eliminating phlegm to relieve cough and preventing and treating ulcers.

CAUTIONS: The recipe belongs to pungent and drying prescriptions, therefore, it is contraindicated in patients suffering from pulmonary tuberculosis with haemoptysis, sticky phlegm due to deficiency of *yin* and bloody phlegm.

Decoction for Clearing Away Gallbladder-heat

(Wendan Tang)

SOURCE: ***Prescriptions Assigned to the Three Categories of Pathogenic Factors of Diseases***

INGREDIENTS:

No. 1 Pinellia tuber, *Rhizoma Pinelliae* 6 g

No. 2 Bamboo shavings, *Caulis Bambusae in Taeniam* 6 g

No. 3 Fruit of immature citron, *Fructus Aurantii Immaturus* (powder-fried) 6 g

No. 4 Tangerine peel, *Pericarpium Citri Reticulatae* 9 g

No. 5 Prepared licorice root, *Radix Glycyrrhizae Praeparata* 5 g

No. 6 Tuckahoe, *Poria* 5 g

No. 7 Fresh ginger, *Rhizoma Zingiberis Recens* 5 pcs.

No. 8 Chinese-dates, *Fructus Ziziphi Jujubae* 1 pc.

DIRECTIONS: All the drugs are to be decocted in water for oral administration.

FUNCTIONS: Regulating the flow of *qi* and resolving phlegm, clearing away heat from gallbladder and regulating the stomach.

气消痰；复用少许乌梅收敛肺气，为佐药。甘草调和诸药，兼润肺和中，为使药。

现代研究证实，本方具有健胃止呕、祛痰止咳作用，尚能防治溃疡病。

【使用注意】 本方属辛燥之剂，凡肺痨咯血、阴虚燥痰、痰中带血者忌用。

温 胆 汤

【来源】 《三因极一病证方论》

【组成】 半夏、竹茹、枳实(面炒)各6克，陈皮9克，甘草(炙)3克，茯苓5克。

【用法】 生姜五片，大枣一枚，水煎服。

【功用】 理气化痰，清胆和胃。

INDICATIONS: Incoordination between the gallbladder and the stomach with stirring up of phlegm-heat marked by vertigo, vomiting, gastric discomfort with acid regurgitation, palpitation, insomnia due to vexation, epilepsy, bitter taste in the mouth, slight thirst, yellow greasy fur of the tongue, and slippery, rapid pulse or taut rapid pulse.

Disorder of vegetative nerve, menopausal syndrome, neurosism, cerebral arteriosclerosis and chronic gastritis marked by the symptoms of incoordination between the gallbladder and the stomach with stirring up of phlegm-heat can be treated by the modified recipe.

INTERPRETATION: No.1 in the recipe lowers adverse flow of *qi* to regulate the stomach, eliminates dampness to resolve phlegm, as a pricipal drug. No.2 clears away heat and resolves phlegm to arrest vomiting and relieve restlessness; No.3 promotes the circulation of *qi* to remove phlegm and renders phlegm to come downward with *qi*, used as an assistant drug. As adjuvant drugs, No.4 regulates *qi* to eliminate dampness, and No.6 strengthens the spleen to excrete dampness and get the dampness and phlegm cleared away. No.7, No.8 and No.5 tonify the spleen and regulate the stomach, coordinating the effects of other drugs in the recipe.

Modern researches have proved that the recipe has the effects of tranquilizing the mind, coordinating the functions of vegetative nerve and arresting vomiting.

CAUTIONS: Since it is a heat-clearing and phlegm-elimintaing one, the recipe is not indicated for insomnia due to deficiency of heart, palpitation due to deficiency of blood, vertigo due to deficiency of *yin*, vomiting due to cold of the stomach, etc.

【主治】 胆胃不和，痰热上扰证，表现为眩晕，呕吐，嘈杂，心悸，虚烦不眠，癫痫，口苦微渴，苔黄腻，脉滑数或弦数。

植物神经失调、更年期综合征、神经衰弱、脑动脉硬化病、慢性胃炎等表现为胆胃不和、痰热上扰证者，可用本方加减治疗。

【方解】 方中半夏降逆和胃，燥湿化痰，为主药。竹茹清热化痰，止呕除烦；枳实行气消痰，使痰随气下，为辅药。陈皮理气燥湿，茯苓健脾渗湿，使湿去痰消，为佐药。生姜、大枣、甘草益脾和胃而协调诸药。

现代研究证实，本方具有镇静、调整植物神经系统功能以及制吐等作用。

【使用注意】 本方为清热祛痰之剂，凡心虚失眠、血虚心悸、阴虚眩晕、胃寒呕吐等，均非所宜。

Section 2

Heat-clearing and Phlegm-eliminating Recipes

This group of recipes is mainly composed of heat-clearing and phlegm-eliminating drugs, effective in clearing and dissolving heat-phlegm. They are indicated for heat-phlegm syndrome.

Bolus for Clearing *Qi* and Phlegm

(Qingqi Huatan Wan)

SOURCE: ***Textual Research on Prescriptions***

INGREDIENTS:

No. 1 Trichosanthes seed, *Semen Trichosanthis* 30 g
No. 2 Tangerine peel, *Pericarpium Citri Reticulatae* 30 g
No. 3 Skullcap root, *Radix Scutellariae* 30 g
No. 4 Apricot kernel, *Semen Pruni Armentiacae* 30 g
No. 5 Fruit of immature citron, *Fructus Aurantii Immaturus* 30 g
No. 6 Tuckahoe, *Poria* 30 g
No. 7 Arisaema with bile, *Arisaema cum Bile* 45 g
No. 8 Pinellia tuber, *Rhizoma Pinelliae* 45 g

DIRECTIONS: The above drugs are mixed with ginger juice to make boluses. Take 6 g each time with warm boiled water.

FUNCTIONS: Clearing away heat, dissolving phlegm, regulating *qi* and relieving cough.

INDICATIONS: Stagnation of phlegm and heat in the lung marked by cough with thick yellowish sputum, fullness and stuffiness sensation in the chest and hypochondrium, rapid breath, nausea, vomiting, red tongue, yellowish greasy fur and

第二节　清热化痰剂

清热化痰剂主要由清热化痰药组成，有清化热痰作用，适用于热痰证。

清气化痰丸

【来源】《医方考》

【组成】瓜蒌仁、陈皮、黄芩、杏仁、枳实、茯苓各30克，胆南星、半夏各45克。

【用法】姜汁为丸，每服6克，温开水送下。

【功用】清热化痰，理气止咳。

【主治】痰热内结证，表现为咳嗽痰黄，粘稠难咯，胸膈痞满，甚则气急呕恶，舌质红，苔黄腻，脉滑数。

slippery and rapid pulse.

Chronic bronchitis, pneumonia marked by the syndrome of stagnation of phlegm and heat in the lung can be treated with the recipe.

INTERPRETATION: No.7, with a bitter taste and cold nature and effective in clearing heat and resolving phlegm, is indicated for obstruction due to phlegm and fire of excess type, used as a principal drug in the recipe. As assistant drugs, No.3 and No.1 purge lung-fire, resovle heat-phlegm, strengthen the effect of No.7; and No.5 and No.2 keep the adverse *qi* flowing downward and relieve flatulence, clear away phlegm and remove obstruction. No.6 strengthens the spleen to remove dampness, No.4 smooths circulation of lung-*qi* and No.8 eliminats dampness to resolve phlegm, all as adjuvant drugs.

Modern researhes have proved that the recipe has the heat-clearing, antibacterial, phlegm-eliminating, cough-relieving and asthma-relieving effects.

CAUTIONS: It is contraindicated in patients with cold-phlegm syndrome and sticky-phlegm syndrome.

Section 3

Recipes for Moistening the Dryness and Resolving Phlegm

The recipe is mainly composed of drugs for moistening the lung and resolving phlegm. It is indicated for sticky-phlegm syndrome.

Powder of Fritillary Bulb and Snakegourd Fruit

(Beimu Gualou San)

SOURCE: ***Medicine Comprehended***

慢性气管炎、肺炎表现为痰热内结证者，可用本方治疗。

【方解】 方中胆南星味苦性凉，清热化痰，治实痰实火之壅闭，为主药。黄芩、瓜蒌仁降肺火，化热痰，助胆星之力；枳实、陈皮下气开痞，消痰散结，为辅药。茯苓健脾渗湿，杏仁宣利肺气，半夏燥湿化痰，为佐药。

现代研究证实，本方具有解热、抗菌、祛痰、镇咳及平喘作用。

【使用注意】 寒痰、燥痰皆禁用。

第三节　润燥化痰剂

润燥化痰剂主要由润肺化痰药组成，适用于燥痰证。

贝母瓜蒌散

【来源】 《医学心悟》

INGREDIENTS:

No. 1 Fritillary bulb, *Bulbus Fritillariae* 5 g

No. 2 Snakegourd fruit, *Fructus Trichosanthis* 3 g

No. 3 Root of trichosanthes, *Radix Trichosanthis* 2 g

No. 4 Tuckahoe, *Poria* 2 g

No. 5 Tangerine peel, *Exocarpium Citri Reticulatae* 2 g

No. 6 Root of Balloonflower, *Radix Platycodi* 2 g

DIRECTIONS: All the drugs should be decocted in water for oral administration.

FUNCTIONS: Nourishing the lung and clearing away heat, regulating *qi* and resoving phlegm.

INDICATIONS: Cough due to dryness of the lung marked by difficulty in expectoration, dryness of the throat, dyspnea, etc.

Chronic bonchitis marked by cough due to dryness of the lung can be treated by the modified recipe.

INTERPRETATION: As a principal drug, No.1 clears away heat and nourishes the lung, resolves phlegm to arrest cough and dispels the stagnation of phlegm and *qi*. No.2 clears away heat and moistens the dryness, regulates *qi* and removes phlegm, and dispels obstruction of *qi* in the chest, used as an asistant drug. No.3 clears heat to resolve sputum, promotes the production of body fluids to moisten dryness. No.4 strengthens the spleen and induces diuresis to inhibit phlegm-producing sources; No.5 regulates *qi* to resolve phlegm, gets the *qi* flowing normally and phlegm cleared away; No.6 disperses the functional disturbance of the lung-*qi*.

Modern researhes have proved that the recipe has the effects of dilating the bronchi, enhancing the secretion of the mucosa of the respiratory tract and the effects of eliminating phlegm and relieving inflammation.

CAUTIONS: Flaring up of deficiency-fire type due to the deficiency of kidney-*yin* marked by cough, dryness of throat, flushing of zygomatic region, night sweat and other symptoms

【组成】 贝母5克，瓜蒌3克，天花粉、茯苓、橘红、桔梗各2克。

【用法】 水煎服。

【功用】 润肺清热，理气化痰。

【主治】 肺燥咳嗽证，表现为咯痰不利，咽喉干燥，上气喘促等。

慢性支气管炎表现为肺燥咳嗽证者，可用本方加减治疗。

【方解】 方中贝母清热润肺，化痰止咳，开痰气之郁结，为主药。瓜蒌清热润燥，理气涤痰，通胸膈之痹塞，为辅药。天花粉清热化痰，且可生津润燥；茯苓健脾利湿，以杜绝生痰之源；橘红理气化痰，使气顺痰消；桔梗宣利肺气。

现代研究证实，本方具有扩张支气管、增强呼吸道粘膜分泌以及祛痰、消炎等作用。

【使用注意】 肾阴不足，虚火上炎而见咳嗽、咽干、颧红、

should be treated with the drugs nourishing *yin* and purging the fire other than this recipe.

Section 4

Recipes for Warming the Lung to Resolve Cold Phlegm

This group of recipes is mainly composed of drugs for warming the lung to resolve phlegm. They are indicated for cold phlegm syndrome.

Decoction of Poria, Licorice, Schisandra, Dried Ginger and Asarum

(Ling Gan Wuwei Jiang Xin Tang)

SOURCE: ***Synopsis of Prescription of the Golden Chamber***

INGREDIENTS:

No. 1 Tuckahoe, *Poria* 12 g
No. 2 Licorice root, *Radix Glycyrrhizae* 6 g
No. 3 Dried ginger, *Rhizoma Zingiberis* 9 g
No. 4 Wild ginger (whole plant), *Herba Asari* 6 g
No. 5 Fruit of Chinese magnolia vine, *Fructus Schisandrae* 6 g

DIRECTIONS: All the drugs should be decocted in water for oral administration.

FUNCTIONS: Warming the lung to reduce phlegm-fluid retention.

INDICATIONS: The phlegm-fluid retention syndrome of cold type marked by cough with copious whitish thin sputum, discomfort in the chest, whitish and moist fur and taut and slippery pulse.

盗汗等证，宜滋阴降火，不宜用本方。

第四节　温化寒痰剂

温化寒痰剂主要由温肺化痰药组成，适用于寒痰证。

苓甘五味姜辛汤

【来源】《金匮要略》

【组成】茯苓12克，甘草6克，干姜9克，细辛6克，五味子6克。

【用法】水煎服。

【功用】温肺化饮。

【主治】寒饮内停证，表现为咳嗽痰多，清稀色白，胸膈不快，舌苔白滑，脉弦滑。

Chronic bronchitis, bronchial asthma and other diseases marked by the above syndrome can be treated by the modified recipe.

INTERPRETATION: No. 3, with a pungent flavor and a hot nature, can not only warm the lung and expel cold to remove phlegm-fluid retention but also warm and activate the spleen-*yang* to eliminate dampness, used as a principal drug. As assistant drugs, No. 4, with a pungent flavor and a dispersing effect, warms the lung to expel cold, assists No. 3 in resolving the cold retention of phlegm-fluid, and No. 1 ,which is sweet and insipid, strengthens the spleen to excrete diuresis. No. 5 astringes the lung-*qi* to arrest cough and when used in combination with No.4 can yield both the expelling and astringing effects, expelling without damaging the body resistance while astringing without retaining the pathogenic factors.

Modern researches have proved that the recipe has the effects of eliminating phlegm, relieving cough and allaying dyspnea.

CAUTIONS: The recipe belongs to pungent, warm, dry and heat prescriptions, it is contraindicated in patients with cough due to lung-heat, lung-dryness, deficiency of *yin*, phlegm-fire and pulmonary tuberculosis.

Decoction of Three Kinds of Seed for the Aged

(Sanzi Yangqin Tang)

SOURCE: ***Han's Book on Medicine***

INGREDIENTS:

No. 1 White mustard seed, *Semen Sinapis Albae* 6 g

No. 2 Perilla fruit, *Fructus Perillae* 9 g

No. 3 Radish seed, *Semen Raphani* 9 g

DIRECTIONS: All the drugs should be decocted in water for oral administration.

慢性支气管炎、支气管哮喘等表现为寒饮内停证者，可用本方加减治疗。

【方解】 方中干姜辛热，既温肺散寒以化饮，又温运脾阳以祛湿，为主药。细辛辛散，温肺散寒，助干姜散寒饮；茯苓甘淡，健脾渗湿，为辅药。五味子敛肺气而止咳，与细辛相配，一散一收，散不伤正，收不留邪。

现代研究证实，本方具有祛痰、镇咳、改善呼吸困难等作用。

【使用注意】 本方为辛温燥热之剂，肺热、肺燥、阴虚、痰火、肺痨所致之咳嗽，均非所宜。

三子养亲汤

【来源】《韩氏医通》

【组成】 白芥子6克，苏子9克，莱菔子9克。

【用法】 水煎服。

FUNCTIONS: Sending down the abnormally ascending *qi* to relieve the discomfort in the chest, and resolving phlegm and promoting digestion.

INDICATIONS: Stagnation of phlegm and *qi* marked by cough, dyspnea, abundant expectoration and feeling of stuffiness in the chest, poor appetite and dyspepsia, whitish greasy tongue fur and slippery pulse.

Chronic bronchitis, bronchiectasis, bronchial asthma, pulmonary emphysema, cardiac asthma and other diseases marked by the syndrome of stagnation of phlegm and *qi* can be treated by the modified recipe.

INTERPRETATION: No. 1 in the recipe warms the lung and promotes the flow of *qi*, relieves chest discomfort and resolves phlegm. No. 2 lowers the adverse flow of *qi* and removes phlegm to arrest cough and relieve asthma. No. 3 promotes digestion to remove food stagnancy, and promotes the circulation of *qi* to eliminate phlegm.

Modern researches have proved that the recipe has the effects of eliminating phlegm, relieving cough and dyspnea, inducing diuresis, promoting gastrointestinal peristalsis and digestive and absorptive functions.

CAUTIONS: When effective result is obtained after administration, the cause of the disease should be taken into consideration in the treatment.

Section 5

Recipes for Dispelling Wind-phlegm

This group of recipes is fit for the treatment of wind-phlegm syndrome, which can be divided into endogenous type and exopathic type. Exopathic wind-phlegm syndrome

【功用】 降气快膈，化痰消食。

【主治】 痰壅气滞证，表现为咳嗽喘逆，痰多胸痞，食少难消，舌苔白腻，脉滑等。

慢性支气管炎、支气管扩张、支气管哮喘、肺气肿、心脏性哮喘等表现为痰壅气滞证者，可用本方加减治疗。

【方解】 方中白芥子温肺利气，快膈消痰；苏子降气行痰，止咳平喘；莱菔子消食导滞，行气祛痰。

现代研究证实，本方具有祛痰、镇咳、改善呼吸困难、利尿促进蠕动、增强消化吸收等作用。

【使用注意】 服后得效，应兼顾其本。

第五节 治风化痰剂

治风化痰剂适用于风痰证。风痰为病，有内外之分。外风生痰，由外感风邪，肺气不宣，痰浊内生所致。治宜疏风化痰，常

is caused by the stagnation of phlegm in the chest resulting from the obstruction of lung-*qi* due to the affection of exopathic wind pathogens, so it should be treated by the recipe composed of the drugs for dispelling pathogenic wind and the drugs for resolving phlegm. Its typical recipe is Cough Powder. Endogenous wind-phlegm syndrome is caused by up-stirring of liver-wind with stagnated phlegm, so it should be treated by the recipe composed of the drugs for calming liver-wind and those for resolving phlegm, the typical recipe being Decoction of Pinellia, Bighead Atractylodes and Gastrodia.

Decoction of Pinellia, Bighead Atractylodes and Gastrodia

(Banxia Baizhu Tianma Tang)

SOURCE: *Medicine Comprehended*

INGREDIENTS:

No. 1 Pinellia tuber, *Rhizoma Pinelliae* 9 g

No. 2 Gastrodia tuber, *Rhizoma Gastrodiae* 6 g

No. 3 Tuckahoe, *Poria* 6 g

No. 4 Tangerine peel, *Pericarpium Citri Reticulatae* 6 g

No. 5 Bighead atractylodes rhizome, *Rhizoma Atractylodis Macrocephalae* 15 g

No. 6 Licorice root, *Radix Glycyrrhizae* 4 g

No. 7 Fresh ginger, *Rhizoma Zingiberis Recens* 1 pc.

No. 8 Chinese-dates, *Fructus Ziziphi Jujubae* 2 pcs.

DIRECTIONS: All the drugs are to be decocted in water for oral administration.

FUNCTIONS: Drying dampness to resolve phlegm, calming the liver to tranquilize the endogenous wind.

INDICATIONS: Up-stirring of wind-phlegm marked by dizziness, headache, feeling of oppression in the chest, nausea,

用宣散风邪药与化痰药配伍成方，代表方为止嗽散。内风挟痰，多因素有痰浊，肝风内动，挟痰上扰所致，治宜熄风化痰，常用平肝熄风药与化痰药配伍组方，代表方为半夏白术天麻汤。

半夏白术天麻汤

【来源】 《医学心悟》

【组成】 半夏 9 克，天麻、茯苓、橘红各 6 克，白术15克，甘草 4 克。

【用法】 生姜一片，大枣二枚，水煎服。

【功用】 燥湿化痰，平肝熄风。

【主治】 风痰上扰证，表现为眩晕头痛，胸闷呕恶，舌苔白

vomiting, whitish and greasy tongue fur, taut and slippery pulse, etc.

Aural vertigo, functional disturbance of vegetative nerve, cerebral arteriosclerosis, chronic gastroenteritis, vestibular neuritis, cerebrovascular accident and other disorders marked by the syndrome of up-stirring of wind-phlegm can be treated by the modified recipe.

INTERPRETATION: No. 1 in the recipe eliminates dampness to resolve phlegm, and lowers the adverse flow of *qi* to arrest vomiting. No. 2 resolves phlegm and calms endopathic wind to relieve vertigo. The combined use of the two drugs plays a very important role in the treatment of vertigo with headache due to wind-phlegm syndrome. They are principal drugs. No. 5, as an assistant drug, reinforces the spleen to eliminate dampness, and when combined with No. 1 and No.2, it can eliminate dampness to resolve sputum. No.3 strengthens the spleen to excrete dampness; No. 4 regulates *qi* to resolve phlegm; No. 7 and No. 8 regulate *ying* and *wei*, all acting as adjuvant drugs. No. 6 regulates the stomach and coordinates the effects of the other drugs as a guiding drug.

CAUTIONS: The recipe has warming, drying and wind-calming effects, so it is not fit for the treatment of dizziness or headache caused by up-stirring of the liver-*yang*, hyperactivity of the liver-*yang*, hyperactive liver-*qi* due to deficiency of liver-*yin*, and deficiency of both liver-*yin* and kidney-*yin*.

Cough Powder

(Zhisou San)

SOURCE: ***Medicine Comprehended***

INGREDIENTS:

No. 1 Balloonflower root, *Radix Platycodi* (parched) 1000 g
No. 2 Schizonepeta, *Herba Schizonepetae* 1000 g
No. 3 Tatarian aster root, *Radix Asteris* (steamed) 1000 g

腻，脉弦滑等。

耳源性眩晕、植物神经失调、脑动脉硬化病、慢性胃肠炎、前庭神经炎、脑血管意外等表现为风痰上扰证者，可用本方加减治疗。

【方解】 方中半夏燥湿化痰，降逆止呕；天麻化痰熄风而止头眩；二者合用，为治风痰眩晕头痛之要药，为主药。白术健脾燥湿，与半夏、天麻配伍，祛湿化痰，为辅药。茯苓健脾渗湿；橘红理气化痰；姜枣调和营卫，为佐药。甘草和中而调药性，为使药。

【使用注意】 本方属温燥熄风之剂，凡肝阳上扰、肝阳上亢、阴虚肝旺、肝肾阴虚所致之眩晕、头痛，皆非所宜。

止 嗽 散

【来源】《医学心悟》

【组成】 桔梗(炒)、荆芥、紫菀(蒸)，百部(蒸)、白前(蒸)

No. 4 Stemona tuber, *Radix Stemonae* (steamed) 1000 g

No. 5 Swallowwort rhizome, *Rhizoma Cynanchi Vincetoxici* 1000 g

No. 6 Prepared licorice root, *Radix Glycyrrhizae Praeparata* (parched) 375 g

No. 7 Tangerine peel, *Pericarpium Citri Reticulatae* 500 g

DIRECTIONS: Grind the above drugs into fine powder. Take 6 grams each time with warm boiled water or with ginger juice. The drugs can also be decocted in water for oral use, with the dosage reduced proportionally according to the original recipe.

FUNCTIONS: Arresting cough and resolving phlegm, and inducing diaphoresis and ventilating the lung.

INDICATIONS: Attack of pathogenic wind on the lung marked by cough, itching throat, slight chills and fever, white and thin tongue fur, etc.

The common cold, influenza, bronchitis, attack of chronic bronchitis, pulmonary tuberculosis and others marked by the symptoms of attack of pathogenic wind on the lung can be treated by the modified recipe.

INTERPRETATION: No. 3, No. 4 and No.5 arrest cough and resolve phlegm. No. 1 and No. 7 facilitate and check the flow of lung-*qi* to arrest cough and resolve phlegm. No. 2 expels wind and induces diaphoresis while No. 6 coordinates the effects of the other drugs, and the combined use of the two drugs with No. 1 can relieve sore throat more effectively.

Modern researches have proved that the recipe has relatively curative effects of relieving cough and eliminating phlegm, not to mention its effects of inducing diaphoresis and clearing away heat.

CAUTIONS: Phthisical cough due to *yin* deficiency should not be treated with this recipe. Cough due to lung-heat and phlegm-fire must be treated with the recipe very carefully.

各1000克，甘草(炒)375克，陈皮500克。

【用法】 共为末，每服6克，温开水或姜汤送下。亦可水煎服，用量按原方比例酌减。

【功用】 止咳化痰，疏表宣肺。

【主治】 风邪犯肺证，表现为咳嗽咽痒，或微有恶寒发热，舌苔薄白等。

感冒、流行性感冒、支气管炎、慢性支气管炎发作、肺结核等表现为风邪犯肺证者，可用本方加减治疗。

【方解】 方中紫菀、百部、白前止咳化痰；桔梗、橘红（陈皮去白）宣降肺气，止咳消痰；荆芥祛风解表，甘草调和诸药，二者与桔梗配合，更能清利咽喉。

现代研究证实，本方镇咳、祛痰作用较强，也有发汗、解热效果。

【使用注意】 阴虚劳嗽者不宜使用；肺热或痰火咳嗽，亦宜慎用。

Chaper XVI

Dampness-eliminating Prescriptions

Those mainly composed of dampness-eliminating drugs, functioning in dispelling dampness and promoting diuresis, treating stranguria and turbid urine and for the treatment of damp diseases are generally known as dampness-eliminating prescriptions.

Damp disease is caused either by attack of pathogenic dampness from the exterior or by retention of dampness due to functional disturbance in fluid transport. If exopathic dampness attacks the superficial channels and collaterals, the patients will have such symptoms as chills, fever, feeling of fullness in the head, heavy sensation in the body or arthroncus and limited movement of the joints; while endogenous dampness affects the spleen, lung, kidney and tri-warmer, causing dysfunction of the urinary bladder in micturition, which leads to drainage disturbance of fluid and dampness, as a result, retention of fluid and phlegm or edema will occur. But since the superficial channels and collaterals, and the *zang*-and-*fu* organs, the exterior and the interior, are interrelated, exopathic dampness can transmit inwards to the *zang*-and-*fu* organs, and endogenous dampness can transmit outwards to the superficial muscle and skin, in other words, exopathic and endogenous dampness can influence each other in causing diseases.

Pathogenic dampness often causes illness in combination either with pathogenic wind, cold, summer-heat or heat. The human bodies differ in deficiency and excess, sturdiness and weakness. The affected parts differ in the upper

第十六章

祛 湿 剂

凡以祛湿药物为主组成，具有化湿利水、通淋泄浊等作用，治疗水湿病证的一类方剂，统称为祛湿剂。

湿邪为病，有从外袭，有自内生。如外湿侵犯肌表经络，则见恶寒发热，头胀身重，或关节肿胀，屈伸不利；内湿则影响脾肺肾三焦，膀胱气化不行，致使水湿排泄障碍，停聚为饮、为痰、为肿。然肌表与脏腑，表里相关，表湿可以内传脏腑，里湿亦可外溢肌肤，故外湿内湿，亦可相兼为病。

湿邪为病，常有风、寒、暑、热相兼，人体有虚实强弱之别，所犯部位又有上下表里之分，病情亦有寒化、热化之异。因此，

and the lower, the exterior and the interior, and the diseases also differ in cold-transformation and heat-transformation. Therefore, pathogenic dampness in the upper and exterior parts of the body can be dispelled by inducing slight diaphoresis, pathogenic dampness in the lower and interior parts of the body can be removed by means of aromatic, bitter, and desiccant drugs, or removed by means of sweet, insipid, and diuretic drugs. Cold syndrome should be treated by warming the *yang* and dispersing dampness; heat syndrome should be treated by clearing away heat and eliminating dampness; debilitated patients with excessive dampness should be treated by both dispelling dampness and strengthening the body resistance. Therefore the dampness-eliminating prescriptions can be divided into the following five kinds.

Section 1

Recipes for Eilminating Dampness and Regulating the Stomach

This group of recipes is mainly composed of drugs bitter in taste, warm in nature, with dampness-eliminating effect and aromatics with turbid-dispelling effect, suitable for the treatment of wind-cold syndrome caused by exopathogen with damp stagnancy due to internal injury.

Peptic Powder

(Pingwei San)

SOURCE: ***Prescription of Peaceful Benevolent Dispensary***

INGREDIENTS:

No. 1 Atractylodes rhizome, *Rhizoma Atractylodis* (rough bark

祛湿之法，大抵湿邪在上在外者，可表散微汗以解之；在内在下者，可芳香苦燥以化之，或甘淡渗利以除之；从寒化者，宜温阳化湿；从热化者，宜清热祛湿；体虚湿盛者，又当祛湿扶正兼顾。祛湿剂可分以下五类。

第一节　燥湿和胃剂

燥湿和胃剂主要由苦温燥湿与芳香化浊药物组成，适用于外感风寒、内伤湿滞证。

平　胃　散

【来源】 《太平惠民和剂局方》

【组成】 苍术(去粗皮，米泔浸二日)15克，厚朴(去粗皮，姜

discarded, soaked in rice-washed water for two days) 15 g

No. 2 Magnolia bark, *Cortex Magnoliae Officinalis* (bark removed, ginger juice prepared, fried) 9 g

No. 3 Tangerine peel, *Pericarpium Citri Reticulatae* 9 g

No. 4 Licorice root, *Radix Glycyrrhizae* (fried) 4 g

DIRECTIONS: Grind the above drugs into fine powder Take 3 to 5 grams each time with the decoction of fresh ginger and Chinese-dates; or decoct them in water for oral adiministration.

FUNCTIONS: Drying dampness and strengthening the spleen, promoting the circulation of *qi* and regulating the stomach.

INDICATIONS: Stagnancy of dampness in the stomach and spleen marked by feeling of fullness in the abdomen, anorexia, tastelessness, nausea, vomiting, eructation, acid regurgitation, heavy sensation of the body, lassitude and sleepiness, frequent diarrhea, white, greasy and thick tongue fur and slow pulse.

Acute gastroenteritis, catarrhal gastritis, gastrointestinal neurosis and acute indigestion marked by the syndrome of stagnancy of dampness in the stomach and spleen can be treated by the modified recipe.

INTERPRETATION: No. 1, used in large dosage as a principal drug, dispels dampness to promote the function of the spleen. No. 2 promotes the circulation of *qi* and eliminates dampness to relieve distension and fullness in the abdomen, acting as an assistant drug. No 3 regulates *qi* and eliminates dampness, as an adjuvant drug. No. 4, sweet in taste and mild in nature, regulates the stomach and coordinates the effects of the other drugs in the recipe. Fresh ginger and Chinese-dates regulate the functions of the spleen and the stomach.

Modern researches have proved that the recipe has the effects of regulating gastrointestinal function and eliminating

汁制，炒香)、陈皮(去白)各9克，甘草(炒)4克。

【用法】 共为细末，每服3～5克，姜、枣煎汤送下；或作汤剂水煎服。

【功用】 燥湿健脾，行气和胃。

【主治】 脾胃湿滞证，表现为脘腹胀满，不思饮食，口淡无味，呕吐恶心，嗳气吞酸，肢体沉重，怠惰嗜卧，常多自利，舌苔白腻而厚，脉缓。

急性胃肠炎、胃卡他性炎症、胃肠神经官能症、急性消化不良等表现为脾胃湿滞证者，可用本方加减治疗。

【方解】 方中苍术重用除湿运脾，为主药。厚朴行气化湿，消胀除满，为辅药。陈皮理气化湿，为佐药。甘草甘缓和中，调和诸药；生姜、大枣调和脾胃。

现代研究证实，本方可调整胃肠机能、祛除多余的水分。

excessive water from the body.

CAUTIONS: The recipe, bitter in taste, pungent in flavor, warm and dry in nature, tends to consume *yin* and blood. Therefore, it is contraindicated in patients suffering from deficiency of the spleen without dampness or patients with deficiency-*yin* marked by red tongue with little fur, bitter taste in the mouth with thirst or rapid pulse.

Powder of Agastachis for Restoring Health

(Huoxiang Zhengqi San)

SOURCE: ***Prescription of Peaceful Benevolent Dispensary***

INGREDIENTS:

No. 1 Shell of areca nut, *Pericarpium Arecae* 30 g
No. 2 Dahurian angelica root, *Radix Angelicae Dahuricae* 30 g
No. 3 Leaf of purple perilla, *Folium Perillae* 30 g
No. 4 Tuckahoe, *Poria* 30 g
No. 5 Pinellia tuber, *Rhizoma Pinelliae* 60 g
No. 6 Bighead atractylodes rhizome, *Rhizoma Atractylodis Macrocephalae* 60 g
No. 7 Tangerine peel, *Perticarpium Citri Reticulatae* 60 g
No. 8 Magnolia bark, *Cortex Magnoliae Officinalis* (bark removed, ginger-juice-fried) 60 g
No. 9 Root of balloonflower, *Radix Platycodi* 60 g
No.10 Wrinkled gianthyssop, *Herba Agastachis* 90 g
No.11 Prepared licorice root, *Radix Glycyrrhizae Praeparata* 75 g

DIRECTIONS: Grind the drugs into fine powder. Take 6 grams each time with decoction of fresh ginger and Chinese-dates, or decoct them in water for oral administration.

FUNCTIONS: Relieving exterior syndrome, eliminating dampness and regulating *qi* and the stomach.

INDICATIONS: Vomiting and diarrhea due to exterior

【使用注意】 本方苦辛温燥，易耗伤阴血，故脾虚无湿或阴虚之人，症见舌红少苔，口苦而渴或脉数者忌用。

藿香正气散

【来源】《太平惠民和剂局方》

【组成】 大腹皮、白芷、紫苏、茯苓各30克，半夏曲、白术、陈皮(去白)、厚朴(去粗皮、姜汁炒)，苦桔梗各60克，藿香90克，甘草(炙)75克。

【用法】 共为细末，每服6克，姜、枣煎汤送服，或作汤剂水煎服。

【功用】 解表化湿，理气和中。

【主治】 表寒里湿吐泻证，表现为恶寒发热，头痛，胸脘满

cold with interior dampness marked by chills, fever, headache, fullness sensation and oppressed feeling in the chest and abdomen, vomiting, diarrhea, borborygmus and abdominal pain, and thick and greasy tongue fur.

The common cold of gastrointestinal type, influenza, acute gastroenteritis, gastroduodenal ulcer, chronic colitis, food poisoning, epidemic parotitis and other diseases belonging to exterior cold with endogenous dampness can be treated with the modified recipe.

INTERPRETATION: No.10 is administered in large dosage as a principal drug, with a pungent flavor and aromatic smell. It can not only dispel wind-cold but also expel the turbid pathogen and regulate the stomach to arrest vomiting; meanwhile it can send up the lucid *qi* and send down the turbid, clear away summer-heat and filthy pathogens. No. 3 and No.2, pungent in flavor, aromatic in smell and effective in dispersing exopathogens, assist No.10 in dispersing wind and cold from the body surface and eliminate dampness concurrently by means of its aroma. No. 5 and No. 7 dry dampness and regulate the stomach, lower the adverse flow of *qi* to arrest vomiting. No. 6 and No. 4 strengthen the spleen and the stomach and regulate the middle-warmer to arrest diarrhea. No. 1 and No. 8 promote the circulation of *qi*, dispel dampness, regulate the middle-warmer to relieve fullness sensation in the abdomen. No. 9, which can facilitate the flow of the lung-*qi* and relieve fullness in the chest and hypochondrium, is helpful in dispersing dampness as well as in relieving the exterior syndrome. Fresh ginger, Chinese-dates and No. 11 regulate the functions of the spleen and the stomach and coordinate the effects of the other drugs in the recipe.

Modern researches have proved that the recipe has better effects of regulating gastrointestinal function, arresting vomiting and diarrhea and reinforcing the stomach; meanwhile, it has the effects of inducing diaphoresis, allaying fever, relieving

闷，呕吐，腹泻，肠鸣腹痛，舌苔厚腻。

胃肠型感冒、流行性感冒、急性胃肠炎、胃及十二指肠溃疡、慢性结肠炎、食物中毒、流行性腮腺炎等证属表寒里湿者，可用本方加减治疗。

【方解】 方中藿香重用，既能辛散风寒，又可芳香化浊，和胃止呕，且兼升清降浊，解暑辟秽，为主药。配以苏叶、白芷辛香发散，助藿香外解风寒，兼可芳香化浊。半夏、陈皮燥湿和胃降逆止呕。白术、茯苓健运脾胃，和中止泻。大腹皮、厚朴行气化湿，畅中除满。桔梗宣肺利膈，既利于解表，又益于化湿。生姜、大枣、甘草调和脾胃，且调和药性。

现代研究证实，本方调整胃肠机能、制吐、止泻、健胃等作用较强，且具有发汗、解热、镇痛、抗菌、抗病毒、祛痰、镇咳、

pain, resisting bacteria and virus, eliminating phlegm, relieving cough, inducing diuresis.

CAUTIONS:

1. Since mainly composed of pungent, aromatic, warm-natured and desiccant drugs, the recipe is contraindicated in patients with excessive fire due to deficiency of *yin*. In addition, patients with thirst and yellow and greasy tongue fur should use the recipe with great care.

2. When used in the form of decoction, the drugs should be decocted for a shorter time to prevent the decrease in effect.

Section 2

Heat-clearing and Dampness-eliminating Recipes

This kind of recipes is mainly composed of heat-clearing and dampness-drying drugs, indicated for dampness-heat syndrome.

Oriental Wormwood Decoction

(Yinchenhao Tang)

SOURCE: ***Treatise on Febrile Diseases***

INGREDIENTS:

No. 1 Oriental wormwood, *Herba Artemisiae Capillaris* 30 g
No. 2 Capejasmine fruit, *Fructus Gardeniae* 15 g
No. 3 Rhubarb, *Radix et Rhizoma Rhei* 9 g

DIRECTIONS: All the above drugs are to be decocted in water for oral administration.

FUNCTIONS: Clearing away heat and eliminating dampness to treat jaundice.

INDICATIONS: Jaundice due to damp-heat characterized by bright yellow coloration of the skin and eyes, slight fullness

利尿等作用。

【使用注意】

1. 本方药多辛香温燥，阴虚火旺者忌用；若口渴而苔黄腻者慎用。

2. 作汤剂，不宜久煎，以免药性耗散，影响疗效。

第二节 清热祛湿剂

清热祛湿剂主要由清热利湿药组成，适用于湿热证。

茵陈蒿汤

【来源】《伤寒论》

【组成】茵陈30克，栀子15克，大黄9克。

【用法】水煎服。

【功用】清热，利湿，退黄。

【主治】湿热黄疸证，表现为一身面目俱黄，黄色鲜明，腹

sensation in the abdomen, thirst, disturbance in urination, yellow and greasy tongue fur and deep and rapid pulse.

Patients with acute infectious icteric hepatitis, cholecystitis, cholelithiasis and acute pancreatitis marked by the syndrome of jaundice due to damp-heat can be treated by the modified recipe.

INTERPRETATION: No. 1 in the recipe is used in large dosage as a principal drug to clear away heat and dampness for the treatment of jaundice. No. 2 removes obstruction in the tri-warmer, guides dampness and heat downward and eliminates dampness and heat through urination, as an assistant drug. No. 3 purges away heat, removes blood stasis and relieves constipation, as an adjuvant drug.

Modern researches have proved that the recipe is effective in normalizing the function of the gallbladder, nourishing the liver, allaying fever, relieving inflammation and inducing diuresis and has, in addition, the purgative, antibacterial, antiviral and bleeding-arresting effects.

CAUTIONS: The recipe is contraindicated in patients with jaundice of *yin* type.

Decoction of Three Kinds of Kernel

(Sanren Tang)

SOURCE: ***Treatise on Differentiation and Treatment of Epidemic Febrile Diseases***

INGREDIENTS:

No. 1 Bitter apricot kernel, *Semen Armeniacae Amarum* 15 g
No. 2 Talc, *Talcum* 18g
No. 3 Rice-paper pith, *Tetrapanacis* 6 g
No. 4 Round cardamon seed, *Semen Amoni Cardamoni* 6 g
No. 5 Lophatherum, *Herba Lophatheri* 6 g
No. 6 Magnolia bark, *Cortex Magnoliae Officinalis* 6 g
No. 7 Coix seed, *Semen Coicis* 18 g

微满，口中渴，小便不利，舌苔黄腻，脉沉数。

急性传染性黄疸型肝炎、胆囊炎、胆石症、急性胰腺炎等表现为湿热黄疸症者，可用本方加减治疗。

【方解】 方中茵陈重用清热利湿，退黄，为主药。栀子通利三焦，导湿热下行，引湿热自小便出，为辅药。大黄泻热逐瘀，通利大便，为佐药。

现代研究证实，本方具有利胆、保肝、解热、消炎、利尿、泻下、抗菌、抗病毒、止血等作用。

【使用注意】 阴黄证不宜使用。

三 仁 汤

【来源】 《温病条辨》

【组成】 杏仁 15 克，飞滑石 18 克，白通草 6 克，白蔻仁 6

No. 8 Pinellia tuber, *Rhizoma Pinelliae* 10 g

FUNCTIONS: Promoting the functional activities of *qi* and eliminating dampness and heat.

INDICATIONS: Initial stage of infectious febrile disease due to dampness and heat marked by headache, chills, pain and heavy sensation of the body, slight yellow complexion, fullness in the chest and anorexia, afternoon fever, white fur, absence of thirst, and taut, thready and feeble pulse.

Acute gastroenteritis, acute hepatitis, influenza, pyelitis, typhoid fever and other cases related to the above syndrome with more dampness than heat can be treated by the modified recipe.

INTERPRETATION: No. 1 facilitates the flow of lung-*qi* in the upper-warmer. No. 4, as an aromatic, dispels dampness and promotes the circulation of *qi* to remove the stagnation in the middle-warmer. No.7, sweet in taste and cold in nature, excretes dampness and heat to strengthen the spleen. No. 2, No. 3 and No. 5, sweet in taste, cold and bland in nature, strengthen the effects of excreting dampness and clearing heat. No. 8 and No. 6 can promote the circulation of *qi* to dispel dampness and relieve feeling of fullness in the upper abdomen.

Modern researches have proved that the recipe is effective in strengthening the actions of allaying fever, regulating the function of the stomach and intestine, arresting vomiting and diarrhea, inducing diuresis, relieving inflammation and resisting bacteria.

CAUTIONS: The recipe is contraindicated in patients with deficiency of *yin*-fluid, or fever due to *yin* deficiency. Damp-heat diseases with more manifestations of heat than dampness should be treated with great care.

Eight Health Restoring Powder

(Bazheng San)

SOURCE: ***Prescription of Peaceful Benevolent Dispensary***

克，竹叶6克，厚朴6克，生薏苡仁18克，半夏10克。

【功用】 宣畅气机，清利湿热。

【主治】 湿温初起，表现为头痛恶寒，身重疼痛，面色淡黄，胸闷不饥，午后身热，苔白不渴，脉弦细而濡。

急性胃肠炎、急性肝炎、流行性感冒、肾盂炎、肠伤寒等证属湿温初起、湿重热轻者，可用本方加减治疗。

【方解】 方中杏仁宣利上焦肺气；白蔻仁芳香化湿，行气宽中；薏苡仁甘淡性寒，渗利湿热而健脾；滑石、通草、竹叶甘寒淡渗，增强利湿清热之功；半夏、厚朴行气化湿，散结除痞。

现代研究证实，本方具有增强散热、调整胃肠、制吐、止泻、利尿、消炎、抗菌等作用。

【使用注意】 阴亏津少或阴虚发热者禁用。湿温病热重于湿者，慎用。

八 正 散

【来源】《太平惠民和剂局方》

INGREDIENTS:

No. 1 Plantain seed, *Semen Plantaginis* 500 g
No. 2 Chinese pink herb, *Herba Dianthi* 500 g
No. 3 Prostrate knotweed, *Herba Polygoni Avicularis* 500 g
No. 4 Talc, *Talcum* 500 g
No. 5 Capejasmine fruit, *Fructus Gardeniae* 500 g
No. 6 Prepared licorice root, *Radix Glycyrrhizae Praeparata* 500 g
No. 7 Fiveleaf akebia (stem), *Caulis Akebiae* 500 g
No. 8 Rhubarb, *Radix et Rhizoma Rhei* (coated with flour paste and then roasted, sliced after removal of the coat and then baked) 500 g
No. 9 Rush pith, *Medulla Junci* 3 g

DIRECTIONS: Grind the drugs into powder, and then decoct 6 to 9 grams of the powder and No. 9 with water until 70% of the water remains for oral use; or all the above drugs are directly decocted in water for oral use, with the dosage modified in proportion to the original recipe.

FUNCTIONS: Clearing away heat and purging fire, inducing diuresis for treating stranguria.

INDICATIONS: Stranguria due to dampness and heat marked by subjective sensation of spasmatic distension and fullness of the lower abdomen, distending pain in the loins and abdomen, dribbling urination, difficulty in micturition, cloudy and dark urine, frequent and urgent micturition or retention of urine, dryness of mouth and throat, red tongue with yellow fur, and slippery forcefull pulse.

Acute urethritis, cystitis, pyelitis, stone or infection in urinary system marked by stranguria due to dampness and heat can be treated with the modified recipe.

INTERPRETATION: No. 7, No. 4, No. 1, No. 2 and No. 3 induce diuresis for treating stranguria and clear away dampness and heat. No.5 purges dampness and heat from the tri-warmer. No. 8 clears away heat and purges fire. No. 9 promotes heat downward by inducing diuresis. No. 6 coordinates the effects

【组成】 车前子、瞿麦、萹蓄、滑石、山栀子仁、甘草(炙)、木通、大黄(面裹煨，去面切，焙)各500克。

【用法】 为散，每用6～9克，水一盏，入灯芯3克煎至七分，去滓温服；亦可作汤剂，水煎服，用量按原方比例酌情增减。

【功用】 清热泻火，利水通淋。

【主治】 湿热淋证，表现为小腹急结，腰腹胀痛，小便淋涩混赤，尿频尿急，甚或癃闭不通，口燥咽干，舌红苔黄，脉滑实

急性尿道炎、膀胱炎、肾盂炎、泌尿系结石、感染等表现为湿热淋证者，可用本方加减治疗。

【方解】 方中木通、滑石、车前子、瞿麦、萹蓄利水通淋，清利湿热；山栀仁清泻三焦湿热；大黄泄热降火；灯芯导热下行；

of the other drugs in the recipe and relieves spasm.

Modern researches have proved that the recipe has the effects of relieving inflammation and pain and allaying fever.

CAUTIONS: Bitter in taste and cold in nature, the recipe is indicated for stranguria. It is contraindicated in the debilitated and in pregnancy. In treating stranguria complicated by chyluria, stranguria induced by overstrain and stranguria caused by disorder of *qi*, great care should be taken.

Recipe No.II for Removing Gallstones

(Dandao Paishi Erhao Fang)

SOURCE: Qingdao Municipal Hospital

INGREDIENTS:

No. Lysimachia, *Herba Lysimachiae* 30 g

No. 2 Oriental wormwood, *Herba Artemisiae Capillaris* (to be decocted later) 30 g

No. 3 Curcuma root, *Radix Curcumae* 30 g

No. 4 Honeysuckle flower, *Flos Lonicerae* 30 g

No. 5 Forsythia fruit, *Fructus Forsythiae* 30 g

No. 6 Aucklandia root, *Radix Aucklandiae* 18 g

No. 7 Fruit of immature citron or trifoliate orange, *Fructus Aurantii Immaturus* 12 g

No. 8 Rhubarb, *Radix et Rhizoma Rhei* (to be decocted later) 30 g

No. 9 Mirabilite, *Natrii Sulphas* (taken after being infused in boiling water) 6 g

DIRECTIONS: All the drugs listed above should be decocted in water for oral administration.

FUNCTIONS: Clearing away heat, normalizing the function of the gallbladder, soothing the liver and regulating the circulation of *qi* to remove gallstones.

INDICATIONS: Cholelithiasis of damp-heat type marked by fever, pain in the right hypochondrium, fullness sensation in the abdomen, bitter taste, sticky mouth, dark urine, constipation, jaundice, red tongue with yellow and greasy fur, and taut,

甘草调和诸药，缓急。

现代研究证实，本方具有消炎、镇痛、解热等作用。

【使用注意】 本方苦寒通淋，若体虚者及孕妇忌用。膏淋、劳淋、气淋均宜慎用。

胆道排石II号方

【来源】 青岛市立医院方

【组成】 金钱草30克，茵陈蒿（后下）30克，郁金30克，金银花30克，连翘30克，木香18克，枳实12克，大黄（后下）30克，芒硝（冲服）6克。

【用法】 水煎，茵陈蒿后下，芒硝冲服。

【功用】 清热利胆，疏肝理气，排石。

【主治】 湿热型胆石症，表现为发热，右胁痛，腹满，口苦，

slippery rapid pulse.

Cholelithiasis, infection of the biliary tract and other diseases marked by the above-mentioned syndrome of damp-heat type can be treated by the modified recipe.

INTERPRETATION: As a principal drug, No. 1, sweet and salty in taste and cold in nature, produces the effects of clearing away heat and toxins, eliminating dampness-heat, subduing jaundice, and normalizing the functioning of the gallbladder to remove gallstones. No. 2, bitter in taste and slight cold in nature, clears away heat and dampness and normalizes the functional activities of the gallbladder for treating jaundice. No. 4 and No. 5 dispel heat and clear away toxins, assist No. 1 and No. 2 to normalize the functioning of the gallbladder and cure jaundice. No. 3, No. 6 and No. 7 regulate *qi*. No. 8 and No. 9 clear the bowels to purge fire and relieve constipation. All the above drugs assist No. 1 in normalizing the functioning of the gallbaldder and removing gallstones.

Modern researches have proved that the recipe has the effects of normalizing the function of the gallbladder, relieving inflammation and pain, relaxing Oddi's sphincter, contracting the gallbladder, removing gallstones, relieving constipation and inducing diuresis.

CAUTIONS: The recipe is contraindicated in pregnancy.

Recipe for Removing Urinary Tract Stone

SOURCE: Beijing Guanganmen Hospital

INGREDIENTS:

No. 1 Turtle shell, *Carapax Trionycis* 9 to 30 g

No. 2 Selfheal spike, *Spica Prunellae* 9 to 15 g

No. 3 Job's tear seed, *Semen Coicis* 15 to 30 g

No. 4 Dahurian angelica root, *Radix Angelicae Dahuricae* 9 to 15 g

No. 5 Lysimachia, *Herba Lysimachiae* 30 to 60 g

No. 6 Climbing fernspore, *Spora Lygodii* (wrapped in a piece of

口粘，尿赤，便秘，甚则出现黄疸，舌红，苔黄腻，脉弦滑数。

胆石症、胆道感染等表现有上述湿热证候者，可用本方加减治疗。

【方解】 方中金钱草为主药，甘咸微寒，清热解毒，祛湿热，退黄疸，利胆排石。茵陈蒿苦微寒，清热除湿，利胆退黄；银花、连翘清热解毒，助金钱草、茵陈利胆退黄；郁金、木香、枳实理气，大黄、芒硝清肠泻火通便。以上共助利胆排石。

现代研究证实，本方具有利胆、消炎、镇痛、松弛奥狄氏括约肌、收缩胆囊、排除胆石、泻下、利尿等作用。

【使用注意】 孕妇忌服。

泌尿系结石方

【来源】 北京广安门医院

【组成】 鳖甲9～30克，夏枯草9～15克，薏苡仁15～30

cloth before it is decocted) 9 g

No. 7 talc, *Talcum* 15 to 30 g

No. 8 Atractylodes rhizome, *Rhizoma Atractylodis* 9 to 15 g

DIRECTIONS: All the drugs listed above are to be decocted in water for oral administration.

FUNCTIONS: Clearing away heat, inducing diuresis, softening and resolving hard stone.

INDICATIONS: Urinary tract stone marked by paroxysmal lumbago or pain in one side of the abdomen often radiating to pudendum, or accompanied by fever, hematuria, urodynia, dysuria, discontinuance of urination, yellow fur of the tongue and taut pulse.

INTERPRETATION: No. 5, No. 3, No. 6, and No. 7 clear away heat and toxins and induce diuresis to remove stone. No. 1, No. 2 soften and resolve hard masses to assist in removing urinary stone. No. 4 and No. 8, with a pungent and warm property and the effects of eliminating dampness and relieving pain, can not only prevent the excessive cold and cool of the other drugs but also help the other drugs induce diuresis and remove urinary stone.

Modern researches have proved that the recipe has the effects of resolving urinary stone, inducing diuresis, and relieving pain, spasm and inflammation.

CAUTIONS: The decoction may be taken in combination with drinking a large amount of water, diuretic medication, electric needle therapy, exercise and so on so as to promote the removal of the stones.

Decoction for Chyluria

(Ruminiao Tang)

SOURCE: Shandong Medical University

INGREDIENTS:

No. 1 Hypoglauca yam, *Rhizoma Dioscoreae Hypoglaucae* 30 g

克，白芷 9～15 克，金钱草 30～60 克，海金砂(包煎)9 克，滑石 15～30 克，苍术 9～15 克。

【用法】 水煎服。

【功用】 清热利湿，软坚散结。

【主治】 泌尿系结石(石淋)，表现为发作性腰痛或腹部一侧痛，多放射至阴部，或兼发热、血尿、排尿痛、排尿难、排尿中断等，舌苔黄，脉弦。

【方解】 方中金钱草、薏苡仁、海金砂、滑石清热解毒，利尿排石；鳖甲、夏枯草软坚散结，以助排石；白芷、苍术其性辛温，而化湿止痛，既可防他药寒凉之偏，又可助其利尿排石。

现代研究证实，本方具有溶解结石、利尿、镇痛、镇痉、消炎等作用。

【使用注意】 服药时可配合大量饮水、口服利尿药、电针、活动等，以促使结石排出。

乳糜尿汤

【来源】 山东医科大学方

No. 2 Prostrate knotweed, *Herba Polygoni Avicularis* 15 g
No. 3 Climbing fern spore, *Spora Lygodii* 30 g
No. 4 Pyrrosia leaf, *Folium Pyrrosiae* 30 g
No. 5 Tuckahoe, *Poria* 18 g
No. 6 Fruit of glossy privet, *Fructus Ligustri Lucidi* 12 g
No. 7 Safflower, *Flos Carthami* 9 g
No. 8 Dried rehmannia root, *Radix Rehmanniae* 15 g
No. 9 Yellow corktree bark, *Cortex Phellodendri* 6 g

DIRECTIONS: All the above drugs are to be decocted in water for oral administration.

FUNCTIONS: Clearing heat and dampness, nourishing *yin* and promoting blood circulation.

INDICATIONS: Chyluria.

INTERPRETATION: No. 1, No. 2, No. 3 and No. 4 can clear away heat and promote diruesis to treat stranguria, as principal drugs for the treatment of cloudy urine. No. 9, with a bitter taste, cold nature and purgative effect, tends to purge kidney-fire and clear away damp-heat from the lower-warmer. No. 5, sweet and bland in taste and neutral in nature, contributes to the removal of dampness and promotion of diuresis, and can replenish the spleen. No. 8 and No. 6 are sweet and bitter in taste and cold in nature, effective in clearing away heat from the blood and nourishing the liver and kidney. No. 7, with a pungent nature for dispersion and the warm nature, functions in removing blood stasis to arrest pain. The joint use of all the drugs produces the effects of clearing away heat and dampness and relieving chyluria.

Modern researches have proved that the recipe has the effects of inducing diruesis and relieving inflammation.

CAUTIONS:

1. The recipe is contraindicated in patients suffering from disturbance in urination due to deficiency of *qi* in the middle-warmer without dampness and heat.

2. With drastic drugs, the recipe has the effect of removing

【组成】 萆薢 30 克，萹蓄 15 克，海金砂 30 克，石苇 30 克，茯苓 18 克，女贞子 12 克，红花 9 克，生地 15 克，黄柏 6 克。

【用法】 水煎服。

【功用】 清热利湿，滋阴活血。

【主治】 乳糜尿(膏淋)。

【方解】 方中萆薢、萹蓄、海金砂、石苇清热利尿通淋，为治白浊之主药。黄柏苦寒沉降，长于泻肾家之火，清下焦湿热；茯苓甘淡而平，利水渗湿，兼能益脾；生地、女贞子甘苦而寒，清热凉血，滋补肝肾；红花辛散温通，以活血祛瘀止痛。诸药合用，共奏清热利湿、分清化浊之效。

现代研究证实，本方具有利尿、消炎等作用。

【使用注意】

1. 凡无湿热，而因中气不足小便不利者，忌用。

2. 本方有破血作用，故孕妇忌用。

blood stasis, therefore it is contraindicated in pregnancy.

Section 3

Recipes for Removing Dampness by Promoting Diuresis

This group of recipes is mainly composed of diuretics and has the effect of removing dampness by promoting diuresis, so it is indicated for the syndrome of fluid-retention within the body.

Powder of Five Drugs with Poria

(Wuling San)

SOURCE: ***Treatise on Febrile Diseases***

INGREDIENTS:

No. 1 Umbellate pore fungus, *Polyporus Umbellatus* 9 g

No. 2 Oriental water plantain rhizome, *Rhizoma Alismatis* 15 g

No. 3 Bighead atractylodes rhizome, *Rhizoma Atractylodis Macrocephalae* 9 g

No. 4 Tuckahoe, *Poria* 9 g

No. 5 Cassia twig, *Ramulus Cinnamomi* 6 g

DIRECTIONS: All the drugs should be made into pulvis and taken 3 to 6 grams each time, or decocted in water for oral administration.

FUNCTIONS: Removing dampness by promoting diuresis and warming *yang* to promote the functions of *qi*.

INDICATIONS: Syndrome of fluid retention within the body marked by headache, fever, thirst with vomiting after drinking water, disturbance in urination, white greasy fur or white and thick fur and floating pulse; or edema, diarrhea,

第三节　利水渗湿剂

利水渗湿剂主要由利水渗湿药组成，有渗利水湿作用，适用于水湿停留证。

五　苓　散

【来源】《伤寒论》

【组成】 猪苓9克，泽泻15克，白术9克，茯苓9克，桂枝6克。

【用法】 做散剂，每服3～6克，或作汤剂水煎服。

【功用】 利水渗湿，温阳化气。

【主治】 水湿内停证，表现为头痛发热，渴欲饮水，水入即吐，小便不利，舌苔白腻或白厚，脉浮；或为水肿，泄泻，痰饮，

fluid-retention syndrome, dizziness and a feeling of palpitation in the lower abdomen.

Acute gastroenteritis, cyclic vomiting, pseudocholera, urticaria of cold type, initial stage of acute nephritis, edema of scrotum, and retention of urine belonging to the syndrome of fluid-retention within the body can be treated by the modified recipe.

INTERPRETATION: No. 2 in the recipe is used in large dosage as a principal drug with sweet and bland taste and cold nature for removing dampness by promoting diuresis. No. 4 and No. 1, as diuretics, strengthen the effect of removing excessive fluid and No. 3 enriches the spleen to transport and transform water and dampness, both being used as assistant drugs. No. 5 can relieve the exterior syndrome by dispelling pathogenic cold and warm *yang* to expel *qi*, acting as an adjuvant drug.

Modern researches have proved that the recipe has the effects of promoting blood circulation and inducing diuresis.

CAUTIONS:

1. The recipe is aimed at inducing diuresis, so patients with deficiency of the spleen-*qi* and with insufficiency of the kidney-*qi* should be treated with the recipe in combination with tonics for reinforcing the spleen-*qi* . It is contraindicated in patients with oliguria due to *yin* deficiency.

2. As the recipe tends to excrete dampness and induce diuresis, long-term administration of it should be avoided.

Umbellate Pore Decoction

(Zhuling Tang)

SOURCE: ***Treatise on Febrile Diseases***

INGREDIENTS:

No. 1 Umbellate pore fungus, *Polyporus Umbellatus* 9 g

No. 2 Tuckahoe, *Poria* 9 g

眩晕，脐下动悸。

急性胃肠炎、周期性呕吐、假性霍乱、寒性荨麻疹、急性肾炎初期、阴囊水肿、尿潴留等证属水湿内停者，可用本方加减治疗。

【方解】 方中泽泻重用为主药，其味甘淡性寒，利水渗湿。茯苓、猪苓淡渗，增强利水蠲饮之功；白术健脾而运化水湿，为辅药。桂枝既解表散寒，又温阳化气，为佐药。

现代研究证实，本方具有促进血液循环、利尿等作用。

【使用注意】

1．本方为淡渗利水之剂，若脾气虚弱，肾气不足者，宜与补脾益气药同用；阴虚小便不利者忌用。

2．本方偏于渗利，不宜久服。

猪 苓 汤

【来源】 《伤寒论》

【组成】 猪苓、茯苓、泽泻、阿胶、滑石各9克。

No. 3 Oriental water plantain rhizome, *Rhizoma Alismatis* 9 g
No. 4 Donkey-hide gelatin, *Colla Corri Asini* 9 g
No. 5 Talc, *Talcum* 9 g

DIRECTIONS: All the drugs except No. 4 should be decocted in water for oral administration. No. 4 should be taken after being melted by the finised decoction in two separate doses.

FUNCTIONS: Clearing away heat, inducing diruesis and nourishing *yin* to arrest bleeding.

INDICATIONS: Retention of fluid in the body with impairment of *yin* due to pathogenic heat marked by difficulty and pain in micturition or blood urine, distention and fullness sensation in the lower abdomen, or insomnia with restlessness, thirst, diarrhea, cough, etc.

Gastroenteritis, mild urinary infection, lithangiuria and nephritis marked by the above syndrome can be treated with the modified recipe.

INTERPRETATION: As principal drugs in the recipe, No. 1 and No. 2 tend to act on the channels of the kidney and urinary bladder. No. 1 is sweet, insipid, slightly bitter in taste, with the bitter component able to descend directly to the *shaoyin* channels, and the sweet and insipid able to remove dampness and induce diuresis; No. 2 strengthens the spleen to excrete dampness. No. 3, as diuretics, induces diuresis. No. 5 clears away heat to treat stranguria. No. 4 nourishes *yin* and moistens dryness to relieve restlessness of deficiency type.

Modern researches have proved that the recipe has antibacterial, antiinflammatory, diuretic and strengthening and tonifying effects.

CAUTIONS: If the patients have high fever, hyperhidrosis due to excessive pathogenic heat causing severe impairment of *yin*, the recipe should be used very carefully.

【用法】 水煎服，阿胶分两次烊化。

【功用】 清热利水，养阴止血。

【主治】 水热伤阴证，表现为小便不利、涩痛或尿血，小腹胀满，或心烦不眠，渴欲饮水，下利，咳嗽等。

肠胃炎、轻型泌尿系炎症、尿路结石、肾炎等表现为湿热伤阴者，可用本方加减治疗。

【方解】 方中猪苓、茯苓入肾、膀胱二经，猪苓甘淡微苦，苦能下降直达少阴，甘淡能渗利水湿，茯苓健脾渗湿，共为主药。泽泻渗利小便，滑石清热通淋，阿胶滋阴润燥，除虚烦。

现代研究证实，本方具有抗菌、消炎、利尿、滋养强壮等作用。

【使用注意】 若邪热炽盛，汗出过多，伤阴严重者，应慎用。

Tetrandra and Astragalus Decoction

(Fangji Huangqi Tang)

SOURCE: ***Synopsis of Prescriptions of the Golden Chambhr***

INGREDIENTS:

No. 1 Tetrandra root, *Radix Stephaniae Tetrandrae* 12 g

No. 2 Milkvetch root, *Radix Astragali seu Hedysari* 15 g

No. 3 Prepared licorice root, *Radix Glycyrrhizae Praeparata* 6 g

No. 4 Bighead atractylodes rhizome, *Rhizoma Atractylodis Macrocephalae* 9 g

No. 5 Fresh ginger, *Rhizoma Zingiberis* 3 pcs.

No. 6 Chinese-date, *Fructus Ziziphi Jujubae* 3 pcs.

DIRECTIONS: All the dyugs should be decocted in water for oral administration.

FUNCTIONS: Invigorating *qi* and dispelling wind, strengthening the spleen and promoting the circulation of *qi*.

INDICATIONS: Wind-edema or wind-dampness syndrome marked by perspiration, aversion to wind, heavy sensation of the body, oliguria, pale tongue with white fur and floating pulse.

Acute or chronic nephritis, nephrotic syndrome, cardiac edema and renal edema manifested as wind-edema or wind-dampness syndrome can be treated by the modified recipe.

INTERPRETATION: No.1 in the recipe dispels pathogenic wind and promotes diuresis and No. 2 invigorates *qi* and strengthens the body surface resistance, and promotes diuresis to alleviate edema. The combined use of the two principal drugs can strengthen the body resistance to eliminate pathogenic factors. No. 4 invigorates *qi* and strengthens the spleen, assisting the spleen to transport and transform nutrients. When combined with No. 2, it can produce more effect on reinforcing *wei*, acting as an assistant drug. No. 3, as a guiding drug, replenishes the spleen and regulates the stomach, coordinates the effects of the other drugs in the recipe and when used together with

防己黄芪汤

【来源】《金匮要略》

【组成】防己 12 克，黄芪 15 克，甘草(炒)6 克，白术 9 克，生姜 3 片，大枣 3 枚。

【用法】水煎服。

【功用】益气祛风，健脾利气。

【主治】风水或风湿证，表现为汗出恶风，身重，小便不利，舌淡苔白，脉浮。

急性及慢性肾炎、肾病综合征、心脏性水肿、肾性水肿等表现为风水或风湿证者，可用本方加减治疗。

【方解】方中防己祛风行水；黄芪益气固表，且能行水消肿；二药配伍，扶正驱邪，共为主药。白术补气健脾，助脾运化；配黄芪，更有实卫之功，为辅药。甘草益脾和中，调和诸药，加姜、

fresh ginger and Chinese-dates, it can regulate *ying* and *wei.*

Modern researches have proved that the recipe has the effects of inducing diuresis, alleviating edema, relieving pain and spasm, promoting blood circulation, improving immunity and preventing allergic reactions.

CAUTIONS: The recipe is indicated for edema due to *qi*-deficiency but not fit for edema of excess type.

Powder of Peel of Five Drugs

(Wupi San)

SOURCE: ***Huatuo's Treatise on Viscera***

INGREDIENTS:

No. 1 Ginger peel, *Cortex Zingiberis* 9 g

No. 2 Mulberry bark, *Cortex Mori Radicis* 9 g

No. 3 Tangerine peel, *Pericarpium Citri Reticulatae* 9 g

No. 4 Shell of areca nut, *Pericarpium Arecae* 9 g

No. 5 Poria peel, *Cortex Poria* 9 g

DIRECTIONS: All the drugs should be decocted in water for oral administration.

FUNCTIONS: Removing dampness to alleviate edema, regulating the flow of *qi* to strengthen the spleen.

INDICATIONS: Severe edema due to hypofunction of the spleen with excessive dampness, marked by general dropsy, heavy sensation of the limbs or the whole body, distention and fullness in the chest and abdomen, dyspnea, oliguria and edema during pregnancy, white and greasy fur of the tongue and deep and slow pulse.

Edema of abrupt onset, edema during pregnancy, and the initial stage of acute nephritis manifested as syndrome of excessive dampness due to hypofunction of the spleen can be treated by the modified recipe.

INTERPRETATION: No. 5 in the recipe induces diuresis and excretes dampness, and strengthens the spleen to promote

枣调和营卫，为使药。

现代研究证实，本方具有利尿消肿、镇痛、镇痉、促进循环、增强免疫、抗过敏等作用。

【使用注意】 本方用于气虚水肿，若水肿实证，则非本方所宜。

五 皮 散

【来源】《华氏中藏经》

【组成】 生姜皮、桑白皮、陈橘皮、大腹皮、茯苓皮各9克。

【用法】 水煎服。

【功用】 利湿消肿，理气健脾。

【主治】 脾虚湿盛之皮水证，表现为一身悉肿，肢体沉重，心腹胀满，上气喘急，小便不利以及妊娠水肿等，苔白腻，脉沉缓。

突发性水肿、妊娠水肿、急性肾炎初期等表现为脾虚湿盛之皮水者，可用本方加减治疗。

【方解】 方中茯苓皮利水渗湿，兼以补脾助运化；生姜皮辛

its transporting and transforming water and nutrients at the same time. No. 1, pungent in flavor, disperses fluid-retention. No.2 clears away and purges the lung-*qi* to dredge water passage. No. 4 promotes the flow of *qi* and water to relieve distention and fullness in the abdomen. No. 3 regulates the stomach-*qi* and resolves turbid dampness. The combined use of the five drugs produces the effect of inducing diuresis to alleviate edema.

Modern researches have proved that the recipe has the effects of inducing diuresis, regulating intestinal peristalsis, promoting excretion of digestive juice, inducing perspiration and lowering high blood pressure.

CAUTIONS: The recipe tends to induce diuresis to alleviate edema, patients with obvious edema due to excessive deficiency of the spleen or accompanied by wind pathogen should be treated by modifying the original recipe.

Section 4

Recipes for Warming and Resolving Water-dampness

This group of recipes is mainly composed of drugs that warm *yang* and those which promote diuresis, having the effects of warming and resolving water-dampness, and indicated for cold-dampness syndrome.

Decoction of Poria, Bighead Atractylodes, Cinnamon and Licorice

(Ling Gui Zhu Gan Tang)

SOURCE: ***Tretaise on Febrile Diseases***

INGREDIENTS:

No. 1 Tuckahoe, *Poria* 12 g

No. 2 Cinnamon twig, *Ramulus Cinnamoni* 9 g

散水气；桑白皮肃降肺气，以通调水道；大腹皮行水气，消胀满，陈皮和胃气，化湿浊。五皮合用，共奏行水消肿之效。

现代研究证实，本方具有利尿、调整肠道蠕动、促进消化液分泌、发汗、降压等作用。

【使用注意】 本方以行水消肿为主，若脾虚甚，水肿明显，或兼有风邪者，需在本方的基础上加减相应的药物。

第四节　温化水湿剂

温化水湿剂主要由温阳药与利湿药组成，有温化水湿的作用，适用于寒湿证。

苓桂术甘汤

【来源】 《伤寒论》

【组成】 茯苓12克，桂枝 9 克，白术、甘草(炙)各 6 克。

No. 3 Bighead atractylodes rhizome, *Rhizoma Atractylodis Macrocephalae* 6 g

No. 4 Prepared licorice root, *Radix Glycyrrhizae Praeparata* 6 g

DIRECTIONS: All the drugs are to be decocted in water for oral administration.

FUNCTIONS: Strengthening the spleen and excreting dampness, warming and resolving the retention of phlegm and fluid.

INDICATIONS: Syndrome of retention of phlegm and fluid due to deficiency-*yang* marked by distention and fullness in the chest and hypochondrium, palpitation, dizziness, cough with clear thin phlegm, white moist and glossy tongue fur, and taut and slippery pulse.

Disturbance of vegetative nerve, migraine, tinnitus, dizziness, hypotension, chronic gastritis, chronic bronchitis and other disorders marked by the syndrome of retention of phlegm and fluid due to deficiency of *yang* can be treated by the modified recipe.

INTERPRETATION: No. 1 in the recipe is taken as a principal drug for strengthening the spleen, excreting dampness, dispelling phlegm and resolving retention of fluid. No. 2, as an assistant drug, warms *yang* to promote the function of *qi*, and meanwhile, lowers the adverse flow of *qi*. The combination of the two drugs, one being diuretic and the other being of warm nature, can warm, resolve and excrete cold phlegm and excessive fluid. No. 3, as an adjuvant drug, strengthens the spleen to eliminate dampness and assists the spleen in transportation and transformation. No. 4 invigorates *qi* and regulates the stomach as a guiding drug.

Modern researches have proved that the recipe has the effects of promoting digestion and absorption, discharging excessive water from the body and promoting blood circulation.

CAUTIONS: The drugs in the recipe are warm and dry

【用法】 水煎服。

【功用】 健脾渗湿，温化痰饮。

【主治】 阳虚痰饮证，表现为胸胁胀满，心悸，眩晕，咳吐清痰，舌苔白滑，脉弦滑。

植物神经失调、偏头痛、耳鸣、眩晕、低血压病、慢性胃炎、慢性支气管炎等表现为阳虚痰饮证者，可用本方加减治疗。

【方解】 方中以茯苓为主药，健脾渗湿，祛痰化饮。桂枝为辅药，温阳化气，兼平冲降逆；与茯苓相配，一利一温，温化渗利寒饮。白术健脾燥湿，助脾运化，为佐药。甘草益气和中，为使药。

现代研究证实，本方具有促进消化吸收、排泄多余水分、促进循环等作用。

【使用注意】 本方药性温燥，有耗伤津液之弊，对阴虚津亏

in nature and may lead to both the loss and impairment of body fluids. Therefore, the recipe is contraindicated in patients with deficiency-*yin* and insufficiency of the body fluid.

Diuretic Decoction by Strengthening *Yang* of the Spleen and Kidney

(Zhen Wu Tang)

SOURCE: ***Treatise on Febrile Diseases***

INGREDIENTS:

No. 1 Tuckahoe, *Poria* 9 g

No. 2 White peony root, *Radix Paeoniae Alba* 9 g

No. 3 Bighead atractylodes rhizome, *Rhizoma Atractylodis Macrocephalae* 6 g

No. 4 Fresh ginger, *Rhizoma Zingiberis Recens* 9 g

No. 5 Prepared aconite root, *Radix Aconiti Praeparata* (roasted and peel-removed) 9 g

DIRECTIONS: All the drugs should be decocted in water for oral administration.

FUNCTIONS: Warming *yang* to induce diuresis.

INDICATIONS: Retention of fluid in the body due to the *yang*-deficiency of the spleen and kidney marked by oliguria, heavy sensation and pain of the limbs, abdominal pain and diarrhea or edema, white tongue fur, absence of thirst and deep pulse.

Nephrotic syndrome, alimentary edema, cardiac edema, chronic nephritis, hypothyroidism, hypopituitarism, chronic gastroenteritis and other conditions marked by the syndrome of retention of fluid in the body due to deficiency-*yang* can be treated by the modified recipe.

INTERPRETATION: No. 5 ,extremely pungent and hot in nature, warms the kidney and the spleen to invigorate *yang* as a principal drug. No. 1 and No. 4 are used as assistant drugs. The former, sweet and insipid in taste and diuretic in property,

者，禁用。

真武汤

【来源】《伤寒论》

【组成】茯苓9克，芍药9克，白术6克，生姜9克，附子（炮去皮）9克。

【用法】水煎服。

【功用】温阳利水。

【主治】脾肾阳虚，水气内停证，表现为小便不利，四肢沉重疼痛，腹痛下利，或肢体浮肿，苔白不渴，脉沉。

肾病综合征、低蛋白性水肿、心脏性水肿、慢性肾炎、甲状腺机能低下、垂体机能低下、慢性胃肠炎等表现为阳虚水停证者，可用本方加减治疗。

【方解】方中附子大辛大热，温肾暖土，以助阳气，为主药。

can strengthen the spleen in eliminating dampness and alleviating fluid retention and the latter, pungent and warm in nature, can warm *yang*, dispel cold and remove fluid retention. No.3, as an adjuvant drug, can strengthen the spleen and eliminate dampness to assist the spleen in transportation and transformation. No. 2 can relieve spasm to arrest abdominal pain, acting as a guiding drug.

Modern researches have proved that the recipe has the effects of promoting circulation and metabolism.

Section 5

Recipes for Expelling Wind-dampness

This group of recipes is mainly composed of antirheumatics, effective in expelling wind-dampness and indicated for numbness and arthralgia due to pathogenic wind-dampness or rubella with pruritus.

Decoction of Notopterygium for Rheumatism

(Qianghuo Shengshi Tang)

SOURCE: ***Differentiation on Endogenous and Exogenous Diseases***

INGREDIENTS:

No. 1 Notopterygium root, *Rhizoma seu Radix Notopterygii* 6 g
No. 2 Pubescent angelica root, *Radix Angelicae Pubescentis* 6 g
No. 3 Ligusticum root, *Rhizoma et Ligustici* 3 g
No. 4 Ledebouriella root, *Radix Ledebouriellae* 3 g
No. 5 Prepared licorice root, *Radix Glycyrrhizae Praeparata* 3 g
No. 6 Chuanxiong rhizome, *Rhizoma Ligustici Chuanxiong* 3 g
No. 7 Chastetree fruit, *Fructus Viticis* 2 g

茯苓甘淡渗利，健脾渗湿，以利水邪；生姜辛温，温阳祛寒散水气，为辅药。佐以白术健脾燥湿，助脾之运化。白芍缓急止腹痛，为使药。

现代研究证实，本方具有促进循环、改善代谢等作用。

第五节 祛风胜湿剂

祛风胜湿剂主要由祛风湿药组成，有祛除风湿的作用，适用于风湿痹痛或风疹瘙痒证。

羌活胜湿汤

【来源】《内外伤辨惑论》

【组成】羌活、独活各6克，藁本、防风、甘草(炙)、川芎各3克，蔓荆子2克。

DIRECTIONS: All the above drugs should be decocted in water for oral administration.

FUNCTIONS: Expelling wind-dampness, arresting pain and relieving the exterior syndrome.

INDICATIONS: Attack of wind-damp on the body surface marked by heavy sensation and pain of the head and body or general aching and difficulty in turning round or sidewards, slight aversion to wind and cold, white fur of the tongue and floating and slow pulse.

The common cold, influenza, sciatica and chronic rheumatic arthritis ascribed to the syndrome of attack of wind-damp on the body surface can be treated by the modified recipe.

INTERPRETATION: Both as principal drugs, No. 1 can dispel wind-dampness from the upper part of the human body and No. 2 tends to dispel wind-dampness from the lower part. The combined use of the two can expel wind-dampness from the whole body and the joints to treat arthralgia. No. 4 and No. 3, as assistant drugs, can dispel wind-cold to relieve headache. No. 6 promotes blood circulation and expels wind to arrest pain and No. 7 dispels wind to arrest pain, both acting as adjuvant drugs. No. 5, as a guiding drug, coordinates the effects of the other drugs in the recipe.

Modern researches have proved that the recipe has great effect of relieving pain and is effective in inducing diaphoresis, promoting blood circulation, resisting viruses and inducing diuresis.

CAUTIONS: Since the recipe is one for relieving the exterior syndrome by dispelling wind and dampness with drugs pungent in flavor and warm in nature, it is contraindicated in patients with wind-heat syndrome due to invasion of exopathogen or those suffering from the common cold with perspiration.

【用法】 水煎服。

【功用】 祛风胜湿，止痛解表。

【主治】 风湿犯表证，表现头身重痛，或一身尽痛，难以转侧，微恶风寒，苔白脉浮缓。

感冒、流行性感冒、坐骨神经痛、慢性风湿性关节炎证属风湿在表者，可用本方加减治疗。

【方解】 方中羌活能祛上部风湿，独活善祛下部风湿，二者相合，能散周身风湿，舒利关节而通痹，共为主药。防风、藁本为辅药，祛风寒，且止头痛。川芎活血，祛风止痛；蔓荆子祛风止痛，为佐药。甘草调和诸药，为使药。

现代研究证实，本方具有很强的镇痛作用，并且有发汗、促进血液循环、抗病毒、利尿等作用。

【使用注意】 本方为辛温解表、祛风除湿之剂，若系外感风热及感冒汗出者，则非所宜。

Pubescent Angelica and Loranthus Decoction

(Duhuo Jisheng Tang)

SOURCE: ***Prescriptions Worth a Thousand Gold for Emergencies***

INGREDIENTS:

No. 1 Pubescent angelica root, *Radix Angelicae Pubescentis* 9 g
No. 2 Loranthus mulberry mistletoe, *Ramulus Loranthi* 6 g
No. 3 Eucommia bark, *Cortex Eucommiae* 6 g
No. 4 Achyranthes root, *Radix Achyranthis Bidentatae* 6 g
No. 5 Wild ginger, *Herba Asari* 6 g
No. 6 Large-leaf gentian root, *Radix Gentianae Macrophyllae* 6 g
No. 7 Tuckahoe, *Poria* 6 g
No. 8 Cinnamon bark, *Cortex Cinnamoni* 6 g
No. 9 Ledebouriella root, *Radix Ledebouriellae* 6 g
No.10 Chuanxiong rhizome, *Rhizoma Ligustici Chuanxiong* 6 g
No.11 Ginseng, *Radix Ginseng* 6 g
No.12 Licorice root, *Radix Glycyrrhizae* 6 g
No.13 Chinese angelica root, *Radix Angelicae Sinensis* 6 g
No.14 White peony root, *Radix Paeoniae Alba* 6 g
No.15 Dried rehmannia root, *Radix Rehmanniae* 6 g

DIRECTIONS: All the above drugs should be decocted in water for oral administration.

FUNCTIONS: Dispelling wind-dampness, arresting pain due to arthralgia-syndrome, tonifying the liver and kidney, invigorating *qi* and nourishing the blood.

INDICATIONS: Persistent arthralgia-syndrome with deficiency of the liver and kidney marked by cold and pain of loins and knees, limited movement, soreness, weakness or numbness of the joints, preference to warmth and aversion to cold, pale tongue with white fur, and deep and feeble pulse.

Chronic arthritis, chronic lumbago, sciatica, chronic rheu-

独活寄生汤

【来源】《备急千金要方》

【组成】 独活9克，桑寄生、杜仲、牛膝、细辛、秦艽、茯苓、肉桂心、防风、川芎、人参、甘草、当归、芍药、干地黄各6克。

【用法】 水煎服。

【功用】 祛风湿，止痹痛，益肝肾，补气血。

【主治】 痹证日久，肝肾两亏证，表现为腰膝冷痛，肢节屈伸不利，酸软无力，或麻木不仁，畏寒喜暖，舌淡苔白，脉沉弱。

慢性关节炎、慢性腰痛、坐骨神经痛、慢性风湿性关节炎等

matic arthritis marked by deficiency of the liver and kidney can be treated by the modified recipe.

INTERPRETATION: No. 1, as a principal drug, which can dispel insidious wind, tends to expel wind-cold-damp pathogens from the lower-warmer, muscles and joints. No. 5 dispels wind-cold from the *yin* channels and expels wind-dampness from the muscles and joints to arrest pain; No. 9 dispels pathogenic wind and removes dampness. No. 6 disperses wind and dampness to relax the muscles and tendons. No. 2, No. 3 and No. 4 expel wind and dampness and tonify both the liver and the kidney at the same time. No. 13, No. 10, No. 15 and No. 14 nourish the blood and promote blood circulation. No.11 and No. 7 supplement *qi* and stengthen the spleen. No. 8 warms the blood and channels and promotes blood circulation. No. 12 coordinates the effects of the other drugs in the recipe.

Modern researches have proved that the recipe has the effects of strengthening the resistance of the body, tranquilizing the mind, relieving pain and spasm, promoting circulation, relieving inflammation and subduing edema.

表现为肝肾两亏证者，可用本方加减治疗。

【方解】 方中以独活为主药，理伏风，善祛下焦与筋骨间之风寒湿邪。细辛发散阴经风寒，搜剔筋骨风湿而止痛；防风祛风邪以胜湿；秦艽除风湿而舒筋；寄生、杜仲、牛膝祛风湿兼补肝肾；当归、川芎、地黄、白芍养血又兼和血；人参、茯苓补气健脾；桂心温通血脉。甘草调和诸药。

现代研究证实，本方具有增强抵抗力、镇静、镇痛、镇痉、改善循环、消炎、消退水肿等作用。

Chapter XVII

Prescriptions for Inducing Astringency

Those mainly composed of astringents, with the effect of inducing astringency to treat extreme loss and consumption of *qi*, blood and semen are generally known as prescriptions for astringency.

The clinical manifestations of loss and consumption of *qi*, blood and semen vary with the causes and regions of diseases, inducing spontaneous perspiration, night sweat, chronic diarrhea, protracted dysentery, emission, enuresis and metrorrhagia, metrostaxis and leukorrhagia. This kind of prescriptions is, therefore, classified into four types according to the different effects of the drugs: the recipes for consolidating superficial resistance for hidroschesis; the recipes for relieving diarrhea with astringents; the recipes for treating spontaneous emission and enuresis with astringents and the recipes for curing metrorrhagia and leukorrhagia.

Section 1

Recipes for Consolidating Superficial Resistance for Hidroschesis

This kind of recipes is mainly composed of the drugs for restoring *qi* and consolidating superficial resistance to arrest perspiration. It is indicated for the treatment of spontaneous perspiration due to failure of superficial-*qi* to protect the body

第十七章

固涩剂

凡主要由收敛固涩药组成，具有收敛固涩作用，以治气血精液滑脱散失之证的方剂，统称固涩剂。

气血津液的滑脱散失，因其发病原因和发病部位的不同而表现为自汗、盗汗、久泻、久痢、遗精、遗尿、崩漏及带下等。因此，本类方剂根据其不同作用分为固表止汗、涩肠固脱、涩精止遗、固崩止带等四类。

第一节　固表止汗剂

固表止汗剂主要由益气固表药组成，有固表止汗作用，适用

against diseases or for the treatment of night sweat caused by interior heat due to deficiency of *yin*.

Jade-screen Powder

(Yupingfeng San)

SOURCE: ***Danxi's Experimental Therapy***

INGREDIENTS:

No. 1 Ledebouriella root, *Radix Ledebouriellae* 30 g

No. 2 Astragalus root, *Radix Astragali seu Hedysari* 30 g

No. 3 Bighead atractylodes rhizome, *Rhizoma Atractylodis Macrocephalae* 60 g

DIRECTIONS: Grind the drugs into fine powder. Take 6 to 9 grams each time, twice a day, with warm boiled water. The recipe can also be decocted in water for oral administration, with the dosage decreased in proportion to the original recipe.

FUNCTIONS: Invigorating *qi* and consolidating the superficial resistance to arrest perspiration.

INDICATIONS: Failure of superficial-*qi* to protect the body against diseases marked by spontaneous perspiration, excessive sweating, liability to wind pathogen, pale complexion, pale tongue with white fur, and floating, feeble and soft pulse.

Hyperhidrosis, allergic rhinitis, chronic rhinitis and susceptibility to the common cold manifested as failure of superficial-qi to protect the body against diseases can be treated by the modified recipe.

INTERPRETATION: No.2 supplements *qi* and consolidates the superficial-*qi*, acting as a principal drug, and No. 3, as an assistant drug, strengthens the spleen and supplements *qi* and assists No. 2 in reinforcing the effects of restoring *qi* and consolidating the superficial-qi. The combined use of the two drugs ensures the sufficiency of *qi* and the consolidation of superficial resistance, arrests profuse and spontaneous sweating and prevents the invasion of exopathogen into the human body. No. 1

于卫外不固或阴虚有热之自汗、盗汗证。

玉屏风散

【来源】 《丹溪心法》

【组成】 防风、黄芪各30克，白术60克。

【用法】 研末，每日2次，每次6～9克，开水送服。亦可按原方用量比例酌减煎服。

【功用】 益气，固表，止汗。

【主治】 表虚卫阳不固证，表现为自汗，多汗，易感风邪，面色晄白，舌淡苔白，脉浮虚软。

多汗症、过敏性鼻炎、慢性鼻炎、易患感冒者表现为表虚卫阳不固者，可用本方加减治疗。

【方解】 方中黄芪益气固表，为主药；白术健脾益气，助黄芪以加强益气固表之功，为辅药；二药合用，则气旺表实，汗不能外泄，邪亦不易内侵。防风走表祛风，并御风邪，为佐使药。且

runs in the body surface to dispel and prevent wind pathogen, acting as an adjuvant and guiding drug. No. 2, combined with No. 1, consolidates the superficial-*qi* without retaining pathogenic factor; No. 1, combined with No. 2, dispels wind pathogen without impairing *qi*. The combination of the two drugs is virtually characteristic of reinforcing accompanied by dispelling, and dispelling accompanied by reinforcing.

Modern researches have proved that the recipe has the effects of improving blood circulation and the nutrition of skin, regulating the functional activities of the sweat gland, strengthening immunity.

CAUTIONS: The recipe is contraindicated in patients with night sweat due to interior heat caused by deficiency of *yin*.

Oyster Shell Powder

(*Muli San*)

SOURCE: ***Prescription of Peaceful Benevolent Dispensary***

INGREDIENTS:

No. 1 Astragalus root, *Radix Astragali seu Hedysari* 30 g

No. 2 Ephedra root, *Radix Ephedrae* 30 g

No. 3 Oyster shell, *Concha Ostreae* 30 g

DIRECTIONS: Grind the above drugs into rough powder and take 9 grams as a portion and decoct it with light wheat (*Fructus Tritici Levis*), and then remove its residue for oral administration. Or decoct them in water for oral administration, with its dosage decreased in proportion to the original recipe.

FUNCTIONS: Consolidating the superficial-qi to arrest sweating, replenishing the heart to suppress the sthenic *yang*.

INDICATIONS: Spontaneous perspiration due to floating of *yang* manifested as general perspiration, especially during sleep in the night, general weakness and lassitude, vexation and palpitation, dreaminess and susceptibility to fright, shortness

黄芪得防风，固表而不留邪；防风得黄芪，祛邪而不伤正，实寓补中有散、散中有补之意。

现代研究证实，本方具有改善皮肤血液循环和营养状态、调整汗腺机能、增强免疫能力等作用。

【使用注意】 凡属阴虚内热之盗汗，不宜应用本方。

牡 蛎 散

【来源】 《太平惠民和剂局方》

【组成】 黄芪、麻黄根、牡蛎各 30 克。

【用法】 为粗末，每次 9 克，与浮小麦同煮，去渣热服。或按原方比例酌减，作汤剂，水煎服。

【功用】 固表敛汗，养心潜阳。

【主治】 阳浮自汗证，表现为身常汗出，夜卧尤甚，体弱神

of breath and fatigue, pale tongue, and thready and weak pulse.

Hyperhidrosis, night sweat, functional disturbance of vegetative nerve and other chronic consumptive diseases manifested by failure of the superficial-*qi* to protect the body against diseases can be treated by the modified recipe.

NTERPRETATION: No. 3, with a salty and astringent nature for arresting sweating, can tranquilize the mind and suppress the sthenic *yang* and is used as a principal drug. No.1 supplements *qi* to reinforce defending *yang* and consolidates the superficial-*qi* to arrest sweating, acting as an assistant drug. As adjuvant and guiding drugs, light wheat clears away heart-heat to ease mental anxiety and astringes the heart-*qi*, and No. 2 expels pathogens from the superficial muscles and skin, guiding the other drugs in the recipe to arrest sweating.

Modern researches have proved that the recrpe produces anhidrotic effect by inhibiting the sweat centre of the central nervous system.

CAUTIONS: The recipe is contraindicated in patients with night sweat due to hyperactivity of pathogenic fire caused by *yin* deficiency.

Section 2

Recipes for Relieving Diarrhea with Astringents

This kind of recipes is mainly composed of the drugs for relieving diarrhea with astringents and those for warming the spleen and kidney. It produces the effect of treating diarrhea and is fit for the treatment of chronic diarrhea, chronic dysentery and lingering diarrhea due to deficiency and coldness of the spleen and kidney.

疲，心烦心悸，多梦易惊，短气倦怠，舌质淡，脉细弱。

多汗症、盗汗症、植物神经失调及其他慢性消耗性疾患表现为卫表不固者，可用本方加减治疗。

【方解】 方中牡蛎咸涩敛汗，镇静潜阳，为主药。黄芪益气实卫，固表止汗，为辅药。浮小麦清心养神，收敛心气；麻黄根行肌表，引诸药收敛止汗，共为佐使之药。

现代研究证实，本方通过抑制中枢神经系统的发汗中枢而起止汗作用。

【使用注意】 凡阴虚火旺而致的盗汗，不宜应用本方。

第二节 涩肠固脱剂

涩肠固脱剂主要由涩肠止泻药与温补脾肾药组成，有涩肠固脱作用。适用于脾肾虚寒所致之泻痢日久、滑脱不禁等病证。

Decoction for Reinforcing the Viscera

(Zhenren Yang Zang Tang)

SOURCE: ***Prescription of Peaceful Benevolent Dispensary***

INGREDIENTS:

No. 1 Ginseng, *Radix Ginseng* 6 g

No. 2 Chinese angelica root, *Radix Angelicae Sinensis* 9 g

No. 3 Bighead atractylodes rhizome, *Rhizoma Atractylodis Macrocephalae* 12 g

No. 4 Nutmeg, *Semen Myristicae* 12 g

No. 5 Bark of Chinese cassia tree, *Cortex Cinnamomi* 3 g

No. 6 Prepared licorice root, *Radix Glycyrrhizae Praeparata* 6 g

No. 7 White peony root, *Radix Paeoniae Alba* 15 g

No. 8 Aucklandia root, *Radix Aucklandiae* 9 g

No. 9 Myrobalan (fruit), *Fructus Chebulae* 12 g

No.10 Poppy capsule. *Pericarpium Papaveris* 20 g

DIRECTIONS: All the drugs should be decocted in water for oral administration.

FUNCTIONS: Warming and tonifying the spleen-*yang* to arrest diarrhea.

INDICATIONS: Chronic diarrhea or chronic dysentery due to deficiency and coldness of the spleen and kidney manifested as prolonged diarrhea or dysentery, incontinence of the feces due to lingering diarrhea or prolapse of anus which fails to be elevated again, abdominal pain that may be relieved by warmness and pressure, listlessness, poor appetite, pale tongue with whitish fur, and deep and slow pulse.

Chronic enteritis, intestinal tuberculosis, chronic dysentery, prolapse of rectum and other diseases marked by lingering diarrhea due to deficiency of *yang* can be treated by the modified recipe.

INTERPRETATION: No. 10 used in large dosage, relieves diarrhea with astringency, and No. 5 warms the kidney

真人养脏汤

【来源】《太平惠民和剂局方》

【组成】人参6克，当归9克，白术12克，肉豆蔻12克，肉桂3克，炙甘草6克，白芍15克，木香9克，诃子12克，罂粟壳20克。

【用法】水煎服。

【功用】温补脾阳，固肠止泻。

【主治】脾肾虚寒之久泻久痢，表现为泻痢日久，大便滑脱不禁或脱肛不收，腹痛喜温、喜按，神疲食少，舌质淡苔白，脉沉迟。

慢性肠炎、肠结核、慢性痢疾、脱肛等表现为阳虚滑脱者，可用本方加减治疗。

【方解】方中罂粟壳重用涩肠止泻，肉桂温肾暖脾，共为主

and spleen, both acting as principal drugs. As assistant drugs, No. 4 warms the kidney and spleen to act on the intestine with its astringency; No. 9 arrests diarrhea with its astringency; No. 1 and No. 3 invigorate *qi* and strengthen the spleen. No. 2 and No. 7 enrich the blood and regulate *ying*, and No. 8 regulates *qi* to remove stagnancy and arrest pain, acting as adjuvant drugs together. No.6 coordinates the effects of the other drugs in the recipe and regulates the stomach, combined with No. 7, it can relieve spasm to arrest pain as a guiding drug.

Modern researches have proved that the recipe has the effects of strengthening the human body, regulating the gastrointestinal peristalsis, relieving spasm, promoting blood circulation and relieving diarrhea.

CAUTIONS: The recipe is contraindicated in patients with primary symptoms of dysentery still with accumulation of toxic heat.

Pill of Four Mirraculous Drugs

(Sishen Wan)

SOURCE: ***Standards of Diagnosis and Treatment***

INGREDIENTS:

No. 1 Nutmeg, *Semen Myristicae* 60 g

No. 2 Psoralea fruit, *Fructus Psoraleae* 120 g

No. 3 Magnolia vine fruit, *Fructus Schisandrae* 60 g

No. 4 Evodia fruit, *Fructus Evodiae* (saturated and fried) 30 g

DIRECTIONS: Add 240 grams of fresh ginger (*Rhizoma Zingiberis Recens*) and 100 pieces of Chinese-dates (*Fructus Ziziphi Jujubae*) to the above-mentioned drugs. Grind them into powder to make pills for oral administration. Take 9 to 12 grams each time before going to bed with light salty water or warm boiled water. If the drugs are to be used in the form of decoction, the dosage can be decreased in proportion to the original recipe.

药。肉豆蔻温肾暖脾而涩肠；诃子涩肠止泻；人参、白术益气健脾，共为辅药。当归、白芍养血和营，木香调气导滞，并能止痛，共为佐药。甘草调药和中，配白芍，又能缓急止痛，为使药。

现代研究证实，本方具有滋养强壮、调整胃肠蠕动、解痉、促进血液循环、收涩止泻等作用。

【使用注意】 下痢初起，积滞热毒未去者，禁用本方。

四 神 丸

【来源】《证治准绳》

【组成】 肉豆蔻60克，补骨脂120克，五味子60克，吴茱萸（浸炒）30克。

【用法】 上药加生姜240克，红枣100枚，和末为丸，每服9～12克，临睡时淡盐汤或白开水送下。若作汤剂，用量可按原方比例酌减。

FUNCTIONS: Warming and tonifying the spleen and kidney to relieve diarrhea with astringency.

INDICATIONS: Diarrhea due to deficiency of the kidney-*yang* manifested as diarrhea before dawn, anorexia, loose stools with undigested food, abdominal pain, lumbago, coldness of the limbs, listlessness, pale tongue with whitish fur, and deep, slow and feeble pulse.

Patients with chronic enteritis, intestinal tuberculosis, ulcerative inflammation of large intestine and other chronic diseases, or old people, manifested by diarrhea before dawn due to *yang*-deficiency of the spleen and kidney can be treated by the modified recipe.

INTERPRETATION: No. 2, with a pungent flavor, bitter taste, warm nature and having the effect of invigorating the gate of life (kidney-*yang*), is an important drug for strengthening physiological fire (motive force of life) and replenishing earth (the spleen), used as a principal drug. No. 1 warms the spleen and kidney and relieves diarrhea with astringency, and No. 4 warms the spleen and stomach to dispel cold and dampness, both acting as assistant drugs. No. 3 is a warm-natured and astringent drug, fresh ginger dispels dampness and promotes the flow of water and Chinese-dates nourishes the spleen and stomach. They are all used as adjuvant and guiding drugs.

Modern researches have proved that the recipe has the effects of protecting the mucosa of stomach and intestine, arresting diarrhea and allergic reaction.

CAUTIONS: The recipe is contraindicated in the patients with diarrhea due to indigestion or accumulation of heat in the stomach and intestine.

【功用】 温补脾肾，涩肠止泻，

【主治】 五更肾泻证，表现为黎明前腹泻，不思饮食，利下清谷，腹痛，腰酸肢冷，神疲乏力，舌质淡，苔薄白，脉沉迟无力。

慢性肠炎、肠结核、溃疡性大肠炎、其他慢性疾病及老人，表现为脾肾阳虚、五更泄泻者，可用本方加减治疗。

【方解】 方中补骨脂辛苦性热而补命门，为壮火益土之要药，为主药。肉豆蔻温脾肾而涩肠止泻；吴茱萸暖脾胃而散寒除湿，并为辅药。五味子为温涩之品；生姜散寒行水；大枣滋养脾胃，并为佐使药。

现代研究证实，本方具有保护胃肠粘膜、收敛止泻、抗过敏等作用。

【使用注意】 食滞不化或肠胃积热所致的泄泻，禁用本方。

Section 3

Recipes for Treating Spontaneous Emission and Enuresis with Astringents

The sort of recipes is mainly composed of the drugs for nourishing the kidney to treat seminal emission and the drugs for reinforcing the kidney to arrest enuresis. It has the effect of treating emission and enuresis, and is indicated for emission and spermatorrhea due to deficiency of the kidney causing the decline of its reserving function and unconsolidation of essence gate; or enuresis and frequent urination due to deficiency of the kidney causing its lack of receiving function and loss of controlling function of the bladder.

Golden Lock Pill for Keeping the Kidney Essence

(Jinsuo Gujing Wan)

SOURCE: ***Collections of Prescriptions with Notes***

INGREDIENTS:

No. 1 Flatstem milkvetch seed, *Semen Astragali Complanti* 60 g

No. 2 Gordon euryale, *Semen Euryales* 60 g

No. 3 Lotus stamen, *Stamen Nelumbinis* 60 g

No. 4 Lotus seed, *Semen Nelumbinis* 60 g

No. 5 Dragon's bone, *Os Draconis Fossilia Ossis Mastodi* (fried) 30 g

No. 6 Oyster shell, *Concha Ostreae* (calcined) 30 g

DIRECTIONS: Grind the above-mentioned drugs into fine powder, mix it with decoction of No.4 to make paste pills for oral administration. Take 9 grams each time with light

第三节　涩精止遗剂

涩精止遗剂主要由补肾涩精药和固肾止遗药组成，有涩精止遗作用。适用于肾虚失藏，精关不固之遗精滑泄；或肾虚不摄，膀胱失约之遗尿、尿频。

金锁固精丸

【来源】《医方集解》

【组成】 沙苑蒺藜、芡实、莲须、莲肉各60克，龙骨(酥炙)，牡蛎(煅)各30克。

【用法】 上药共为细末，莲肉煮粉糊丸，每服 9 克，空腹时

salty water on an empty stomach. The drugs can also be decocted in water for oral administration with the dosage decreased in proportion to the original recipe.

FUNCTIONS: Consolidating the kidney to treat emission.

INDICATIONS: Unconsolidation of the essence gate due to deficiency of the kidney manifested as emission, spermatorrhea, lumbago, tinnitus, lassitude, pale tongue with whitish fur and thready and feeble pulse.

Nocturnal emission, spermatorrhea, insomnia, and dreaminess due to neurasthenia manifested as unconsolidation of the essence gate can be treated by the modified recipe.

INTERPRETATION: No.1 in the recipe tonifies the kidney to arrest emission as a principal drug. No.4 and No.2, as assistant drugs, assist No.1 to tonify the kidney for the treatment of emission. Together as adjuvant drugs, No.3, No.5 and No.6, astringent in nature, are specific for treating emission.

CAUTIONS: The recipe is contraindicated in patients with emission due to downward flow of damp-heat from the liver channel or hyperactivity of pathogenic fire due to *yin*-deficiency.

Mantis Egg-case Powder

(Sangpiaoxiao San)

SOURCE: ***Amplified Materia Medica***

INGREDIENTS:

No. 1 Mantis egg-case, *Oötheca Mantidis* 30 g

No. 2 Polygala root, *Radix Polygalae* 30 g

No. 3 Grassleaved sweetflag rhizome, *Rhizoma Acori Graminei* 30 g

No. 4 Dragon's bone, *Os Draconis Fossilia Ossis Mastodi* 30 g

No. 5 Poria with hostwood, *Poria cum Ligno Hospite* 30 g

No. 6 Chinese angelica root, *Radix Angelicae Sinensis* 30 g

No. 7 Tortoise plastron, *Plastrum Testudinis* (vinegar-fried) 30 g

淡盐汤下。若作汤剂，用量按原方比例酌减。

【功用】 固肾涩精。

【主治】 肾虚精关不固，表现为遗精滑泄，腰酸耳鸣，神疲乏力，舌淡苔白，脉细弱。

神经衰弱之梦遗、滑精、失眠、多梦等表现为精关不固证者，可用本方加减治疗。

【方解】 方中沙苑蒺藜补肾涩精，为主药。莲肉、芡实助主药以补肾涩精，为辅药。莲须、煅龙骨、煅牡蛎性涩收敛，专以涩精为用，共为佐使药。

【使用注意】 肝经湿热下注或阴虚火旺而致遗精者，则非本方所宜。

桑螵蛸散

【来源】《本草衍义》

【组成】 桑螵蛸、远志、菖蒲、龙骨、人参、茯神、当归，龟板(醋炙)各30克。

DIRECTIONS: Grind the drugs into powder. Take 6 grams of powder before going to bed after being mixed with the decoction of pilose asiabell root (*Radix Codonopsis Pilosulae*). All the above drugs can also be decocted in water for oral administration, with the dosage decreased in proportion to the original recipe.

FUNCTIONS: Regulating and tonifying the heart and the kidney to treat emission and enuresis.

INDICATIONS: Deficiency of both the heart and kidney causing loss of controlling function of the urinary bladder manifested as frequent urination or enuresis, emission, absent-mindedness, amnesia, dreaminess, pale tongue with whitish fur, and thready, slow and faint pulse.

Enuresis in children, frequent urination, insomnia and amnesia due to neurasthenia as well as polyuria, diuresis, frequency of urination or diabetes insipidus due to some disorders of endocrine function manifested as deficiency of both the heart and the kidney causing loss of controlling function of the urinary bladder can be treated by the modified recipe.

INTERPRETATION: No.1 in the recipe tonifies the kidney to replenish the vital essence to arrest emission and enuresis with astringency, acting as a principal drug. No.4 tranquilizes the mind and consolidates the vital essence and No.8 replenishes the vital essence and tonifies the kindey and heart, both acting as assistant drugs. As adjuvant drugs, No.5 strengthens *qi* of the middle-warmer, No.7, nourishes the heart and blood and No.6 tranquilizes the mind. No.2 and No.3 tranquilize the mind to restore the normal coordination between the heart (fire) and the kidney (water), acting as adjuvant and guiding drugs.

Modern researches have proved that the recipe has tranquilizing, strengthening and antidiuretic effets.

CAUTIONS: The recipe is contraindicated in patients with frequent urination, enuresis, spontaneous emission due

【用法】 研末，睡前党参汤调下6克。亦可按原方用量比例酌减，水煎服。

【功用】 调补心肾，固精止遗。

【主治】 心肾两虚，膀胱失约证，表现为小便频数或遗尿遗精，心神恍惚，健忘多梦，舌淡苔白，脉细迟弱。

小儿遗尿证，神经衰弱所致的尿频、失眠健忘以及某些内分泌失调的多尿、尿频或尿崩等表现为心肾两虚、膀胱失约证者，可用本方加减治疗。

【方解】 方中桑螵蛸补肾益精，固涩止遗，为主药。龙骨敛心神而涩精气；龟板益阴气而补心肾，并为辅药。人参补中气，当归养心血，茯神安心神，为佐药。远志、菖蒲，安神定志而交通心肾，是佐而兼使之用。

现代研究证实，本方具有镇静、强壮、抗利尿等作用。

【使用注意】 若由下焦火盛或湿热困扰所致的小便频数及遗

to fire-hyperactivity or affection of damp-heat in the lower-warmer.

Section 4

Recipes for Curing Metrorrhagia and Leukorrhagia

This group of recipes is mainly composed of drugs effective in curing metrorrhagia and leukorrhagia, and fit for the treatment of metrorrhagia and dripping with leukorrhea.

Pill for Arresting Uterine Bleeding

(Gujing Wan)

SOURCE: ***Elementary Medicine***

INGREDIENTS:

No. 1 Baikail Skullcap root, *Radix Scutellariae* 30 g
No. 2 White Peony root, *Radix Paeoniae Alba* 30 g
No. 3 Tortoise Plastron, *Plastrum Testudinis* 30 g
No. 4 Ailanthus bark, *Cortex Ailanthi* 21 g
No. 5 Yellow-corktree bark, *Cortex Phellodendri* 9 g
No. 6 Nutgrass flatsedge rhizome, *Rhizoma Cyperi* 7.5 g

DIRECTIONS: Grind the drugs into powder first and then mix it with liquor to make paste pills as big as the seed of Chinese parasol tree. Take 9 grams each time, one or two times a day with warm boiled water. All the above drugs can also be decocted in water for oral administration with the dosage modified in proportion to the original recipe.

FUNCTIONS: Nourishing *yin*, clearing away heat and arresting bleeding to cure metrorrhagia.

尿失精等证，则非本方所宜。

第四节　固崩止带剂

固崩止带剂主要由固崩止带药组成，有固崩止带作用，适用于妇人崩漏及带下淋漓等证。

固　经　丸

【来源】《医学入门》

【组成】 黄芩、白芍、龟板各30克，椿根皮21克，黄柏9克，香附7.5克。

【用法】 为末，酒糊丸梧子大，每日1～2次，每次9克，温开水送服。亦可按原方用量比例酌定，水煎服。

【功用】 滋阴清热，止血固经。

INDICATIONS: Metrorrhagia and metrostaxis or menorrhagia due to interior heat caused by *yin*-deficiency manifested as metrorrhagia and metrostaxis marked by dark red blood with purple and black stagnated blood masses, irritable feverish sensation in the chest, abdominal pain, red urine, red tongue and taut and rapid pulse.

Irregular menstruation, menorrhagia due to inflammation of the genital system and dysfunctional uterine bleeding manifested as the above-mentioned symptoms can be treated by the modified recipe.

INTERPRETATION: No.3 in the recipe nourishes *yin*, purges away fire and tonifies the kidney. No.2 reserves *yin*, replenishes the blood to soften the liver. No.1 and No.5 clear away heat and purge fire to arrest bleeding. No.4, with astringent effect and cold nature, cures metrorrhagia and leukorrhagia and eliminates dampness and heat. No.6 regulates *qi*, allevates mental depression and regulates blood flow.

Decoction for Morbid Leukorrhagia

(Wandai Tang)

SOURCE: ***Fu Qingzhu's Obsterics and Gynecolology***

INGREDIENTS:

No. 1 Bighead atractylodes rhizome, *Rhizoma Atractylodis Macrocephalae* (sand-fried) 30 g

No. 2 Chinese yam, *Rhizoma Dioscoreae* (fried) 30 g

No. 3 Ginseng, *Radix Ginseng* 6 g

No. 4 White peony root, *Radix Paeoniae Alba* (wine-fried) 15 g

No. 5 Plantain seed, *Semen Plantaginis* (wine-fried) 9 g

No. 6 Atractylodes rhizome, *Rhizoma Atractylodis* 9 g

No. 7 Licorice root, *Radix Glycyrrhizae* 3 g

No. 8 Tangerine peel, *Pericarpium Citri Reticulatae* 1.5 g

No. 9 Schizonepeta spike, *Spica Schizonepetae* 1.5 g

【主治】 阴虚内热之崩漏或月经过多证，表现为经行不止，崩中漏下，血色深红，或夹紫黑瘀块，心胸烦热，腹痛溲赤，舌质红，脉弦数者。

生殖系炎症引起的月经不调、月经过多以及功能性子宫出血表现为上述症状者，可用本方加减治疗。

【方解】 方中龟板滋阴降火而益肾；白芍敛阴益血以柔肝；黄芩、黄柏清热泻火以止血；椿根皮收涩性寒，固经止带，并能燥湿清热；香附调气解郁而和血。

完 带 汤

【来源】《傅青主女科》

【组成】 白术(土炒)30克，山药(炒)30克，人参6克，白芍(酒炒)15克，车前子(酒炒)9克，苍术9克，甘草3克，陈皮1.5克，黑芥穗1.5克，柴胡1.8克。

No.10 Bupleurum root, *Radix Bupleuri* 1.8 g

DIRECTIONS: All the above drugs are to be decocted in water for oral administration.

FUNCTIONS: Strengthening the spleen, soothing the liver and resolving dampness to cure leukorrhagia.

INDICATIONS: Leukorrhagia due to deficiency of the spleen manifested as white or yellowish colour, thin discharge without foul smell, physical fatigue, loose stools and pale complexion, pale tongue with white fur, soft and feeble pulse.

Excessive leukorrhea due to inflammation of the genital system belonging to insufficiency of the spleen with over abundance of dampness can be treated with the modified recipe.

INTERPRETATION: As principal drugs, No.3, No.1 and No.2 are all drugs for invigorating *qi* and strengthening the spleen. No.1 can eliminate dampness and No.2 can arrest spontaneous emission. Acting as assistant drugs, No.6 and No.8 eliminate dampness, activate the spleen and promote the circulation of *qi* with their aroma, thus rendering the principal drugs not only to function in tonifying without retention but also to keep the *qi* flowing normally to get the pathogenic dampness eliminated; No.5, being a diuretic drug induces diuresis to eliminate dampness through urination. Acting as adjuvant drugs, No.4 soothes the liver and reinforces the spleen. No.10 ascends the *yang-qi* to prevent the dampness from flowing downward. No.9 enters the blood system, disperses pathogenic wind-dampness to cure leukorrhagia. No.7 coordinates the other drugs and regulates the stomach as a guiding drug.

CAUTIONS: The recipe is not fit for the treatment of leukorrhagia with yellowish discharge or with redish discharge due to downward flow of damp-heat.

【用法】 水煎服。

【功用】 健脾疏肝，化湿止带。

【主治】 脾虚带下证，表现为带下色白或淡黄，清稀无臭，体倦便溏，面色㿠白，舌淡苔白，脉濡弱。

妇女生殖系统慢性炎症引起的白带过多证属脾虚湿盛者，可用本方加减治疗。

【方解】 方中人参、白术、山药均为补气健脾之品，白术并能燥湿，山药兼可涩精，为主药。苍术、陈皮燥湿运脾，芳香行气，既使君药补而不滞，又气行湿自去；车前子淡渗利湿，使水湿从小便而去，共为辅药。白芍舒肝扶脾，柴胡升阳，使湿气不致下流入里；芥穗入血分祛风胜湿以止带，共为佐药。甘草调药和中，为使药。

【使用注意】 湿热下注所致的带下色黄或带下赤白等证，本方不宜使用。

Chapter XVIII

Tonic Prescriptions

Tonic prescriptions concern the tonifying drugs for treating deficiency syndrome by means of tonifying the vital energy, blood, *yin* and *yang* of the human body.

Since syndromes of bodily deficiency and impairment fall into four types called deficiency of *qi*, deficiency of blood, deficiency of *yin*, and deficiency of *yang*, tonic prescriptions have four kinds: recipes as *qi*-tonics, recipes as blood-tonics, recipes as *yin*-tonics and recipes as *yang*-tonics.

Section 1

Recipes as *Qi*-Tonics

This kind of recipes is chiefly made up of *qi*-tonics with the effect of strengthening the function of the spleen and lung and is indicated in the treatment of *qi*-deficiency syndrome of the spleen and lung.

Decoction of Four Noble Drugs

(Si Junzi Tang)

SOURCE: ***Prescription of Peaceful Benevolent Dispensary***

INGREDIENTS:

No. 1 Ginseng, *Radix Ginseng* 10 g

第十八章

补 益 剂

凡以补益药物为主组成，具有补益人体气、血、阴、阳不足，以治各种虚证的方剂，称为补益剂。

人体虚损不足诸证，归纳起来有气虚、血虚、阴虚、阳虚四类。因此，补益剂分为补气剂、补血剂、补阴剂、补阳剂等四种。

第一节 补 气 剂

补气剂主要由补气药组成，能增强脾肺功能，适用于脾肺气虚证。

四 君 子 汤

【来源】 《太平惠民和剂局方》

No. 2 Bighead atractylodes rhizome, *Rhizoma Atractylodis Macrocephalae* 9 g

No. 3 Poria, *Poria* 9 g

No. 4 Prepared licorice root, *Radix Glycyrrhizae Praeparata* 6 g

DIRECTIONS: All the ingredients are to be decocted in water for oral administration.

FUNCTIONS: Replenishing *qi* and strengthening the spleen.

INDICATIONS: *Qi*-deficiency syndrome of the spleen and stomach with symptoms such as poor appetite, watery stool, pale complexion, low and weak voice, lassitude of limbs, thready weak or deep and loose pulse.

The recipe can be modified to treat deficiency of *qi* of the spleen and stomach as seen in cases of indigestion, chronic gastroenteritis, anemia, hypoproteinemia, chronic dysentery and various chronic disorders.

INTERPRETATION: Of the four ingredients in the recipe, No.1, sweet in flavor and warm in nature, possesses the effect of invigorating primordial *qi* and acts as a principal drug to strengthen the spleen and nourish the stomach. No.2, having a bitter flavor and warm nature, is effective for strengthening the spleen and eliminating dampness and is considered as an assistant drug. No.3, sweet and insipid in flavor, exerts the part of an adjuvant drug in achieving the effect of strengthening the spleen. No.4, sweet in flavor and warm in nature, is used as a guiding drug for regulating the middle-warmer.

Modern studies have confirmed that the recipe is effective for stimulating the central nervous system, facilitating the functional activities, promoting metabolism, digestion and absorption, regulating gastrointestinal functions, arresting diarrhea, and relieving swelling and inducing diuresis.

CAUTIONS:

1. Prolonged administration of the recipe may lead to symptoms of dry mouth and tongue, thirst, restlessness and

【组成】 人参10克，白术、茯苓各9克，甘草(炙)6克。

【用法】 水煎服。

【功用】 益气健脾。

【主治】 脾胃气虚证，表现为食少，便溏，面色萎白，语言低微，四肢无力，脉细弱或沉缓等。

消化不良、慢性胃肠炎、贫血、低蛋白血症、慢性痢疾、各种慢性疾患等表现为脾胃气虚证者，可用本方加减治疗。

【方解】 方中人参，甘温大补元气，健脾养胃，为主药。白术苦温健脾燥湿，为辅药。茯苓甘淡渗湿健脾，为佐药。炙甘草，甘温调中，为使药

现代研究证实，本方具有增强中枢兴奋性、促进机能及新陈代谢、增强免疫机能、调整胃肠机能、促进消化吸收、止泻、消肿、利尿等作用。

【使用注意】

1．本方久服可出现口舌干燥、口渴、烦躁等现象。

so on.

2. The recipe should be administered with great care or not at all administered to those with high fever, or hyperactivity of fire due to *yin* deficiency, or fullness due to stagnated *qi*, or insufficiency of body fluid, or excessive thirst and constipation.

Powder of Ginseng, Poria and Bighead Atractylodes

(Shen Ling Baizhu San)

SOURCE: ***Prescription of Peaceful Benevolent Dispensary***

INGREDIENTS:

No. 1 Lotus seed, *Semen Nelumbinis* 500 g

No. 2 Job's-tears seed, *Semen Coicis* 500 g

No. 3 Amomum fruit, *Fructus Amomi* 500 g

No. 4 Platycodon root, *Radix Platycodi* (stir-baked to deep yellowish) 500 g

No. 5 White hyaciath bean, *Semen Dolichoris Album* (macerated in ginger juice, bark removed and stir-baked to just dry) 750g

No. 6 Poria, *Poria* 1000 g

No. 7 Ginseng, *Radix Ginseng* (stem removed) 1000 g

No. 8 Licorice root, *Radix Glycyrrhizae* 1000 g

No. 9 Bighead atractylodes rhizome, *Rhizoma Atractylodis Macrocephalae* 1000 g

No.10 Chinese yam, *Rhizoma Dioscoreae* 1000 g

DIRECTIONS: All the above drugs may be decocted in water for oral administration. The dosage can be decided in proportion to the original recipe.

FUNCTIONS: Nourishing *qi* and strengthening the spleen, regulating the stomach and eliminating dampness.

INDICATIONS: Stagnation of dampness due to deficiency of the spleen marked by lassitude of extremities, general

2．凡高热、阴虚火盛、积滞气胀、津液不足、烦渴便秘，均宜慎用或不用。

参苓白术散

【来源】《太平惠民和剂局方》

【组成】莲子肉500克，薏苡仁500克，缩砂仁 500 克。桔梗(炒令深黄色)500克，白扁豆(姜汁浸，去皮，微炒)750克，白茯苓1000克，人参(去芦)1000克，甘草(炒)1000克，白术1000克，山药1000克。

【用法】水煎服。用量可按原方比例酌定。

【功用】补气健脾，和胃渗湿。

【主治】脾虚湿停证，表现为四肢乏力，形体虚羸，饮食不化，

debility, dyspepsia, vomiting or diarrhea, epigastric distension and fullness, sallow complexion, whitish and greasy coating on the tongue, and feeble and moderate pulse.

In addition, the recipe can be modified to deal with such cases as indigestion, chronic gastroenteritis, anemia, nephrotic syndrome, chronic nephritis and other chronic disorders that are ascribable to stagnation of dampness due to deficiency of the spleen.

INTERPRETATION: In the recipe, Nos. 6,7,8 and 9 with mild effect for tonifying *qi* of the spleen and stomach play together the leading role. Nos.5, 2, 10 and 1 are administered to assist No.9 in strengthening the spleen, eliminating dampness to arrest diarrhea. No.3, acrid in flavor and warm in property, is used to enliven the spleen by means of aroma to assist the principal drugs in promoting the function of the spleen and stomach, and to arrest vomiting and diarrhea. No.4 carries the other drugs in the recipe ascendingly to reach the upper-warmer for replenishment of the lung.

Modern studies have ascertained that the recipe has the efficacies in regulating gastrointestinal functions, promoting digestion and absorption, arresting diarrhea, relieving swelling, norishing the organs and so on.

CAUTIONS: The recipe should be carefully administered to patients with hyperactivity of fire due to *yin* deficiency; and should be used with discretion by patients associated with deficiency of both *qi* and *yin*, or deficiency of *yin* complicated with deficiency of the spleen.

Decoction for Reinforcing Middle-warmer and Replenishing *Qi*

(Buzhong Yiqi Tang)

SOURCE: ***Treatise on the Spleeh and Stomach***

INGREDIENTS:

或吐或泻，胸脘痞闷，面色萎黄，苔白腻，脉虚缓。

消化不良、慢性胃肠炎、贫血、肾病综合征、慢性肾炎和其他慢性疾患表现为脾虚湿停证者，可用本方加减治疗。

【方解】 方中四君子平补脾胃之气，为主，配扁豆、苡仁、山药、莲子辅助白术健脾，渗湿止泻。加砂仁辛温芳香醒脾，佐四君促进脾胃运化，止吐泻。桔梗载药上行，达于上焦以益肺。

现代研究证实，本方具有调整胃肠机能、促进消化吸收、止泻、消肿、营养等作用。

【使用注意】 阴虚火旺者宜慎用；气阴两虚，或阴虚兼有脾虚者，应酌情运用。

补中益气汤

【来源】 《脾胃论》

【组成】 黄芪15克，甘草(炙)5克，人参10克，当归(酒焙

No. 1 Astragalus root, *Radix Astragali seu Hedysari* 15 g

No. 2 Prepared licorice root, *Radix Glycyrrhizae Praeparata* 5 g

No. 3 Ginseng, *Radix Ginseng* 10 g

No. 4 Chinese angelica root, *Radix Angelicae Sinensis* (baked with wine to dry or dried in the sun) 10 g

No. 5 Tangerine peel, *Pericarpium Citri Reticulatae* 6 g

No. 6 Cimicifuga rhizome, *Rhizoma Cimicifugae* 3 g

No. 7 Bupleurum root, *Radix Bupleuri* 3 g

No. 8 Bighead atractylodes rhizome, *Rhizoma Atractylodis Macrocephalae* 10 g

DIRECTIONS All the ingredients can either be decocted in water for oral administration; or ground into powder for making pills. Take 10—15 grams of pills each time with warm boiled water, 2—3 times a day.

FUNCTIONS: Invigorating the spleen, replenishing *qi* and elevating the spleen-*yang* to treat *qi* collapse.

INDICATIONS: Syndrome due to deficiency of the spleen and stomach manifested by fever with perspiration, headache with aversion to cold, thirst with desire for hot drink, short breath and disinclination to talk; or loss of appetite, lassitude of the extremities, pale tongue with whitish coating, deficient and weak pulse as well as hysteroptosis, gastroptosis, protracted diarrhea and protracted dysentery due to the sinking of spleen-*qi*.

Moreover, the recipe can be modified to treat many other diseases attributable to deficiency of *qi* of the spleen and stomach such as hypotension, chronic headache, functional disturbance of the vegetative nerve, chronic gastroenteritis, myasthenia gravis, gastroatonia, prolapse of the rectum, prolapse of the uterus, floating kidney, chronic bleeding, postpartum subinvolution of the uterus, menorrhagia, allergic purpura, thrombocytopenic purpura, chronic low fever and other chronic disorders, and to facilitate recovery after illness or operation.

INTERPRETATION: Of all the ingredients, No.1 acts

干，或晒干）10克，橘皮6克，升麻3克，柴胡3克，白术10克。

【用法】 水煎服。或作丸剂，每服10～15克，每日2～3次，温开水送服。

【功用】 补中益气，升阳举陷。

【主治】 脾胃气虚证，表现为身热有汗，头痛恶寒，渴喜热饮，少气懒言，或饮食无味，四肢乏力，舌质淡苔白，脉虚软无力及气虚下陷之子宫脱垂、胃下垂、久泻、久痢等。

低血压病、慢性头痛、植物神经失调、慢性胃肠炎、重症肌无力、胃弛缓、脱肛、子宫脱垂、游走肾、慢性出血、产后子宫恢复不全、月经过多、过敏性紫斑病、血小板减少性紫斑、慢性低热、病后或术后恢复期及其他慢性疾患，表现为脾胃气虚证者，可用本方加减治疗。

【方解】 方中黄芪益气升阳，为主药。人参、白术、炙甘草

as a principal drug with the effects of replenishing *qi* and elevating *yang*; Nos. 2, 3 and 8, as assistant drugs, share the efforts of invigorating the spleen and replenishing *qi*. Functioning as an adjuvant drugs, No.5 produces the effect of promoting the flow of *qi* while No.4 provides the effect of tonifying blood. No.6 and No.7 are used together as guiding drugs for sending up lucid *yang*.

Modern studies have confirmed that the recipe has the efficacies in improving the cellular immune function promoting metabolism, improving the excitement of cerebral cortex, promoting the tension of skeletal muscles, smooth muscles and supporting tissues; and promoting digestion and absorption.

CAUTIONS: Patients with internal heat due to *yin* deficiency is prohibited from taking this recipe, and for those with the impairment of body fluid and *qi* after illness, it's better to prescribe this recipe together with other drugs.

Pulse-activating Powder

(Shengmai San)

SOURCE: ***Differentiation on Endogenous ond Exogenous Diseases***

INGREDIENTS:

No. 1 Ginseng, *Radix Ginseng* 10 g

No. 2 Ophiopogon root, *Radix Ophiopogonis* 15 g

No. 3 Schisandra fruit, *Fructus Schisandrae* 6 g

DIRECTIONS: All the above drugs are to decocted in water for oral administration.

FUNCTIONS: Supplementing *qi*, promoting the production of body fluid, astringing *yin*-fluid and arresting sweat.

INDICATIONS: Syndrome of impairment of both *qi* and *yin* manifested by general debility, shortness of breath, disinclination to talk, thirst with profuse sweat, dry tongue and throat, deficient and weak pulse, or impairment of the

健脾益气，为辅药。陈皮理气，当归补血，均为佐药。升麻、柴胡升举清阳，为使药。

现代研究证实，本方具有提高机体细胞免疫机能，促进新陈代谢，提高大脑皮层的兴奋性，加强骨骼肌、平滑肌、支撑组织的张力，促进消化、吸收等作用。

【使用注意】 阴虚内热者禁用。病后津气两伤者，亦不宜单用本方。

生 脉 散

【来源】《内外伤辨惑论》

【组成】 人参10克，麦冬15克，五味子6克。

【用法】 水煎服。

【功用】 益气生津，敛阴止汗。

【主治】 气阴两伤证，表现为体倦气短懒言，口渴多汗，咽

lung due to chronic cough, dry cough with shortness of breath, spontaneous perspiration or palpitation, and faint pulse with tendency to exhaustion.

The recipe can be modified to deal with dehydrant shock caused by heat stroke, bleeding, severe vomiting or diarrhea, dramatic injury, scald; or syndrome of impairment of both *qi* and *yin* as seen in cases at recovery stage of febrile diseases or at postoperation, or in cases with chronic disorders; or syndrome of deficiency of both *qi* and *yin* as seen in such cases as tuberculosis, chronic bronchitis, bronchiectasis, etc.

INTERPRETATION: Of the three ingredients in the recipe, the first which is sweet in flavor and warm in property, acts as a principal drug for replenishing *qi* and promoting the production of body fluid, and invigorating primordial *qi*; the second, sweet in flavor and cold in property, is used as an assistant drug for tonifying *yin* and promoting the production of body fluid, and clearing away deficient heat, to get rid of restlessness; the last one, sour in flavor and warm in nature, is used as an adjuvant and guiding drug for astringing the lung to stop sweat. The three drugs, tonifying, removing and astringing respectively, are used jointly to achieve the result of replenishing *qi*, clearing away pathogenic heat and astringing *yin*.

Clinically and experimently, it has been ascertained that the recipe is effective for reinforcing the function of the heart, ascending blood pressure, promoting digestion and absorption, strengthening the general functions, inducing diuresis, arresting sweat, maintaining the body fluid, and nourishing the organs to consolidate constitution.

CAUTIONS: Since it has an astringing effect, it is neither fit for patients whose exopathogen has not been dispelled, nor for those with hyperactivity of heat due to summer-heat diseases, but without impairment of *qi* and body fluid.

干舌燥，脉虚弱，或久咳伤肺，干咳短气，自汗或心悸，脉微欲绝等。

中暑、出血、剧吐、剧泻、创伤、烫伤等所致的脱水性休克，或热病恢复期、手术后、慢性疾患等出现的气阴两伤证，以及肺结核、慢性支气管炎、支气管扩张等出现气阴两虚证者，均可用本方加减治疗。

【方解】 方中以人参甘温，益气生津，大扶元气，为主药。麦冬甘寒，养阴生津，清虚热而除烦，为辅药。五味子酸温，敛肺止汗，为佐使药。三药合用，一补，一清，一敛，而获益气、清热、敛阴之效。

现代研究证实，本方具有强心、升压、促进消化吸收、提高全身机能、抗利尿、止汗、保持体内水分、滋养强壮等作用。

【使用注意】 本方具有收敛作用，若外邪未解或暑病热盛，气津未伤者，均不宜使用。

Section 2

Recipes as Blood-Tonics

This group of recipes is composed of traditional Chinese drugs with the effect of enriching the blood and is indicated in the treatment of deficiency of *ying* and blood.

Decoction of Four Ingredients

(Siwu Tang)

SOURCE: ***Prescription of Peaceful Benevolent Dispensary***

INGREDIENTS;

No. 1 Chinese angelica root, *Radix Angelicae Sinensis* (prepared by soaking in wine and stir-frying) 10 g

No. 2 Chuanxiong rhizome, *Rhizoma Ligustici Chuanxiong* 8 g

No. 3 White peony root, *Radix Paeoniae Alba* 12 g

No. 4 Prepared rhizome of rehmannia, *Radix Rehmanniae Praeparata* (prepared by steaming in wine) 12 g

DIRECTIONS: All the above drugs are to be decocted in water for oral administration.

FUNCTIONS: Nourishing and regulating the blood.

INDICATIONS: Syndrome of deficiency and stagnation of blood with symptoms such as menstrual disorders, abdominal pain, metrorrhagia and metrostaxis accompanied by blood masses and frequent pain, threatened abortion or with vaginal bleeding, as well as postpartum retaining of lochia resulting in a mass or swelling in the abdomen, muscular rigidity and pain in the hypogastrium and alternate attacks of chills and fever.

In addition, the above syndrome occurring in other di-

第二节 补 血 剂

补血剂主要由补血养血药组成，适用于营血亏虚证。

四 物 汤

【来源】 《太平惠民和剂局方》

【组成】 当归(酒浸炒)10克，川芎8克，白芍12克，熟地黄(酒蒸)12克。

【用法】 水煎服。

【功用】 补血调血。

【主治】 血虚血滞证，表现为月经不调，小腹疼痛，崩中漏下，血瘕块硬，时发疼痛，妊娠胎动不安，胎漏下血不止，及产后恶露不下，结生瘕聚，少腹坚痛，时作寒热等。

营养不良、植物神经失调、更年期综合征、月经稀少、闭经、

seases such as malnutrition, vegetative nerve functional disturbance, menopausal syndrome, scanty menstruation, amenorrhea, dysmenorrhea and hypoplasia of uterus can also respond well to the modified recipe.

INTERPRETATION: Of the four ingredients in the recipe, the first provides the effect of tonifying and activating the blood and the last is mainly used as hematic tonic. No.2 is used to promote flow of *qi* and blood circulation while No.3 to preserve *yin* to nourish the blood. The four ingredients working in combination yield the result of tonifying the blood without causing stagnation and promoting the flow of blood without breaking the blood thereby the recipe is worthy one for tonifying and activating the blood.

Modern studies have confirmed that the recipe has the therapeutic effects in tranquilizing the mind, relieving muscle spasm, regulating menstruation, etc.

CAUTIONS: As No.3 and No.4 are of *yin* type with mild effect which are liable to cause stagnation of *qi* and impairment of *yang*, the recipe is not advisable for patients with *yang* deficiency of the spleen and stomach marked by anorexia and watery stool.

Decoction for Invigorating the Spleen and Nourishing the Heart

(Guipi Tang)

SOURCE: ***Prescriptions for Succouring the Sick***

INGREDIENTS:

No. 1 Bighead atractylodes rhizome, *Rhizoma Atractylodis Macrocephalae* 30 g

No. 2 Poria with hostwood, *Poria cum Ligno Hospite* 30 g

No. 3 Astragalus root, *Radix Astragali seu Hedysari* 30 g

No. 4 Longan aril, *Arillus Longan* 30 g

子宫发育不全、痛经等表现为血虚血滞证者，可用本方加减治疗。

【方解】 方中当归补血、活血；熟地补血为主；川芎行气活血；芍药敛阴养血。本方补血而不滞，行血而不破血，实为补血活血要剂。

现代研究证实，本方具有镇静、镇痉、调整月经等作用。

【使用注意】 方中地、芍为阴柔之品，易于滞气伤阳，如平素脾胃阳虚，食少便溏者，不宜使用。

归脾汤

【来源】《济生方》

【组成】 白术30克，茯神30克，黄芪30克，龙眼肉30克，酸

No. 5 Wild jujuba seed, *Semen Ziziphi Spinosae* (stir-fried, shell removed) 30 g

No. 6 Ginseng, *Radix Ginseng* 15 g

No. 7 Aucklandia root, *Radix Aucklandiae* 15 g

No. 8 Prepared licorice root, *Radix Glycyrrhizae Praeparata* 8g

No. 9 Chinese angelica toot, *Radix Angelicae Sinensis* 3 g

No.10 Polygala root, *Radix Polygalae* (honey-parched) 3 g

DIRECTIONS: With the addition of fresh ginger 6 g and Chinese-dates 3—5 pcs., all the drugs are decocted in water for oral administration. The dosage can also be increased proportionately according to the above recipe to make honeyed boluses. Each bolus weighs 9 grams. One bolus is to be taken each time with boiled water on an empty stomach, three times a day.

FUNCTIONS: Replenishing *qi* and tonifying the blood, invigorating the spleen and nourishing the heart.

INDICATIONS: Weakness of both the spleen and heart marked by palpitation or severe palpitation, amnesia, insomnia, night sweat, fever of deficient type, anorexia, general debility, sallow complexion, pale tongue with thin and whitish coating, and thready and loose pulse; hemafecia due to dysfunction of the spleen in governing the blood, metrorrhagia, metrostaxis, preceded menstrual period with excessive blood loss in light colour, and continuous dripping of menstruation or morbid leukorrhagia, etc.

Moreover, the recipe can be modified to treat other cases such as disturbance of the vegetative nerve, menopausal syndrome, cardiac neurosis, insomnia, amnesia, anemia, thrombocytopenia, hypoproteinemia, chronic gastroenteritis, nervous gastritis, uterine functional bleeding that are ascribed to insufficiency of both the spleen and heart.

INTERPRETATION: In the recipe, No.3 and No.6, as principal drugs, have the effects of tonifying *qi* and invigorating the spleen; No.1 and No.8, sweet in flavor and warm in

枣仁(炒，去壳)30克，人参15克，木香15克，甘草(炙)8克，当归3克，远志(蜜炙)3克。

【用法】 加生姜6克，红枣3～5枚，水煎服。或按上述比例加大剂量，炼蜜为丸，每丸重9克，空腹时，每次服1丸，开水送下，日服3次。

【功用】 益气补血，健脾养心。

【主治】 心脾两虚证，表现为心悸怔忡，健忘失眠，盗汗虚热，食少体倦，面色萎黄，舌质淡，苔薄白，脉细缓。或脾不统血之便血，妇女崩漏，月经提前，量多色淡，或经血淋漓不止，或带下等证。

植物神经失调、更年期综合征、心脏神经官能症、失眠、健忘症、贫血、血小板减少、低蛋白血症、慢性胃肠炎、神经性胃炎、子宫功能性出血等表现为心脾两虚证者，可用本方加减治疗。

【方解】 方中人参、黄芪补气健脾，为主药；白术、甘草甘

nature, assist the principal drugs in enriching the source of the production of *qi* and blood by reinforcing the spleen and replenishing *qi*. No.9, with a sweet and acrid flavor and warm property, is good at enriching the liver to promote the generation of heart-blood; Nos. 2,4 and 5, all being sweet in flavor and neutral in nature, function in nourishing the heart and tranquilizing the mind; No.10 has the effect of relieving mental stress by means of restoring normal coordination between the heart (fire) and the kidney (water); No.7 has the effect of regulating the flow of *qi* and enlivening the spleen and is used to prevent *qi*-replenishing drugs and blood tonics from causing stagnation of *qi* and interfering the functions of the spleen and stomach.

Recent studies have proved that this recipe is effective for promoting digestion and absorption, strengthening metabolism, consolidating the constitution by nourishing the body, regulating the excitement of the cerebrum, promoting gastrointestinal peristalsis as well as arresting diarrhia.

CAUTIONS: The recipe should not be administered to those with heat-evil hidden interiorly and those with rapid pulse due to *yin* deficiency.

Decoction of Prepared Licorice

(Zhi Gancao Tang)

SOURCE: ***Treatise on Febrile Diseases***

INGREDIENTS:

No. 1 Prepared licorice root, *Radix Glycyrrhizae Praeparata* 12 g

No. 2 Fresh ginger, *Rhizoma Zingiberis* 9 g

No. 3 Ginseng, *Radix Ginseng* 6 g

No. 4 Dried rehmannia root, *Radix Rehmanniae* 30 g

No. 5 Cinnamon twig, *Ramulus Cinnamomi* 9 g

No. 6 Donkey-hide gelatin, *Colla Corii Asini* 6 g

No. 7 Ophiopogon root, *Radix Ophiopogonis* 10 g

温补脾益气，助主药以资气血生化之源；当归甘辛温养肝而生心血；茯神、枣仁、龙眼肉甘平养心安神；远志交通心肾而定志宁心；木香理气醒脾，以防益气补血药滋腻滞气，有碍脾胃运化功能。

现代研究证实，本方具有促进消化吸收、加强代谢、滋养强壮、调整大脑的兴奋性、促进胃肠蠕动以及止泻等作用。

【使用注意】 邪热内伏及阴虚脉数者忌用。

炙甘草汤

【来源】 《伤寒论》

【组成】 甘草（炙）12克，生姜9克，人参6克，生地黄30

No. 8 Hemp seed, *Fructus Cannabis* 10 g
No. 9 Chinese dates, *Fructus Ziziphi Jujubae* 10 g

DIRECTIONS: With the exception of donkey-hide gelatin, all the other drugs in the recipe are to be mixed and decocted in water for a fixed period of time and, then the liquid part is separated from the residue and mixed with 10ml of rice wine. Donkey-hide gelatin, separately melted in boiling water, is divided into three portions and one portion is mixed with 1/3 of the decoction just before oral administration. One dose is decocted three times. The decoction is to be taken in three separate doses in one day.

FUNCTIONS: Replenishing *qi*, enriching the blood and nourishing *yin* to restore pulse.

INDICATIONS: Deficiency of both *qi* and blood manifested by intermittent pulse, i.e. a slow and weak pulse pausing at regular intervals, or knotted pulse, or slow pulse with irregular intervals, palpitation, amaciation, shortness of breath, pallor, coat on the tongue with reduced saliva, frequent fever of deficiency type with unproductive cough, or with little expectoration of bloody sputum, insomnia due to vexation, spontaneous perspiration, or night sweat, dry mouth and throat, obstipation, and weak and rapid pulse.

Equally, other cases such as ventricular premature beat, primary stage of atrioventricular block, functional arrhythmia, auricular fibrillation, cardiovascular neurosis, hyperthyroidism, rheumatic heart disease and others that pertain to the deficiency of both *qi* and blood, can respond well to the modified recipe.

INTERPRETATION: Acting as a principal drug in the recipe, the first ingredient gives the effect of enriching *qi*, replenishing the stomach and restoring the pulse. No.3 together with the last one, is capable of nourishing the heart and spleen by way of replenishing *qi*. Nos. 4,6,7 and 8, all sweet in taste and moist in nature for nourishing *yin* and

克，桂枝9克，阿胶6克，麦冬10克，麻仁10克，大枣10克。

【用法】 除阿胶外，其余各药混合煎煮，取汁倒出，加入清酒10毫升。另将阿胶略加开水炖化，分三次入药汁搅匀服。1剂煎服3次，1天服完。

【功用】 益气养血，滋阴复脉。

【主治】 气虚血少，症见脉结代，心动悸，体羸气短，面皖色淡，舌苔少津，或虚热时发，干咳无痰，或咯痰不多，痰中带血丝，虚烦不得眠，自汗或盗汗，咽干口燥，大便难，脉虚数者。

室性期前收缩、房室传导阻滞初期、功能性心律不齐、心房颤动、心脏神经官能症、甲状腺机能亢进、风心病等表现为气虚血少者，可用本方加减治疗。

【方解】 方中炙甘草补气益胃复脉，为主药。人参、大枣益气以补心脾。生地、麦冬、阿胶、麻仁甘润滋阴，养心补血，润

the heart, supplement the blood, moisten the lung and promote the production of body fluid. No.2, No.5 and rice wine, acrid in taste and warm in property, are used for activating *yang* and restoring pulse, and in compatibility with drugs for replenishing *qi* and nourishing *yin*, they can gain the superiority of warmness without dryness, beneficial to promoting the flow of *qi* and the blood and easing the blood vessels.

Modern studies have ascertained that this recipe has the efficacies in increasing cerebral excitement, strengthening the function of heart, dilating the coronary artery.

CAUTIONS: As the recipe has the effects of moistening dryness and relaxing the bowels, it is not suitable for patients with weakness of gastrointestine or with diarrhea.

Section 3
Recipes as *Yin*-Tonics

Recipes as *yin*-tonics refer to those that consist of *yin*-nourishing drugs and are indicated in the treatment of *yin*-deficiency of the liver and kidney.

Bolus of Six Drugs Including Rehmannia

(Liuwei Dihuang Wan)

SOURCE: ***Key to Therapeutics of Childen's Diseases***

INGREDIENTS:

No. 1 Prepared rhizome of rehmannia, *Rhizoma Rehmanniae Praeparata* 240 g

No. 2 Dogwood fruit, *Fructus Corni* 120 g

No. 3 Dried Chinese yam, *Rhizoma Dioscoreae* 120 g

No. 4 Oriental water plantain, *Rhizoma Alismatis* 90 g

No. 5 Poria, *Poria* 90 g

肺生津。姜、桂、酒性味辛温，通阳复脉，与益气滋阴药相配，温而不燥，流通气血，通利脉道。

现代研究证实，本方具有提高脑的兴奋性、加强心脏的驱血功能、扩张冠状动脉等作用。

【使用注意】 本方具有润燥通便作用，凡胃肠虚弱或腹泻下利者不宜用。

第三节 补 阴 剂

补阴剂主要由滋阴药组成，适用于肝肾阴虚证。

六味地黄丸

【来源】《小儿药证直诀》

【组成】 熟地黄240克，山萸肉、干山药各120克，泽泻、茯

No. 6 Moutan bark, *Cortex Moutan Radicis* 90 g

DIRECTIONS: Grind the drugs intɔ fine powder and mix with honey to make boluses as big as the seed of Chinese parasol, to be administered orally 6-9 grams each time with warm boiled water or slight salt water, 2-3 times a day. The drugs can also be decocted in water for oral administration with the dosage reduced in proportion as the original recipe.

FUNCTIONS: Nourishing and enriching the liver and kidney.

INDICATIONS: Syndrome due to the deficiency of vital essence of liver and kidney with symptoms of weakness and soreness of waist and knees, vertigo, tinnitus, deafness, night sweat, emission as well as persistant opening of fontanel. Or the flaring up of sthenic fire resulting in symptoms such as hectic fever, feverish sensation in the palms and soles, diabetes or toothache due to fire of deficiency type, dry mouth and throat, red tongue with little fur, and thready and rapid pulse.

In addition, the above recipe can be modified to treat many other diseases indicating the syndrome due to the deficiency of vital essence of liver and kidney such as vegetative nerve functional disturbance, hypertension, arteriosclerosis, diabetes, chronic nephritis, hyperthyroidism, pulmonary tuberculosis, chronic urinary infection, bronchial asthma, amenorrhea, scanty menstruation, or infantile dysplasis and interlectual hypoevolutism.

INTERPRETATION: The first drug, as the principal one, possesses the effect of nourishing the kidney-*yin* and supplementing the essence of life. As assistant drugs, No.2, sour in flavor and warm in nature, is used for nourishing the kidney and replenishing the liver, while No.3 for nourishing the kidney-*yin* and tonifying the spleen. The rest ingredients collectively play the role of adjuvant drugs. No.4 coordinates with the principal drug in clearing the kidney and purging

苓、丹皮各90克。

【用法】 研细末，炼蜜为丸，如梧子大，每次6～9克，每日2～3次，温开水或淡盐汤送服。亦可水煎服，用量按原方比例酌减。

【功用】 滋补肝肾。

【主治】 肝肾阴虚证，表现为腰膝酸软，头目眩晕，耳鸣耳聋，盗汗遗精，以及小儿囟开不合之症。或虚火上炎而致骨蒸潮热，手足心热，或消渴，或虚火牙痛，口燥咽干，舌红少苔，脉细数。

植物神经失调、高血压病、动脉硬化、糖尿病、慢性肾炎、甲状腺机能亢进、肺结核、慢性泌尿系感染、支气管哮喘、经闭、月经过少等，或小儿、乳幼儿发育不良及智力发育迟缓表现为肝肾阴虚证者，可用本方加减治疗。

【方解】 方中熟地重用滋肾阴，益精髓，为主药；山萸肉酸温滋肾益肝，山药滋肾阴补脾，为辅药；泽泻配熟地而泻肾降

turbid evils, No.6 cooperates with No.2 in purging liver fire, and No.5 shares the effort together with No.3 to excrete dampness from the spleen. The whole recipe acts as both tonics and purgatives with tonifying effect dominant.

Clinically and experimentally, the recipe has the effects of nourishing the body and consolidating the constitution, inhibiting hypercatabolism, reducing excitement of the brain, adjusting endocrine function and vegetative nerve, lowering blood pressure and blood sugar, inducing diuresis, improving the function of the kidney as well as promoting the epithelial hyperplasia of the esophagus and preventing cancer, etc.

CAUTIONS: Since it tends to be greasy tonics, the recipe should be administered carefully to patients with weakened function of the spleen in transporting and distributing nutrients and water.

Bolus as Kidney-*Yin*-Tonic

(Zuogui Wan)

SOURCE: ***Complete Works of Zhang Jing yue***

INGREDIENTS:

No. 1 Prepared rhizome of rehmannia, *Rhizoma Rehmanniae Praeparata* 240 g

No. 2 Chinese yam, *Rhizoma Dioscoreae* (parched) 120g

No. 3 Wolfberry fruit, *Fructus Lycii* 120 g

No. 4 Dogwood fruit, *Fructus Corni* 120 g

No. 5 Cyathula root, *Radix Cyathulae* (rinsed in wine and well steamed) 90 g

No. 6 Dodder seed, *Semen Cuscutae* 120 g

No. 7 Antler glue, *Colla Cornus Cervi* (broken into pieces and parched into pearls) 120 g

No. 8 Tortoise-plastron glue, *Colla Plastri Testudinis* (cut into pieces and parched into pearls, but not prescribed in case the patient shows no pathogenic fire) 120 g

浊；丹皮配山茱萸泻肝火；茯苓配山药而渗脾湿，共为佐药。全方补泻并用，以补为主。

现代研究证实，本方具有滋养强壮、抑制异化作用亢进、降低脑的兴奋性、调整内分泌机能、调整植物神经、降压、降血糖、利尿、改善肾功能及促进食管上皮细胞增生、抗癌等作用。

【使用注意】 本方性偏滋腻，脾虚运化无力者应慎用。

左 归 丸

【来源】《景岳全书》

【组成】 熟地黄240克，山药(炒)120克，枸杞120克，山茱萸120克、川牛膝(酒洗蒸熟)90克，菟丝子120克，鹿胶(敲碎，炒珠)120克，龟胶(切碎，炒珠，无火者，不必用)120克。

DIRECTIONS: The boluses are made out of the powdered drugs with honey. Each bolus weighs 9 g. One bolus is to be taken each time with slightly salty liquid in the early morning and before bed time on an empty stomach.

FUNCTIONS: Nourishing *yin* and tonifying the kidney.

INDICATIONS: Syndrome of deficiency of genuine *yin* marked by vertigo, lassitude in the loins and legs, seminal emission or spermatorrhea, spontaneous perspiration, night sweat, dry mouth and throat, thirst with desire for drinks, smooth tongue with little coating, and thready or rapid pulse.

Besides, syndrome of deficiency of genuine *yin* occurring in cases of debilitated constitution due to advanced age, chronic disorders, or recovery stage of febrile diseases can be treated with the modified recipe.

INTERPRETATION: In the recipe, No. 1, great in dosage, is used to nourish the kidney-*yin*; No. 3 is to supplement the essence of life and improve acuity of vision; and No. 4 is to astringe seminal emission and sweating. Both No. 7 and No.8, which have close relation to health, are used in combination for replenishing and tonifying the essence, with the former tending to tonify *yang* and the latter tending to nourish *yin*. No. 6, assisted by No. 5, has the effect of strengthening the waist and knees and reinforcing the muscles and joints. No.2 gives the effect of nourishing and replenishing the spleen and kidney.

CAUTIONS: Prolonged administration of the recipe is liable to obstruct the function of the spleen and stomach, for this reason, it is advisable to add into the recipe tangerine peel, amomum fruit or other drugs so as to regulate the flow of *qi* to enliven the spleen and to avoid any disturbance with tonification.

【用法】 制为蜜丸，每丸约重9克。早、晚空腹时各服一丸，淡盐汤送下。

【功用】 滋阴补肾。

【主治】 真阴不足证，表现为头目眩晕，腰酸腿软，遗精滑泄，自汗，盗汗，口燥咽干，渴欲饮水，舌光少苔，脉细或数。

年老体衰、慢性疾患、热病恢复期等表现为真阴不足证者，可用本方加减治疗。

【方解】 方中熟地重用滋肾阴，枸杞益精明目，山萸肉涩精敛汗。龟鹿二胶为血肉有情之品，鹿胶偏于补阳，龟板偏于滋阴，两胶合力，益精填髓。菟丝子配牛膝，强腰膝，健筋骨。山药滋补脾肾。

【使用注意】 本方久服，每易滞脾碍胃，故在运用时，宜加入陈皮、砂仁等以理气醒脾，防止进补妨运之弊。

Bolus for Replenishing Vital Essence

(Da Buvin Wan)

SOURCE: ***Danxi's Experiential Therapy***

INGREDIENTS:

No. 1 Phellodendron bark, *Cortex Phellodendri* (parched) 120 g
No. 2 Wind-weed rhizome, *Rhizoma Anemarrhenae* (Macerated in rice wine and then parched) 120 g
No. 3 Prepared rhizome of rehmannia, *Rhizoma Rehmanniae Praeparata* (steamed in rice wine) 180 g
No. 4 Tortoise plastron, *Plastrum Testudinis* (friedwith honey to crisp) 180 g

DIRECTIONS: Grind the four ingredients into fine powder, make boluses out of the mixture of the powder and the paste of steamed spinal cord of pig and mix with honey. Weighing 9 grams, one bolus is taken each time with slightly salty water in the early morning and before bed time. Or the drugs can be decocted, each dosage being correspondingly reduced in proportion to the original recipe.

FUNCTIONS: Nourishing *yin* and purging pathogenic fire.

INDICATIONS: Syndrome of hyperactivity of fire due to *yin* deficiency manifested as hectic fever, night sweat, spermatorrhea, productive bloody cough, heamatemesis, irritability with inclination to anger, feverish and sore knees and feet with flaccidity, red tongue with little coating, and rapid and forceful *chi* pulse.

Equally, the above syndrome seen in cases of hyperthyroidism, renal tuberculosis, bone tuberculosis and diabetes can respond well to the treatment with the modified recipe.

INTERPRETATION: Dominant in dosage, the last two ingredients of the recipe are administered to nourish *yin* and suppress hyperactive *yang*, and invigorate water to control

大补阴丸

【来源】《丹溪心法》

【组成】黄柏(炒)、知母(酒浸炒)各120克，熟地黄(酒蒸)、龟板(酥炙)各180克。

【用法】上四味，碾为细末，猪脊髓适量蒸，捣如泥状，炼蜜，混合拌匀和药粉为丸，每丸约重9克。每日早晚各服1丸，淡盐水送服，或按原方比例酌减，水煎服。

【功用】滋阴降火。

【主治】阴虚火旺证，表现为骨蒸潮热，盗汗遗精，咳嗽咯血，吐血，心烦易怒，足膝痛热痿软，舌红少苔，尺脉数而有力。

甲状腺机能亢进、肾结核、骨结核及糖尿病表现为阴虚火旺者，可用本方加减治疗。

【方解】方中重用熟地、龟板滋阴潜阳，壮水制火。黄柏，

fire. The first two drugs with a bitter flavor and cold property are used to purge pathogenic fire to protect genuine *yin*. As excipients, the spinal cords of pig and honey both possess a sweet moist property and not only provide the effect of tonifying the essence to reinforce its resistance to pathogenic factors, but are able to restrict the overdryness and bitterness of the first two drugs. The combination of all the drugs in the recipe gains the result of nourishing *yin* and purging the ministerial fire.

Clinically and experimentay, it is ascertained that the above recipe possesses the efficacies of allaying fever, relieving inflammation, tranquilizing the mind, restraining the excitement of vegetative nerve, and nourishing the body to build up the constitution.

CAUTIONS: The recipe is not advisable for patients with watery stool after meal.

Decoction for Nourishing the Liver and Kidney

(Yiguan Jian)

SOURCE: ***Supplement to the Classified Medical Records of Well-known Physicians***

INGREDIENTS:

No. 1 Glehnia root, *Radix Glehniae* 10 g
No. 2 Ophiopogon root, *Radix Ophiopogonis* 10 g
No. 3 Chinese angelica root, *Radix Angelicae Sinensis* 10 g
No. 4 Dried rehmannia root, *Radix Rehmanniae* 30 g
No. 5 Wolfberry fruit, *Fructus Lycii* 10 g
No. 6 Sichuan chinaberry, *Fructus Mediae Toosendan* 5 g

DIRECTIONS: All the above drugs are to be decocted in water for oral administration.

FUNCTIONS: Nourishing the liver and kidney, soothing the liver and regulating the circulation of *qi*.

知母苦寒泄火以保真阴。更以猪脊髓、蜂蜜甘润之品，既能滋补精髓以培其本，又能制约知、柏过于苦燥。诸药合用，共奏滋阴精而泻相火之功。

现代研究证实，本方具有解热、消炎、镇静、抑制植物神经兴奋、滋养强壮作用。

【使用注意】 若食后便溏者，忌用本方。

一 贯 煎

【来源】 《续名医类案》

【组成】 北沙参、麦冬、当归身各10克，生地黄30克，枸杞子10克，川楝子 5 克。

【用法】 水煎服。

【功用】 滋养肝肾，疏肝理气。

INDICATIONS: Hypochondriac and thoracic pain due to deficiency of *yin* of the liver and kidney with stagnancy of the liver-*qi*, manifested by hypochondriac and thoracic fullness and pain, acid regurgitation, dry mouth and throat, reddened tongue with reduced saliva, thready and feeble or feeble and taut pulse, as well as hernia and abdominal mass.

Moreover, other cases attributed to deficiency of *yin* of the liver and kidney such as chronic hepatitis, primary stage of cirrhosis, fatty liver, chronic gastritis, gastric ulcer, diabetes, hypertension as well as other chronic disorders can respond well to the treatment with the modified recipe.

INTERPRETATION: Being the largest in dosage, No. 4 is preferred to as a principal drug used to tonify the insufficiency of genuine *yin* of the liver and kindey by way of nourishing *yin* and enriching the blood. Nos. 1,2,3 and 5, possessing the effects of supplementing *yin* and soothing the liver, share the part of an assistant drug along with No. 4 which has the effects of nourishing *yin*, enriching the blood and promoting the production of body fluid. Functioning as an adjuvant and guiding drug, No. 6 is used in small amount to sooth the liver and regulate the circulation of *qi*, and though bitter and dry in property, its dry property can be restrained and the effect of relieving the depressed liver remained when it is decocted together with a large amount of *yin*-tonifying drugs with a sweet flavor and cold property.

Modern studies have confirmed that this recipe has the efficacies of protecting the liver, lowering the level of blood sugar, strengthening immunity, tranquilizing the mind, relieving inflammation, allaying fever, arresting pain, regulating vegetative nerve, etc.

CAUTIONS: Since there are more greasy drugs for nourishment in the recipe, it is better not to be administered for those with sputum and stagnation of body fluid.

【主治】 肝肾阴虚，气郁胁痛，表现为胸胁胀痛，吞酸吐苦，咽干口燥，舌红少津，脉细弱或虚弦以及疝气瘕聚等。

慢性肝炎、肝硬变初期、脂肪肝、慢性胃炎、胃溃疡、糖尿病、高血压及其他慢性疾患表现为肝肾阴虚者，可用本方加减治疗。

【方解】 方中生地重用，滋阴养血以补肝肾真阴不足，为主药。沙参、麦冬、当归、枸杞子益阴柔肝，合生地滋阴养血生津，为辅药。配少量川楝子，疏肝解郁，其性虽苦燥，但配入大量甘寒养阴药中，燥性即被抑制，而疏泄肝气之功尤存，为方中佐使药。

现代研究证实，本方具有保肝、降血糖、增强免疫能力、镇静、消炎、解热、镇痛、调整植物神经等作用。

【使用注意】 方中滋腻药物较多，对于停痰积饮者，忌用本方。

Section 4

Recipes as *Yang*-Tonics

This sort of recipes is mainly composed of the drugs for warming and tonifying the kidney-*yang* and applied to syndrome of weakness of kidney-*yang*.

Bolus for Tonifying the Kidney-qi

(Shenqi Wan)

SOURCE: ***Synopsis of Prescriptions of the Golden Chamber***

INGREDIENTS:

No. 1 Dried rehmannia root, *Radix Rehmanniae* 240 g
No. 2 Chinese yam, *Rhizoma Dioscoreae* 120 g
No. 3 Dowgood fruit, *Fructus Corni* 120 g
No. 4 Oriental water plantain, *Rhizoma Alismatis* 90 g
No. 5 Poria, *Poria* 90g
No. 6 Moutan bark, *Cortex Moutan Radicis* 90 g
No. 7 Cinnamon twig, *Ramulus Cinnamomi* 30 g
No. 8 Prepared aconite root, *Radix Aconiti Praeparata* (stir-baked at high temperature) 30 g

DIRECTIONS: Grind drugs into very fine powder and then mix them with honey to make boluses weighing 9g each. One bolus is to be taken in the morning and another in the evening with warm boiled water. Or instead, the drugs are decocted proportionately with reference to the dosage of the original recipe.

FUNCTIONS: Warming and tonifying the kidney-*yang*.

INDICATIONS: Insufficiency of the kidney-*yang* manifested by lassitude in the loins, legs and feet, cold feeling in the lower part of the body, stiffness in the lower abdomen, dysphoria with smothery sensation resulting in inability to lie

第四节 补 阳 剂

补阳剂主要由温补肾阳药物组成，适用于肾阳虚弱证。

肾 气 丸

【来源】《金匮要略》

【组成】干地黄240克，薯蓣(山药)120克，山茱萸120克，泽泻90克，茯苓90克，牡丹皮90克，桂枝30克，附子(炮)30克。

【用法】混合辗细，炼蜜为丸，每丸重9克，早、晚各服1丸，开水送下。或根据原方用量比例酌情增减，水煎服。

【功用】温补肾阳。

【主治】肾阳不足证，表现为腰腿脚弱，下半身常有冷感，少腹拘急，烦热不得卧而反倚息，小便不利或小便反多，舌质淡

flat but rest against bed instead, dysuria or polyuria, bulgy and pale tongue, feeble pulse or deep and faint pulse, as well as phlegm-retention syndrome, diabetes, flaccidity of lower limbs, etc.

Equally, the above syndrome occurring in chronic nephritis, diabetes, vegetative nerve disturbance, senile dementia, primary stage of prostatic hyperplasia, infertility, amenorrhea and other chronic disorders, or urinary dysfunction may be treated with the modified recipe.

INTERPRETATION: Of all the ingredients in the recipe, the first three are all used as tonics, the first replenishing the kidney-*yin* while the second and the third nourishing the liver and spleen to reinforce the effect of the first one. The last two drugs which are dosed the least are used to warm and replenish the kidney-*yang*. No. 4 and No. 5 play their part in removing dampness and promoting diuresis. No. 6 has the effect of removing liver-fire and is coordinated with the invigorators for kidney-*yang* to produce the consequence of coexistance of both invigorating and purging action for the purpose of getting rid of the greasy side involved in the invigorating action.

Modern researches have proved that this recipe has the efficacies in improving hypophysis-adrenocortical function, promoting blood circulation, tranquilizing the mind, lowering blood pressure, strengthening kidney function, protecting the liver and so on.

CAUTIONS: It is not advisable to administer this recipe for patients with hyperactivity of fire due to *yin* deficiency and impairment of body fluid due to dryness-heat.

而胖，脉虚弱尺部沉微，以及痰饮、消渴、脚气等。

慢性肾炎、糖尿病、植物神经失调、老年性痴呆、前列腺肥大初期、不孕症、经闭、其他慢性疾患或排尿机能异常等表现为肾阳不足者，可用本方加减治疗。

【方解】 方中干地黄滋补肾阴，山茱萸、山药滋补肝脾，以助干地黄滋补肾中之阴；并以少量桂枝、附子温补肾中之阳。泽泻、茯苓利水渗湿，丹皮清泻肝火，与温补肾阳药相配，意在补中寓泻，以使补而不腻。

现代研究证实，本方具有改善垂体-肾上腺皮质功能、促进血液循环、镇静、降压、改善肾功能、保肝等作用。

【使用注意】 凡阴虚火旺、燥热伤津之病证，均不宜运用本方。

Chapter XIX

Resolving Prescriptions

The resolving prescriptions are chiefly made up of digestives and resolvents with the effects of promoting digestion and removing stagnated food, disintegrating masses and relieving distension and fullness. They are grouped into two kinds: the recipes for promoting digestion and removing stagnated food and the recipes for disintegrating masses and relieving distension and fullness.

Section 1

Recipes for Promoting Digestion and Removing Stagnated Food

This group of recipes is composed of the digestives with the effects of promoting digestion and removing stagnated food and applied to the treatment of impairment by overeating.

Lenitive Pill

(Baohe Wan)

SOURCE: ***Danxi's Experiential Therapy***
INGREDIENTS:
No. 1 Hawthorn fruit, *Fructus Crataegi* 180 g
No. 2 Medicated leaven, *Massa Fermentata Medicinalis* 60 g

第十九章

消 导 剂

凡以消导药为主组成，具有消食导滞、消痞化积作用，以治积滞痞块的方剂，称为消导剂。

消导剂分为消食导滞和消痞化积两类。

第一节 消食导滞剂

消食导滞剂主要由消食药组成，有消食导滞作用，适用于伤食证。

保 和 丸

【来源】《丹溪心法》

【组成】 山楂180克，神曲60克，半夏、茯苓各90克，陈皮、

No. 3 Pinellia tuber, *Rhizoma Pinelliae* 90 g
No. 4 Poria, *Poria* 90g
No. 5 Tangerine peel, *Pericarpium Citri Reticulatae* 30 g
No. 6 Forsythia fruit, *Fructus Forsythiae* 30 g
No. 7 Seed of radish, *Semen Raphani* 30 g

DIRECTIONS: The pills are prepared by grinding all the above drugs into very fine powder first and then refining powdered drugs with water, to be taken 6—9g each time with warm boiled water. The drugs may also be decocted in water for oral administration, with the dosage being one tenth of the original recipe.

FUNCTIONS: Promoting digestion and regulating the stomach.

INDICATIONS: Retention of food due to improper diet with symptoms such as stuffiness and fullness in the epigastrium, distention in the abdomen with pain at times, acid regurgitation and eructation with fetid odor, loss of appetite, nausea, vomiting, or diarrhea, intermittent fever or dysentery due to retention of food, greasy and yellowish coating of the tongue, and slippery pulse.

Equally, the above syndrome occurring in cases such as indigestion and gastroenteritis and others may be treated with the modified recipe.

INTERPRETATION: In the recipe, the first drug, considered as the principal drug, can be used to remove all kinds of food stagnancy. It is especially good at removing the stagnancy of greasy food. The second and the last drugs act in combination as assistant drugs, with former being effective for promoting digestion and strengthening the spleen, especially for removing stagnated food related to immoderate drinking, while the latter being contributive to keeping the adverse *qi* downward and promoting digestion, especially to removing the stagnated grain food. The rest act together as adjuvant drugs, of which No. 3 and No. 5 have the effect of promoting

连翘、萝卜子各30克。

【用法】 共为末，水泛为丸，每服6～9克，温开水送下。亦可水煎服，用量按原方十分之一即可。

【功用】 消食和胃。

【主治】 食积停滞证，表现为胸脘痞满，腹胀时痛，嗳腐吞酸，厌食呕恶，或大便泄泻，食疟下痢，舌苔腻而黄，脉滑。

消化不良、胃肠炎等表现为食积停滞证者，可用本方加减治疗。

【方解】 方中山楂可消一切饮食积滞，尤善消肉食油腻之积为主药。神曲消食健脾，更化酒食陈腐之积；萝卜子下气消食，长于消谷面之积，共为辅药。半夏、陈皮行气化滞，和胃止呕；

the flow of stomach-*qi* and removing the stagnated food, regulating the functions of stomach to arrest vomiting; No. 4 has the effects of strengthening the spleen and inducing diuresis, regulating the stomach and spleen to arrest diarrhea; and No.6 has the effects of clearing away heat and scattering stagnancy.

Modern studies have proved that this recipe possesses the efficacies for promoting digestion and peristalsis of the stomach and intestines, arresting vomiting, subduing inflammation and resisting bacteria.

CAUTIONS: The recipe should be administered with great care to patients with the insufficiency of spleen. Greasy and spicy food is prohibited during administration.

Pill of Immature Bitter Orange for Removing Stagnancy

(Zhishi Daozhi Wan)

SOURCE: ***Treatise on Differentiation of Internal and External Injuries***

INGREDIENTS:

No. 1 Rhubarb root, *Radix et Rhizoma Rhei* 30 g
No. 2 Immature bitter orange, *Fructus Aurantii Immaturus* 15 g
No. 3 Medicated leaven, *Massa Fermentata Medicinalis* 15 g
No. 4 Poria, *Poria* 9 g
No. 5 Scutellaria root, *Radix Scutellariae* 9 g
No. 6 Coptis root, *Rhizoma Coptidis* 9 g
No. 7 Bighead atractylodes rhizome, *Rhizoma Atractylodis Macrocephalae* 9 g
No. 8 Oriental water plantain rhizome, *Rhizoma Allismatis* 6 g

DIRECTIONS: The drugs are ground into particles and then made into pills by refining powder with water, to be taken 6–9g each time with warm boiled water, twice a day. The drugs may also be decocted in water for oral administration. The dosage is reduced in proportion as the original recipe.

茯苓健脾利湿，和中止泻；连翘清热而散结，共为佐药。

现代研究证实，本方具有助消化、促进肠胃蠕动、镇呕、抗菌、消炎等作用。

【使用注意】 脾虚者应慎用。服药期间禁油腻厚味之品。

枳实导滞丸

【来源】 《内外伤辨惑论》

【组成】 大黄30克，枳实、神曲各15克，茯苓、黄芩、黄连、白术各9克，泽泻6克。

【用法】 水泛为丸，每服6～9克，温开水送下，每日2次。或原方比例酌减，水煎服。

FUNCTIONS: Promoting digestion to remove stagnated food and eliminating dampness-heat.

INDICATIONS: Syndrome due to stagnated food and dampness-heat manifested as epigastric distress and fullness, dysentery and diarrhea, or constipation, scanty and deep-coloured urine, yellow and greasy coating of the tongue and slow and vigorous pulse.

Moreover, other diseases such as acute indigestion, gastroenteritis, bacterial diarrhea and others that indicate stagnancy of food and dampness-heat in the spleen and stomach may be treated with the modified recipe.

INTERPRETATION: In the recipe, No. 1 dominates in dosage and acts as the principal drug used to clean up the stagnancy of food. No. 2 as an assistant drug, promotes the flow of *qi* and scatters food accumulation. The rest all share the role of adjuvant and guiding drugs, of which, No. 5 and No. 6 both contribute their effort in removing heat-dampness, and arresting dysentery; No. 4 and No.8 devote in combination their effects in inducing diuresis, excreting dampness and arresting diarrhea, and No. 7 plays its part in strengthening the spleen and removing dampness.

As modern researches have confirmed, this recipe possesses the efficacies in promoting peristalsis of the stomach and intestines, assisting in digestion and absorption, and functions in arresting diarrhea, inducing diuresis, relieving inflammation, resisting bacteria and others by purgation.

CAUTIONS: Inadvisable for patients with stagnated food due to deficiency of the spleen.

Pill for Invigorating the Spleen

(Jianpi Wan)

SOURCE: *Standards of Diagnosis and Treatment*

INGREDIENTS:

【功用】 消导积滞，清利湿热。

【主治】 湿热食滞证，表现为胸脘痞满，下痢泄泻，或大便秘结，小便短赤，舌苔黄腻，脉沉有力等。

急性消化不良、胃肠炎、细菌性腹泻等表现为食滞、脾胃湿热者，可用本方加减治疗。

【方解】 方中大黄重用，荡涤实积，为主药。枳实行气散结，导滞除痞，为辅药。黄芩、黄连清热燥湿，厚肠止痢；茯苓、泽泻利水渗湿止泻；白术健脾燥湿，共为佐使药。

现代研究证实，本方具有促进胃肠蠕动、帮助消化吸收，通过泻下作用以达止泻、利尿、消炎、抗菌等作用。

【使用注意】 脾虚食滞者忌用。

健脾丸

【来源】《证治准绳》

No. 1 Bighead atractylodes rhizome, *Rhizoma Atractylodis Macrocephalae* (parched) 75 g
No. 2 Aucklandia root, *Radix Aucklandiae* (to be ground seperately from others) 22 g
No. 3 Coptis root, *Rhizoma Coptidis* (wine-parched) 22g
No. 4 Licorice root, *Radix Glycyrrhizae* 22 g
No. 5 Poria, *Poria* 60 g
No. 6 Ginseng, *Radix Ginseng* 45 g
No. 7 Medicated leaven, *Massa Fermetata Medicinalis* (parched) 30 g
No. 8 Tangerine peel, *Pericarpium Citri Reticulatae* 30 g
No. 9 Amomum fruit, *Fructus Amoni* 30 g
No. 10 Germinated barkey, *Fructus Hordei Germinatus* (parched) 30g
No. 11 Hawthorn fruit, *Fructus Crataegi* 30 g
No. 12 Chinese yam, *Rhizoma Dioscoreae* 30 g
No. 13 Nutmeg, *Semen Myristicae* (floured wrapped in paper and beaten by a hand mallet so as to get rid of its oil) 30 g

DIRECTIONS: Make paste pills with starch paste out of powdered drugs or make pills by refining the powder with water. The pills are to be taken 6—9 grams each time with warm boiled water twice a day.

FUNCTIONS: Strengthening the spleen and regulating the stomach, promoting digestion and arresting diarrhea.

INDICATIONS: Retention of food due to deficiency of the spleen marked by poor appetite, indigestion, distention and fullness in the stomach and abdomen, loose bowels, greasy coating of the tongue, and feeble pulse.

The modification of the recipe is advisable for the above syndrome as seen in cases such as chronic enteritis, disturbance of intestinal function, irritable colon, etc.

INTERPRETATION: In the recipe, Nos. 1,4,5 and 6 are considered as four noble ingredients which can provide the effect

【组成】 白术(炒)75克，木香(另研)、黄连(酒炒)、甘草各22克，白茯苓60克，人参45克，神曲(炒)、陈皮、砂仁、麦芽(炒)、山楂、山药、肉豆蔻(面裹纸包槌击去油)各30克。

【用法】 糊丸或水泛为丸，每服6～9克，温开水送下，日2次。

【功用】 健脾和胃，消食止泻。

【主治】 脾虚食积证，表现为食欲不振，消化不良，脘腹胀满，大便溏薄，苔腻，脉虚弱。

慢性肠炎、肠功能紊乱、结肠过敏等表现为脾虚食积者，可用本方加减治疗。

【方解】 方中以四君子汤补气健脾，其中白术，茯苓用量偏

of reinforcing *qi* and the spleen, of which No. 1 and No. 5 are inhibited in larger dosage to reinforce mainly the spleen, excrete dampness and stop diarrhea. To assist the four ingredients, No. 12 and No. 13 are administered to strengthen the efficacies in reinforcing the spleen and stopping the diarrhea. Nos. 7,10 and 11 are used to promote digestion and remove stangated food, Nos. 8, and 9 to regulate *qi* and the stomach; No. 3 to clear away heat and dampness.

As modern researches have confirmed, this recipe has the efficacies in adjusting intestinal function, promoting digestion, relieving inflammation, resisting bacteria, etc.

CAUTIONS: It is not fit for those with retention of food brought about by improper eating, overeating and overdrinking.

Section 2

Recipes for Disintegrating Masses and Relieving Distension and Fullness

This group of recipes mainly consists of drugs effective for promoting the flow of *qi* and blood circulation, resolving dampness and phlegm and softening hard masses, and are usually indicated in the treatment of mass, distension and fullness in the abdomen.

Pill with Immature Bitter Orange for Disintegrating Masses and Relieving Stuffiness

(Zhishi Xiaopi Wan)

SOURCE: ***Secret Record of the Chamber of Orchids***

INGREDIENTS:

多，意在着重补脾渗湿而止泻。佐以山药、肉豆蔻助其健脾止泻之力；山楂、神曲、麦芽消食化滞；砂仁、陈皮理气和胃；黄连清热燥湿。

现代研究证实，本方具有调整肠道机能、促进消化、消炎、抗菌等作用。

【使用注意】 饮食不节，暴饮暴食而引起的食积证，不宜使用本方。

第二节　消痞化积剂

消痞化积剂主要由行气活血、化湿消痰、软坚等药组成，有消痞化积作用，适用于癥积痞块证。

积实消痞丸

【来源】 《兰室秘藏》

No. 1 Dried ginger, *Rhizoma Zingiberis* 3 g
No. 2 Prepared licorice root, *Radix Glycyrrhizae Praeparata* 6 g
No. 3 Medicated leaven of germinated barley, *Fructus Hordei Germinatus* 6 g
No. 4 Poria, *Poria* 6 g
No. 5 Bighead atractylodes rhizome, *Rhizoma Atractylodis Macrocephalae* 6 g
No. 6 Medicated leaven of pinellia tuber, *Rhizoma Pinelliae* 9 g
No. 7 Ginseng, *Radix Ginseng* 9 g
No. 8 Prepared magnolia bark, *Cortex Magnoliae Oflcinalis* 12 g
No. 9 Immature bitter orange, *Fructus Aurantii Immaturus* 15 g
No. 10 Phellodendron bark, *Cortex Phellodendri* 15 g

DIRECTIONS: Make water-pills by refining the powdered drugs with water or make paste pills with starchy paste out of the powdered drugs. The pills are to be taken 6-9 grams each time with warm boiled water, twice a day. Alternatively, the drugs may be decocted in water for oral administration.

FUNCTIONS: Disintegrating masses and relieving distention and fullness, strengthening the spleen and regulating the stomach.

INDICATIONS: Masses or distension and fullness due to deficiency of the spleen marked by epigastric masses, distension and fullness, loss of appetite, general debility, or distension and fullness in the chest and hypochondrium accompanied by poor appetite, indigestion, difficult bowel movement, greasy coating of the tongue and slippery pulse.

The modified recipe is advisable for the above syndrome occurring in cases of chronic gastritis and chronic diarrhea.

INTERPRETATION: In the recipe, Ingredient No. 9 is referred to as a principal drug, giving the effects of promoting the flow of *qi* and disintegrating masses. Acting as an assistant drug, No. 8 has the same effect as No. 9 and is therefore used to reinforce the effect of the principal drug. The combination of the above two drugs results in strengthening the effect of

【组成】 干生姜3克，炙甘草、麦芽曲、白茯苓、白术各6克，半夏曲、人参各9克，厚朴(炙)12克，枳实、黄柏各15克。

【用法】 水泛小丸或糊丸，每服6～9克，温开水送下，日2次。亦可水煎服。

【功用】 消痞除满，健脾和胃。

【主治】 脾虚痞满证，表现为心下痞满，不思饮食，体弱倦怠，或胸腹痞胀，食少不化，大便不畅，苔腻，脉滑。

慢性胃炎、慢性腹泻表现为脾虚痞满证者，可用本方加减治疗。

【方解】 方中枳实行气消痞，为主药；厚朴行气除满，为辅药；二者合用，以加强消痞除满之效。黄柏清热燥湿而除痞，半

relieving distension and fullness. The last drug has the effects of clearing up heat and removing dampness to disintegrate masses. No. 6, pungent and warm in property, has the effects of removing dampness and regulating the stomach. And No. 1 is capable of warming the stomach and spleen to dispel cold. The joining use of No. 1, No. 6 and No.10 brings about best effect of dispersion with pungent property and purgation with bitter property. No. 7 is able to strengthen the body resistance and reinforce the spleen, No. 4 and No. 5 both able to strengthen the spleen and remove dampness, No. 3 able to promote the digestion and regulate the stomach, and No. 2 is used as the temper of all the drugs in the recipe.

CAUTIONS: It is not fit for patients with mass of excess type.

夏曲辛温散湿和胃，又少佐干姜温中祛寒，三味相伍，辛开苦降之力尤佳。人参扶正健脾，白术、茯苓健脾祛湿，麦芽曲消食和胃，甘草调和诸药。

【使用注意】 痞满属实积者，不宜用。

Chapter XX

Prescriptions for Treating Carbuncles

These prescriptions refer to those that mainly consist of the drugs having the effects of clearing away heat and toxins, promoting pus discharge, or of the herbs for warming *yang* and dissolving lumps. With the effects of removing toxic substances and subduing inflammation, they are applied to the treatment of large carbuncle, cellulitis, nail-like boil and furuncle.

Carbuncle has a wide range, but is generalized as two kinds, internal and external. External carbuncle relates to the inflammation distributing on the superficial regions and covers the variety of large carbuncle, cellulitis, nail-like boil, furuncle, erysipelas, multiple abscess, subcutaneous nodule and scrofula, while internal carbuncle relates to the inflammation occurring in the internal organs such as pulmonary abscess and periappendicular abscess. The prescriptions are subdivided into the recipes for treating external carbuncles and the recipes for treating internal carbuncles.

Section 1

Recipes for Treating External Carbuncles

Fairy Decoction for Treating Cutaneous Infections

(Xianfang Huoming Yin)

SOURCE: ***The Revised Complete Effective Prescriptions for***

第二十章

痈疡剂

凡主要由清热解毒、托里排脓或温阳散结药物组成，具有解毒消痈作用，治疗痈、疽、疔、疖的一类方剂，称为痈疡剂。

痈疡的范围很广，但可概括为内、外两大类。外痈指体表部位的痈肿，一般有痈、疽、疔、疖、丹毒、流注、痰核、瘰疬等；内痈是指脏器的痈肿，如肺痈、肠痈。

痈疡剂可分为外痈剂、内痈剂。

第一节 外痈剂

仙方活命饮

【来源】《校注妇人良方》

Diseases of Women..

INGREDIENTS:

No. 1 Dahurian angelica root, *Radix Angelicae Dahuricae* 3 g
No. 2 Fritillary bulb, *Bulbus Fritillariae* 3 g
No. 3 Ledebouriella root, *Radix Ledebouriellae* 3 g
No. 4 Red peony root, *Radix Paeoniae Rubra* 3 g
No. 5 Chinese angelica root, *Radix Angelicae Sinensis* 3 g
No. 6 Licorice root, *Radix Glycyrrhizae* 3 g
No. 7 Chinese honey locust spine, *Spina Gleditsiae* (parched) 3 g
No. 8 Prepared pangolin scales, *Squama Manitis Praeparata* 3 g
No. 9 Trichosanthes root, *Radix Trichosanthis* 3 g
No.10 Frankincense, *Resina Olibani* 3 g
No.11 Myrrh, *Myrrha* 3 g
No.12 Honeysuckle flower, *Flos Lonicerae* 9 g
No.13 Tangerine peel, *Pericarpium Citri Reticulatae* 9 g

DIRECTIONS: All the above drugs are to be decocted in water or in half water and half wine for oral administration.

FUNCTIONS: Clearing away heat and toxic materials, subduing swelling and resolving masses, activating blood flow and alleviating pain.

INDICATIONS: Primary pyogenic infections of skin and subcutaneous tissues, manifested as swelling and pain in the affected part, or feverish body with slight aversion to cold, thin and whitish or mild yellowish coating of the tongue, and rapid and forceful pulse.

Equally, the above syndrome occurring in various purulent inflammations such as phlegmon, impetigo herpetifomis, furuncle, deep abscess, mastadenitis and others that have not yet ulcerated may be treated with the modified recipe.

INTERPRETATION: Of all the ingredients in the recipe, No. 12 is contributive in removing heat and toxins, No. 1 and No.3 in dispelling exogenous pathogens to promote the discharge of heat-toxin; Nos. 4,5,10 and 11 in activating blood flow

【组成】 白芷、贝母、防风、赤芍、生归尾、甘草节、皂角刺(炒)、穿山甲(炙)，天花粉、乳香、没药各3克，金银花、陈皮各9克。

【用法】 水煎服。或水酒各半煎服。

【功用】 清热解毒，消肿溃坚，活血止痛。

【主治】 疮疡肿毒初起证，表现为局部红肿热痛，或身热微恶寒，苔薄白或微黄，脉数有力。

各种化脓性炎症，如蜂窝织炎、脓疱疮、疖肿、深部脓肿、乳腺炎等表现为上述证候而未溃者，可用本方加减治疗。

【方解】 方中银花清热解毒。防风、白芷疏散外邪，使热毒从外透解。归尾、赤芍、乳香、没药活血散瘀，以消肿止痛。贝

and removing blood stasis in order to relieve swelling and alleviating pain; No. 2 and N. 9 in removing heat and resolving lumps; No.7 and No.8 in promoting blood circulation, discharging pus and dissolving lumps; No.13 in regulating *qi* and No. 6 in resolving pathogen and regulating the stomach and spleen.

Modern researches have ascertained that this recipe possesses the efficacies in resisting bacteria, relieving inflammation, activating blood flow to remove blood stasis and alleviating pain.

CAUTIONS: The recipe is not advisable for patients with above syndrome of *yin* type and should be carefully administered to patients with deficiency of the spleen and stomach in origin, and insufficiency of both *qi* and blood.

Decoction of Four Wonderful Drugs for Quick Restoration of Health

(Simiao Yongan Tang)

SOURCE: ***New Compilation of Proved Recipes***

INGREDIENTS:

No. 1 Honeysuckle flower, *Flos Lonicerae* 90 g

No. 2 Scrophularia root, *Radix Scrophulariae* 90 g

No. 3 Chinese angelica root, *Radix Angelicae Sinensis* 30 g

No. 4 Licorice root, *Radix Glycyrrhizae* 15 g

DIRECTIONS: All the above drugs are to be decocted in water for oral administration.

FUNCTIONS: Removing heat and toxins and activating blood flow to alleviate pain.

INDICATIONS: Gangrene of the extremities marked by such symptoms at the affected extremities as deep redness, slight swelling with burning sensation, ulceration with foul smell, severe pain, or accompanied by thirst, fever, reddened tongue

母、花粉清热散结。山甲、皂刺通行经络，透脓溃坚。以酒煎服，是用其活血通络以助药效。陈皮理气。甘草化毒、和中。

现代研究证实，本方具有抗菌、消炎、活血祛瘀、止痛等作用。

【使用注意】 本方对有阴疽见证者不宜使用；脾胃本虚、气血不足者均宜慎用。

四妙勇安汤

【来源】 《验方新编》

【组成】 金银花、玄参各90克，当归30克，甘草15克。

【用法】 水煎服。

【功用】 清热解毒，活血止痛。

【主治】 脱疽证，表现为患肢黯红微肿灼热、溃烂腐臭、疼

and rapid pulse.

Also, the modified recipe is advisable for thromboangiitis obliterans as well as other diseases due to vascular occlusion pertaining to the above syndrome.

INTERPRETATION: Being principal, No. 1 is dosed the most for removing pathogenic heat and toxins. No. 2 plays the supporting part in purging pathogenic fire and toxins. No. 3 is used to activate blood flow and remove blood stasis. The last drug, No. 4, helps the principal drug in removing pathogenic heat and toxic materials.

Modern researches have proved that this recipe may function as antipyretics, anti-inflammatory agents, antitoxins and obvious antibiotics.

CAUTIONS: The recipe is not advisable for patient with vascular occulsion of *yin*-cold or of deficient *qi*-blood types.

Powder for Promoting Pus Discharge

(Tounong San)

SOURCE: ***Orthodox Manual of External Diseases***

INGREDIENTS:

No. 1 Astragalus root, *Radix Astragali seu Hedysari* 12 g
No. 2 Pangolin scales, *Squama Manitis* 3 g
No. 3 Chuanxiong rhizome, *Rhizoma Ligustici Chuanxiong* 9 g
No. 4 Chinese angelica root, *Radix Angelicae Sinensis* 6 g
No. 5 Chinese honey locust spine, *Spina Gleditsiae* 5 g

DIRECTIONS: All the above drugs are to be decocted in water with some yellow rice wine for oral administration.

FUNCTIONS: Replenishing *qi* and enriching the blood, promoting pus discharge and expelling toxins.

INDICATIONS: Carbuncle of *qi* deficiency marked by formation of pus inside which is hardly prone to break, accompanied by shortness of breath, general debility, poor appetite, weak pulse, etc.

痛剧烈，或见发热口渴，舌红脉数。

血栓闭塞性脉管炎及其他血管闭塞病变，表现为上述症状者，可用本方加减治疗。

【方解】 方中重用银花，清热解毒，为主药。玄参泻火解毒，当归活血散瘀，甘草配银花以加强其清热解毒作用。

现代研究证实，本方具有解热、消炎、解毒及较强的抗菌作用。

【使用注意】 对阴寒型、气血两虚型的血管栓塞性病变，皆非本方所宜。

透脓散

【来源】《外科正宗》

【组成】 生黄芪12克，穿山甲3克，川芎9克，当归6克，皂角刺5克。

【用法】 水煎服，加黄酒适量。

【功用】 益气养血，托毒溃脓。

【主治】 痈疡气虚证，表现为内已成脓，不易外溃，伴有气短体倦、食欲不振、脉无力等。

When pus has formed in the carbuncle or deep-rooted boil but is not easy to ulcerate, or when the toxin can not turn into pus nor will operation help, it is favourable to use the modified recipe.

INTERPRETATION: In the recipe, No. 1 is taken raw to replenish *qi* and discharge toxin. No. 3 and No. 4 are used to activate the blood and regulate *ying*. No. 2 and No.5 are used to dispel, penetrate and resolve carbuncle, so that pus can be discharged. Yellow rice wine is used to reinforce the effect of the drugs in promoting circulation and removing stasis. All the above drugs are used jointly to yield the result of dispelling toxin and discharging pus.

Pill of Cow-bezoare

(Xihuang Wan)

SOURCE: ***Life-saving Manual of Diagnosis and Treatment of External Diseases***

INGREDIENTS:

No. 1 Cow-bezoare, *Calculus Bovis* 1 g

No. 2 Musk, *Moschus* 4.5 g

No. 3 Prepared frankincense, *Resina Olibani* 30 g

No. 4 Prepared myrrh, *Myrrha* 30 g

No. 5 Glutinous millet, (cooked) 30 g

DIRECTIONS: The first four ingredients are ground into fine powder seperately and then mixed with cooked millet which has already been pounded. Pills are made and then dried in the air, to be taken 3—6g each time with yellow rice wine or warm boiled water.

FUNCTIONS: Activating blood flow and alleviating pain, removing toxic materials and relieving swelling.

INDICATIONS: Breast cancer, bubo, scrofula, subcutaneous nodule, multiple abscess, pulmonery abscess, periappendicular abscess, etc.

痈疽疮疡在脓成不易外溃，或不能化毒成脓，消之不可，开刀又不适宜的情况下，可用本方加减治疗。

【方解】 方中黄芪生用，以益气托毒；当归、川芎活血和营；山甲、皂角刺消散穿透，软坚溃脓；黄酒通经行瘀，以助药势。合用共奏托毒溃脓之功。

犀黄丸

【来源】《外科全生集》

【组成】 牛黄1克，麝香4.5克，制乳香、制没药、黄米饭各30克。

【用法】 前四味各研末，和匀，米饭捣烂为丸，晾干（忌火烘），每服3～6克，日2次，黄酒或温水送下。

【功用】 活血定痛，解毒消肿。

【主治】 乳癌、横痃、瘰疬、痰核、流注、肺痈、肠痈等证。

Besides, many acute and chronic inflammations, primary angiitis and tumor may be treated with the above recipe.

INTERPRETATION: In the recipe, No. 1 possesses the effects of removing heat and toxic materials, eliminating phlegm and resolving mass and therefore is referred to as the principal drug. No. 2, as an assistant drug, acts as an agent to activate blood flow and remove blood stasis. No. 3 and No. 4 give the effect of activating blood flow and removing blood stasis to relieve swelling and pain and act as adjuvant drugs together with the last ingredient whose functions of regulating and tonifying the stomach–*qi* can prevent the stomach from being impaired. As a guiding drug, yellow rice wine is required to be taken together with the decoction since it has the effects of activating and promoting blood flow to speed up the effects of the drugs.

CAUTIONS: Although what the recipe treats is ascribed to *yin* syndrome, the recipe itself has nothing to do with nourishing and replenishing. For patients with weakness of *qi* and blood, prolonged administration means impairment of the stomach-*qi*. Patients with hyperactivity of fire due to *yin* deficiency are prohibited to take the recipe, nor the women in pregnancy.

Yang-Activating Decoction

(*Yanghe Tang*)

SOURCE: ***Life-saving Manual of Diagnosis and Treatment of External Diseases***

INGREDIENTS:

No. 1 Prepared rehmannia root, *Radix Rehmanniae Praeparata* 30 g

No. 2 Bark of Chinese cassia tree, *Cortex Cinnamomi* (ground into fine powder) 3 g

No. 3 Ephedra, *Herba Ephedrae* 2 g

No. 4 Antler glue, *Colla Cornus Cervi* 9 g

No. 5 White mustard seed, *Semen Sinapis Albae* 6 g

多种急慢性炎症性疾患、脉管炎初起及肿瘤等，可用本方治疗。

【方解】 方中牛黄清热解毒，化痰散结，为主药。麝香窜通消散，活血开壅，为辅药。乳香、没药活血祛瘀，消肿定痛；黄米饭调养胃气，以防伤胃，共为佐药。以酒送服，取其活血行血以加速药效，为使药。

【使用注意】 本方所治虽属阴症，但无补益之功。若气血虚弱，不宜久服，以免损伤胃气。阴虚火旺者禁用。孕妇忌服。

阳 和 汤

【来源】 《外科全生集》

【组成】 熟地30克，肉桂（研粉）3克，麻黄2克，鹿角胶9

No. 6 Baked ginger, *Zingiberis Praeparata* 2 g
No. 7 Licorice root, *Radix Glycyrrhizae* 3 g

DIRECTIONS: All the above drugs are to decocted in water for oral administration.

FUNCTIONS: Warming *yang* and enriching the blood, and removing pathogenic cold and obstruction.

INDICATIONS: *Yin* syndrome due to insufficiency of *yang* which brings about accumulation of cold, manifested as swelling of the affected region without purulent core, absence of fever and thirst, pale tongue with whitish coating and deep and weak pulse.

Moreover, the modified recipe can treat many other diseases marked by the above syndrome such as bone tuberculosis, peritoneal tuberculosis, lymphoid tuberculosis, thromboangiitis obliterans, chronic osteomyelitis, chronic deep-rooted abscess, prolapse of lumbar intervertebral disc, and proliferating arthritis of lumbar vertebrae.

INTERPRETATION: In the recipe, the first ingredient is the largest in dosage and used to warm and tonify *ying* and blood. No. 4 is used to replenish the essence, strengthen the muscles and bones and assist the first ingredient in enriching the blood. No. 2 and No. 6 are used to dispel cold accumulation by way of warming and invigorating the channels. No. 3 dispels pathogens out through the body surface. No. 5 is used to eliminate pathogenic phlegm between interior-exterior. The last drug is for removing toxic materials.

CAUTIONS:

1. The patients marked by *yang* syndrome or syndrome of half *yang* and half *yin* type are prohibited to take the recipe.

2. The recipe is contraindicated in cases of *yin*-deficiency with fever.

3. The Ingredient No. 3 in the recipe should not be overdosed.

克，白芥子6克，姜炭2克，生甘草3克。

【用法】 水煎服。

【功用】 温阳补血，散寒通滞。

【主治】 阳虚寒凝阴证，表现为局部漫肿无头、皮色不变、不热，口不渴，舌淡苔白，脉沉细。

骨结核、腹膜结核、淋巴结核、血栓闭塞性脉管炎、慢性骨髓炎、慢性深部脓肿、腰椎间盘突出症、腰椎肥大等表现为阳虚寒凝阴证者，可用本方加减治疗。

【方解】 方中熟地重用，温补营血。鹿角胶填补精髓，强壮筋骨，助熟地养血。炮姜、肉桂温通经脉以散寒凝。麻黄开腠理以达表。白芥子祛皮里膜外之痰。生甘草解毒。

【使用注意】

1. 阳证或半阳半阴证，均忌用。

2. 阴虚有热者禁用。

3. 方中麻黄应用不可过量。

Section 2

Recipes for Treating Internal Carbuncles

Reed Rhizome Decoction

(Weijing Tang)

SOURCE: ***Prescriptions Worth A Thousand Gold for Emergencies***

INGREDIENTS:

No. 1 Common reed rhizome, *Rhizoma Phragmitis* 30 g
No. 2 Coix seed, *Semen Coicis* 30 g
No. 3 Waxgourd seed, *Semen Benincasae* 24 g
No. 4 Peach kernel, *Semen Persicae* 9 g

DIRECTIONS: All the above drugs are to be decocted in water for oral administration.

FUNCTIONS: Clearing away pathogenic heat and resolving phlegm, removing obstruction and promoting pus discharge.

INDICATIONS: Pulmonary abscess caused by accumulation of phlegm and heat in the lung with symptoms of yellow, blood-stained expectoration with stinking smell as that of rotten fish, vague pain in the chest which aggravates when coughing, red tongue with yellow greasy coating, and slippery and rapid pulse.

The above symptoms seen in pulmonary abscess and pneumonia may also be treated with the modified recipe.

INTERPRETATION: Of all the ingredients, No. 1 acts as a principal drug for removing heat from the lung; No. 2 and No. 3 function in combination as assistant drugs for resolv-

第二节 内痈剂

苇茎汤

【来源】《千金要方》

【组成】苇茎30克，薏苡仁30克，冬瓜子24克，桃仁9克。

【用法】水煎服。

【功用】清热化痰、逐瘀排脓。

【主治】肺痈痰热瘀结证，表现为咳吐腥臭黄痰脓血，胸中隐隐作痛，咳时尤甚，舌红苔黄腻，脉滑数。

肺脓疡、肺炎等出现上述症状者，可用本方加减治疗。

【方解】方中用苇茎清肺泻热，为主药。冬瓜仁、薏苡仁清

ing heat and phelgm, promoting diuresis and pus discharge; and the last one has the effects of activating blood flow and removing blood stasis to eliminate heat accumulation.

Modern studies have proved that this recipe works successfully as anti-inflammatory agent, antipyretic, pus-discharging drug and phlegm-resolvent.

Decoction of Rhubarb Root and Moutan Bark

(Daihuang Mudan Tang)

SOURCE: *Synopsis of Prescriptions of the Golden Chamber*

INGREDIENTS:

No. 1 Rhubarb root, *Radix et Rhizoma Rhei* 18 g
No. 2 Moutan bark, *Cortex Moutan Radicis* 9 g
No. 3 Peach kernel, *Semen Persicae* 12 g
No. 4 Waxgourd seed, *Semen Benincasae* 30 g
No. 5 Mirabilite, *Natrii Sulphas* 9 g

DIRECTIONS: All the above drugs are to be decocted in water for oral administration.

FUNCTIONS: Purging heat and eliminating blood stasis with potent drugs, removing pathogenic accumulation and relieving swelling.

INDICATIONS: Primary periappendicular abscess marked by fever, perspiration, pain and tenderness in the right lower abdomen or with limitation of the right foot to stretch without formation of pus.

In addition, other diseases such as acute appendicitis, acute pelvic inflammation, acute annexitis that are ascribable to the accumulation of dampness and heat can be treated with the modified recipe.

INTERPRETATION: Of the five ingredients in the recipe, the first one is used to purge the accumulated toxins from

化热痰，利湿排脓，为辅药。桃仁活血祛瘀以消热结。

现代研究证实，本方具有消炎、解热、排脓、祛痰等作用。

大黄牡丹汤

【来源】《金匮要略》

【组成】大黄18克，牡丹皮9克，桃仁12克，冬瓜子30克，芒硝9克。

【用法】水煎服。

【功用】泻热破瘀，散结消肿。

【主治】肠痈初起证，表现为发热汗出，右下腹疼痛拒按，或右足屈而不伸，尚未成脓者。

急性阑尾炎、急性盆腔炎及急性附件炎表现为湿热瘀滞证者，可用本方加减治疗。

【方解】方中大黄泻肠中湿热瘀结之毒；芒硝软坚散结，助

dampness and heat in the intestines; the last one softens the masses and dispels accumulation to assist the first one in purgation. No. 2 and No. 3 are used to cool the blood and remove blood stasis; No. 4 to clean the dampness and heat in the intestines, and to discharge pus and remove abscess.

Modern studies have proved that this recipe has the efficacies in relieving inflammation, resisting bacteria, improving circulation, discharging pus, etc.

CAUTIONS:

1. The recipe is only indicated in patients with periappendicular abscess due to obstruction of dampness-heat and phlegm.

2. The recipe should be administered with great care to the old people, pregnant women, and people with weak constitution.

Powder of Coix Seed, Aconite Root and Patrinia

(Yiyi Fuzi Baijiang San)

SOURCE: *Synopsis of Prescriptions of the Golden Chamber*

INGREDIENTS:

No. 1 Coix Seed, *Semen Coicis* 30 g

No. 2 Prepared aconite root, *Radix Aconiti Praeparata* 6 g

No. 3 Patrinia, *Herba Patriniae* 15 g

DIRECTIONS: All the above drugs are to be decocted in water for oral administration.

FUNCTIONS: Promoting pus discharge and relieving swelling.

INDICATIONS: Periappendicular abscess with pus formed marked by squamous and dry skin, absence of fever, guarding and distention in the right lower abdomen that feels soft when pressing, and rapid pulse.

大黄泻下；桃仁、丹皮凉血祛瘀；冬瓜子清肠中湿热，排脓消痈。

现代研究证实，本方具有消炎、抗菌、改善循环、排脓等作用。

【使用注意】

1. 本方只适用于湿热痰滞肠痈。

2. 老人、孕妇或体质过于虚弱者，宜慎用。

薏苡附子败酱散

【来源】《金匮要略》

【组成】薏苡仁30克，熟附子6克，败酱草15克。

【用法】水煎服。

【功用】排脓消肿。

【主治】肠痈内已成脓证，表现为肌肤甲错，身无热，腹皮急，右下腹胀满，按之濡软，脉数等。

Besides, chronic appendicitis in which pus has already formed and purgation is not suitable for it may be treated with the modified recipe.

INTERPRETATION: As a principal drug, the first ingredient in the recipe is dominant in dosage and has the effects of removing dampness and relieving swelling. The last ingredient, as an assistant drug, is used for promoting pus discharge and removing blood stasis. Being the least in dosage, the second ingredient with a pungent flavor and hot property plays an adjuvant part for dispelling cold-dampness and promoting the *qi*-flow to eliminate depression and obstruction.

CAUTIONS: The recipe should not be administered for patients with acute appendicitis without formation of pus which may be treated by purgation.

慢性阑尾炎脓已成不可下者，可用本方加减治疗。

【方解】 方中薏苡仁重用，利湿消肿，为主药。败酱草排脓破血，为辅药。少佐附子辛热以散寒湿，且行郁滞之气。

【使用注意】 急性阑尾炎，脓未成可下者，忌用本方。

English Index to the Recipes in the Book

E

F

R

S

T

U

W

Y

方剂中文索引

六 画

七 画

八 画

九 画

十 画

Editor's Notes

The book was written by the following authors Jiang Jingxian (the Introduction and part of the Outline); Li Dunqing (Chapter IV to Chapter VII, Chapter XIII to Chapter XV and the part of Outline), Gao Yi (Chapter VIII to Chapter XII); Shi Lanhua (Chapter XVI to XX). The Chinese manuscript of the book was read and revised in succession by Zou Jilong, Zhang Enqin and Zhang Jidong.

The English version of the Introduction, the Outline in Part One, Chapter VIII to Chapter XVII in Part Two and the Index to the recipes were contributed by Cui Jipin and the rest part by Zuo Lianjun. The English version of the book was read and revised in succession by Zhang Enqin, Li Yulin, Yu Wenping, Wen Hongrui and Mr. Howard G. Adams. Zhang Enqin also re-translated part of it.

The final proofs of the Chinese version were checked successively by Qu Jingfeng, Zhang Shaohua and Zhang Enqin, and the English ones by Zhang Shaohua, Wen Hongrui and Zhang Enqin.

编写说明

本册绪论部分由姜静娴编写。总论部分由李敦清、姜静娴编写。各论部分第 4 章至第 7 章及第13章至第15章由李敦清编写；第 8 章至第12章由高毅编写；第16章至第20章由史兰华编写。全部中文稿先后经邹积隆、张恩勤和张继东审定。

绪言、总论、各论第 8 章至第17章及英文索引由崔继聘翻译，其余部分由左连君翻译。译文先后经张恩勤、李玉麟、于文平、温洪瑞和 Howard G. Adams 先生审校。部分内容由张恩勤重译。

本书中文校样由曲京峰、张少华和张恩勤校阅，英文校样先后由张少华、温洪瑞和张恩勤校阅。

PUBLISHED ALONG WITH THE LIBRARY ARE:

- Rare Chinese Materia Medica
- Highly Efficacious Chinese Patent Medicines

《英汉对照实用中医文库》配套书

- 中国名贵药材
- 中国名优中成药

PUBLISHING HOUSE OF SHANGHAI COLLEGE OF TRADITIONAL CHINESE MEDICINE
530 Lingling Road, Shanghai, China

Prescriations of TCM in A Practical English-Chinese Library of TCM
Editor-in-Chief Dr. Zhang Enqin

ISBN 7-81010-112-9/R·111

Printed in Shanghai No. 3 Printing Works.

英汉对照实用中医文库

方 剂 学

主编 张恩勒

上海中医药大学出版社出版发行
(上海零陵路 530 号 邮政编码 200032)
新华书店上海发行所经销
上海市印刷三厂印刷

开本 850×1168 1/32 印张 18.25 插页 6 字数 458 千字
1990 年 4 月第 1 版 1996 年 3 月第 5 次印刷
印数 7501—11500

ISBN 7-81010-112-9/R·111

定价：24.20 元